AMERI... ...

HORMONE IMBALANCE SYNDROME

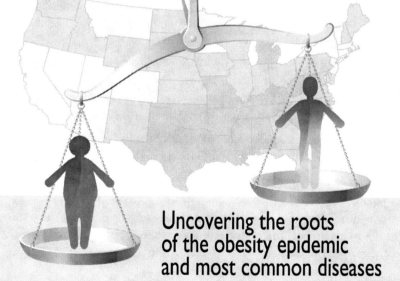

Uncovering the roots
of the obesity epidemic
and most common diseases

BENOIT TANO, M.D., Ph.D.

INTEGRATIVE MEDICAL PRESS

CONTENTS

INTRODUCTION

Obesity is the number one killer in the United States and, increasingly, the world. It kills in silence and indirectly, standing as the root cause of a great many of the diseases treated by healthcare providers, including hyperlipidemia, heart disease, diabetes, hypertension, and malignant tumors, to name only a few. If any other epidemic had caused as many deaths as obesity and its comorbidities, the whole world would be diligently searching for a cure.

Yet most physicians and other healthcare providers take a surprisingly casual attitude toward obesity. In most cases, it is treated as a more or less benign condition easily dealt with if patients would only put forth some effort. This is to say that obesity is often treated as if it were the patient's fault, with healthcare providers frequently assuming that a patient's obesity is the result of poor dietary choices and sedentary lifestyle. When patients present with obesity, hypertension, diabetes, or hyperlipidemia, the recommendation is more often than not to make some lifestyle changes to lose weight and address associated problems. If within three months the patient has not made any progress, medication therapy is plan B.

But this practice, standard in medical offices around the world, actually makes little sense: most patients cannot lose excess weight permanently on their own and almost inevitably end up with medication therapy for their obesity comorbidities. And medication therapy for hypertension and diabetes may compound the problem by causing even more weight gain. From the standpoint of common sense, this is an absurd situation, but the fact is that the orthodox medical community has continued to fight obesity using the same assumptions that have proven to be inadequate in slowing the obesity rate. I think it is time we examine our premises and be open to new possibilities when it comes to understanding the cause of obesity. My research and clinical practice have led me to question the assumption that obesity hinges solely on patients' free will. The evidence strongly suggests that something more sinister is causing the Western World, and particularly America, to be dangerously overweight.

I have come to believe that most of the world's obesity today is due to hormone imbalance. And as the evidence I will present throughout this book amply proves, hormone imbalance, such as hyperestrogenism, is due to pesticides and herbicides used in farmlands and other chemicals used in our daily lives. The organic movement is gaining ground in large part because many people rightly suspect that synthetic chemical (non-organic) farming leads to contamination of farm products and the water sources, and that this lead to diseases such as obesity, cancer and the rest. Frighteningly, this is indeed the case.

Rachel Carson in *Silent Spring* sounded the alarm in the 1960s, but little was done to correct the ill effects of chemicals in our environment. In the 1990s, Theo Colborn and her co-authors in *Our Stolen Future* added more evidence for the detrimental effects of pesticides and herbicides on the environment, and yet neither government nor the scientific community has done much about it. But the evidence has continued to mount. The CDC is at its fourth report about evidence of industrial chemicals in the blood and urine of Americans and yet no firm conclusions are drawn about causality. Most of the damages caused by these chemicals occur in the long run. If the chemicals are found in the blood and urine, should we wait until disease is manifested before taking corrective action or should we prevent diseases from occurring now, to avoid future catastrophe?

The CDC started a survey about obesity trends in 1985 and has published the obesity maps for every year from 1985 to 2010. It is clear from this data that the South and Midwest experience more obesity than the rest of the country, and this prevalence strongly correlates with these regions' heavy use of agricultural chemicals. The CDC's presentation of the data about this obesity prevalence is not accompanied by sound analyses that would clearly establish the connection between agrichemicals and obesity. The survey merely observes the facts without connecting the dots. And those that do try to analyze the data have a hard time persuading researchers to abandon the old argument that fast food and other poor dietary choices are the villains responsible for the obesity epidemic. There is nothing like a national task force with a mandate to seriously study the problem.

At the same time, healthcare providers who see the impact of the obesity epidemic have largely refused to recognize the possible etiologies. Often they are so caught up in the treatment of the symptoms of obesity that they forget about more fundamental issues. Also, the financial pressures imposed on them as employees of big organized medicine largely stifle any motivation to ask the big questions about the causes of the crisis. In medical schools, moreover, there are no courses dedicated to discovering the underlying cause of obesity, the emphasis being on the comorbidities instead of the obesity itself.

But in spite of all these factors working against recognition of obesity's true cause, we might well ask why healthcare workers, with all of their knowledge, training, and experience, seem blind to the reality of the situation. The answer to this question lies in the philosophy of traditional medicine's training and practices.

There has long been a turf battle between different factions of healthcare professionals when it comes to medical education and the basic approach to medicine. Medical schools in the US train two groups of doctors: MDs (Doctors of Medicine), often called allopathic doctors, and DOs (Doctors of Osteopathic Medicine). Like chiropractors, DOs learn musculoskeletal manipulations in addition to their medical training, and they are now allowed to participate in the same residency and fellowship training as MDs. A minority of these two groups of doctors practices what is known as holistic medicine (or alternative medicine), so called because its approach focuses on the individual as a whole instead of compartmentalizing the body into organ systems. The holistic healthcare professional often operates outside the constraints of traditional medicine's established standards. (Henceforth, I will call the traditional healthcare providers "orthodox" medical scientists and the holistic healthcare providers "heterodox" medical scientists.) Although the two groups of healthcare providers study the same problems, they tend to differ over both ethical issues and research methodology.

The methodology favored by orthodox medical scientists includes the *ceteris paribus* technique, which is common to all natural sciences. In Latin, *ceteris paribus* means "other things being equal." Applied to medicine, this means, for example, that the cardiovascular system is studied separately from the pulmonary system, and in general that all the twelve body systems are studied separately from each other. The ceteris paribus technique approach is a form of reductionism. It has led to the "study by organ system" approach taught in medical schools and residency programs. The ceteris paribus technique has allowed medical science to progress; but in the course of all the progress, the big picture has been left aside in medical schools, residency training programs, and therefore in medical practice.

The modern orthodox doctor ends up treating symptoms instead of the root cause of the disease. For example, if a patient is found to have hypertension, medication is given for hypertension; if the same patient suffers from diabetes and hyperlipidemia, each of these conditions is treated separately from the others. The root cause of all three diseases is in hormone imbalance that causes obesity, which in turn causes the three comorbidities. The hormone imbalance aspect is never addressed, and therefore the patients go for years without knowing what is causing their symptoms.

The question often asked of patients is, "What brought you here today?" and the answer leads to a description of symptoms. Healthcare providers then prescribe one or several medications appropriate for the symptoms. Many professionals rarely venture beyond this description to ask why such and such a problem is occurring. Asking why the problem occurs will lead to investigating its root cause, and this, as I have suggested above, healthcare providers are ill-equipped by their training to deal with. Hence they seldom carry out investigations along these lines. But the consequences of this ceteris paribus technique, and its attendant lack of attention to root causes, are serious: polypharmacy and lingering chronic conditions such as obesity, hypertension, diabetes, and cholesterol problems. Currently, many healthcare providers who do want to look at the macro-picture of the human body in disease, and use any means necessary to correct the problems, are crucified by their colleagues who often lack understanding of the big picture because of their reductionist training. For example, adult-onset allergies are on the rise and are more prevalent in women than in men. Yet there are no studies that focus on the root causes. Many epidemiological studies exist and point to women as having more adult-onset asthma, rhinitis, urticaria and the "why women are so vulnerable to these conditions" studies do not follow. Many studies barely touch the subject and mention hormones but the conclusions and connections are lacking.

Healthcare providers are polarized and biased due to their poorly adapted medical education, but health problems in the twenty first century will need analyses adapted to twenty first century technologies. The old dogma of differential diagnosis and treatment is not enough when it comes to solving today's medical problems. The one-symptom, one-medication approach is not adequate, and a macro-medicine approach is desperately needed.

As many holistic medical professionals, and others in the heterodox fold, have come to recognize, Hormone Imbalance Syndrome (HIS) is at the core of the obesity epidemic. But all healthcare providers should learn about hormones and their interactions so as to treat the myriad associated comorbidities. In this case, ignorance is not bliss; as more and more account-ability is demanded of healthcare providers, knowledge is bliss. To acquire knowledge, healthcare providers will have to journey beyond their comfort zones to join those who are looking at the big picture and making a difference in their patients' lives. National organizations such as the NIH, the FDA and the Association of State Medical Boards should encourage healthcare professionals to study endocrine disrupting chemicals and their ill effects on obesity and its comorbidities. The challenge of the twenty first century is hyperestrogenism, hypothyroidism and hypoandrogen-ism leading to obesity and its comorbidities, to cancer and to death. The NIH and FDA should seriously evaluate "bioidenti-cal" hormone therapy that many heterodox scientists claim to do wonders. Prevention is better than cure. If hormone imbalance is wreaking havoc early in patients' lives, why don't we measure these hormones, learn about better ranges and follow them throughout the course of our professional doctor-patient relationship so as to detect and correct the imbalance that leads to disease? Yearly physical exams have incorporated the measurement of thyroid function, but none of the other useful steroid hormones are measured. It is now clear that progesterone deficiency can lead to an underactive thyroid. Progesterone deficiency leads to estrogen dominance that generates many complaints from patients and yet these hormones are hardly ever measured. The healthcare system will be cost-saving if all steroid hormones are measured. Mammograms are done yearly to capture breast cancer, and yet the estrogen that is highly implicated in this cancer is hardly ever measured. It is therefore time for the medical establishment to look at the evidence and tear out the roots of disease.

In the 1930s, a celebrated British economist named John Maynard Keynes wrote a book entitled, *The General Theory of Employment, Interest and Money,* in which he detailed the diagnosis of, and prescribed the treatment for, the Great Depression. He took on the established economic theories and dogma and demonstrated that the cause of the Great Depression of the 1930s was a new phenomenon that called for a different set of solutions. To Keynes, the economists who came before him were "classical and neo-classical economists." In his mind classical and neoclassical meant old fashioned, outdated economic models that were inadequate for solving the new dilemma. In every field there sometimes arises a John Maynard Keynes who starts the revolution that leads to progress. In medicine today there is a need for a John Maynard Keynes who will bring new energy and principles of diagnosis and treatment that will make a difference in people's lives.

Obesity and its comorbidities represent the twenty first century challenge for America. Obesity should be treated aggressively like any other deadly disease. Instead of simply treating the symptoms associated with it, the roots of American obesity should be unearthed and eliminated so as to reduce the associated comorbidities that cause misery and generate billions in healthcare cost every year.

Medicine in America has made progress in terms of the doctor-patient relationship, and the old paternalistic medical practices are being replaced with much better ones. However, many physicians still practice an intrinsically paternalistic medicine. For example, many providers fail to thoroughly explain to patients their deductions and conclusions that justify particular prescriptions. This represents a form of paternalism because providers are indirectly telling the patients, "I know what I am doing, trust me." Many of these providers are frankly just not intellectually honest, and they have hard time admitting that they do not know the answer. To make matters worse, the legal system has forced healthcare providers to practice defensive medicine and many therefore follow blindly the outdated standards of care and wind up providing no care or useless care. Patients become frustrated at the lack of solutions to their problems. Engaging in macro-medicine practice will yield personal and professional satisfaction as patients feel better.

Healthcare professionals should work together for the betterment of the patients instead of letting ego get in the way of cooperation. Patients should not be any provider's private property; concerted efforts of all the providers involved in the care of the patients should be the norm for the sake of patients' well-being. We should all do unto others what we would like done unto us.

The new physician will be a macro-medical scientist and this will not happen without a fight against dogmatic practices. *Si Vis Sanitas Para Bellum:* If you want good health, arm for war.

The book is divided as follows: The first chapter will introduce the obesity model. The second chapter will present obesity comorbidities, associated procedures and mortality in the US so as to shed light on the importance and dimensions of obesity as a disease. This chapter will set the stage to make sense of the obesity statistics. To highlight the importance of obesity as a growing epidemic, the CDC obesity maps are presented in Chapter 3 and analyzed. This chapter also correlates the CDC maps with the USGS (US Geological Survey) pesticides and herbicides maps to make clear the contribution of endocrine-disrupting chemicals to the obesity epidemic. The fourth chapter delves into the effects of the chemicals themselves and why women are more vulnerable than men. This chapter brings attention to the estrogen epidemic and shows how women with higher endogenous estrogen production are at increased risk for obesity and its comorbidities when they are exposed to environmental estrogens. Women develop estrogen dominance when they lose their protective progesterone. Loss of progesterone leads to underactive thyroid. Hence, more women than men have hypothyroidism. The connection between estrogen dominance, leptin resistance, insulin resistance, hypothyroidism and their effects on weight are explored in Chapter 5. Here, readers will learn about endogenous estrogens, xenoestrogens, phytoestrogens and their effects on obesity and its comorbidities. Adult-onset allergies represent a window to overall health and therefore Chapter 6 explores this new phenomenon, pointing out the implications of estrogen as the culprit behind these allergies. Chapter 7 offers a summary of the previous six chapters. Steps to resolving the obesity epidemic are covered in Chapter 8. Finally, a postlogue will offer new directions.

This book uses national data and statistics to show the evidence for the effects of hormone disruption on obesity and its comorbidities. There will be a multitude of tables and maps to convey the information. Naturally, the usual reaction to the viewpoint I advocate has been, "Where's the beef?" or "Show me the proof and I will believe!" In a scientific world filled with many doubting Thomases, proof, proof and more proof is the demand. Throughout this book I have let the overwhelming evidence speak for itself.

Many of our fundamental assumptions have not changed since Galileo. Some of our best scientists are still excoriated for being the first to come up with new ideas that may lead to innovation.

CHAPTER 1

THE OBESITY MODEL

What is a model? A model is a mathematical representation of a theory. What is a theory? A theory is the explanation of the mechanism behind observed phenomena. A theory has definitions, assumptions and hypotheses. The hypotheses can be tested. Obesity by definition is present if an individual has a BMI (Body Mass Index) greater or equal to 30. Overweight is defined as a BMI of 25–29.9. BMI is measured as weight in kg/height in meter squared. The hypothesis commonly postulated is that obesity depends on food consumption and sedentary lifestyles. The quality of the foods is often questioned and the so called "junk foods" are known to be the culprits of the obesity epidemic. Many people assume that low-income individuals have the tendency to consume these junk foods and therefore bear the burden of obesity in the US. To my knowledge, there is no systematic obesity equation that takes into account all the variables that may be contributing to this phenomenon. Hence it is difficult to find adequate solutions. Writing an obesity equation that shows a relationship between obesity and its determinants will help clarify the confusions and allow more effective interventions and predictions of outcomes. Cost effectiveness of various interventions can be measured. In trying to explain the mechanism behind the current obesity phenomenon, I have discovered that the current obesity epidemic may be dependent on foods, chemicals, income, lifestyle choices, genetics, and cultural food preferences.

Foods have three components: carbohydrates, proteins and fats. Chemicals have three components: pesticides, herbicides, and household chemicals including cosmetics and cosmeceuticals. The chemicals produce three effects: they increase estrogen, decrease or increase androgens, and decrease thyroid function. Following the above description of the exogenous variables that affect obesity, a general functional form of the obesity equation can be written as:

OBS = F (carbohydrates, proteins, fat, estrogens, androgens, thyroid, lifestyle choices, genetics, culture, income, ε)   *(1)*

where estrogens are: endogenous production of estradiol and estrone, xenoestrogens due to chemicals and plant derived estrogens known as phytoestrogens. Androgens are: testosterone, dihydrotestosterone, DHEA and androstenedione and thyroid is the thyroid hormone.

Since obesity is often expressed in terms of rate, the specific functional form can be represented by a multiplicative form as follows:

OBS = $A_0 C^{\alpha_1} P^{\alpha_2} F^{\alpha_3} E^{\alpha_4} A^{\alpha_5} T^{\alpha_6} I^{\alpha_7} e^{\varepsilon}$ *(2)*

where **OBS** = Obesity A_0 is a constant term that captures the effects of genetics, lifestyle choices, and cultural food preferences. **C, P, F, E, A, T** and **I,** are carbohydrates, proteins, fats, estrogens, androgens, thyroid, and income, respectively. Epsilon (ε) is the error term that is assumed to be distributed normal with mean zero and variance σ_ε. Epsilon (ε) captures the measurement, omission and specification errors.

Carbohydrates are made up of good carbohydrates and bad carbohydrates; proteins consist of glucogenic proteins, keto-genic proteins and mixed glucogenic and ketogenic proteins. Glucogenic proteins convert to glucogenic amino acids that may increase blood glucose level after consumption and ketogenic proteins convert to ketogenic amino acids that may be stored as fatty acids. Fats consist of saturated, unsaturated, and trans-fats (hydrogenated fats). Estrogens are made up of the endogenous group: estradiol, estrone and estriol; the environmental group known as xenoestrogens and the plant source known as phy-toestrogens. Finally, the androgens consist of Androstenedione, Testosterone, Dihydrotestosterone and Dehydroepiandrosterone commonly known as DHEA.

Taking natural logs of both sides of equation (2) yields:

$$\ln OBS = \ln A_0 + \alpha_1 \ln C + \alpha_2 \ln P + \alpha_3 \ln F + \alpha_4 \ln E + \alpha_5 \ln A + \alpha_6 \ln T + \alpha_7 \ln I + \varepsilon \qquad (3)$$

where α_n, n = 1...7, represent coefficients to be estimated. Each coefficient is the percentage change in the dependent variable, obesity, with respect to the associated percentage change of the corresponding exogenous variable. This equation can be estimated if the amount of total carbohydrates, proteins and fat consumptions in the US is known. The estrogens can be replaced by proxy variables such as discharges for commonly known estrogen related diagnoses such as fibroid tumors, breast cancer, ovarian cancer, uterine cancer... androgen excess can be proxied by discharges for PCOS (polycystic ovarian syndrome) which is highly associated with androgen excess in women. I have seen patients with PCOS who have increased testosterone, DHEA and androstenedione. Many of these patients have acne, ventral obesity, infertility and poor glucose control. Low androgen such as low testosterone can be proxied by decreased libido discharges, male erectile dysfunction discharges and male myocardial infarction discharges. The rationale for myocardial infarction discharges to be used as a proxy for decreased testosterone hinges on the fact that decreased testosterone leads to the ventral obesity in men that is known to have the strongest association with myocardial infarction. The thyroid proxy will be the discharges for hypothyroidism and the income variable will be represented by total disposable income.

How to interpret the coefficients α_n? The coefficient α_1 for example stands for percentage change in obesity per percentage change in carbohydrate consumption. Hence, if carbohydrate consumption decreases by one percent, then obesity may decrease by X% depending on the value of the coefficient α_1. If this coefficient is less than 1, then a decrease in carbohydrate consumption by 1% will decrease obesity by less than 1% and therefore obesity will be inelastic with respect to carbohydrate consumption. If obesity decreases by more than 1%, when carbohydrate consumption decreases by 1%, then obesity is considered to be elastic with respect to carbohydrate consumption. If obesity decreases by exactly 1% when carbohydrate consumption decreases by 1%, then obesity is unitary elastic with respect to carbohydrate consumption. All the coefficients will be interpreted in similar fashion. I have introduced the income variable to capture the idea often expressed without any justification that poor people bear the burden of obesity in the US. The HCUP database analysis in later chapters will show that this idea is not corroborated. We can make this obesity equation more complicated by looking at the chemical effects on the foods as a separate entity. However, since chemical contamination of foods and most household chemicals including cosmetics and cosmeceuticals lead to increased estrogens, increase or decreased androgens and decreased thyroid, a simultaneous equation modeling is not necessary. Although equation (3) is not estimated in this book, inferences are made and conclusions are drawn based on this equation. The evidence of pesticide effects on obesity is presented in Chapter 4.

The next chapter offers a rationale for why we should care about the obesity epidemic. This chapter will demonstrate that obesity and its comorbidities represent the greatest danger for optimal life in the US today.

CHAPTER 2

MAKING SENSE OF OBESITY STATISTICS

To set the stage, this chapter shows the evidence on obesity and its comorbidities. The following tables will depict statistics, as well as procedures associated with morbid obesity and overweight conditions. These statistics are drawn from the HealthCare Cost and Utilization Project. If a patient presents with morbid obesity as principal reason for the office visit, or emergency room visit or hospitalization, what other diagnoses are found that associate with morbid obesity. The tables below summarize the secondary diagnoses associated with morbid obesity and overweight conditions. Procedures associated with morbid obesity are also presented. The tables shed light on the obesity and associated comorbidities and associated procedures. In 2006, morbid obesity discharges were associated with: hypertension, esophageal reflux, type II diabetes, obstructive sleep apnea, depression, asthma without status Asthmaticus (493.90), pure hypercholesterolemia, hyperlipidemia, osteoarthritis, hypothyroidism, female stress incontinence, chronic liver disease, tobacco abuse, peritoneal adhesions, diaphragmatic hernia, arthropathy, lumbago and back pain. The 2008 morbid obesity discharges were related for the most part to the same comorbidities as in 2006 and also to nutritional, endocrine, and metabolic disorders and connective tissue disorders. Tables 1 and 2 present the morbid obesity discharge comorbidities and their ICD-9 codes. Tables 3 and 4 present procedures associated with morbid obesity and overweight conditions. The following procedures: Respiratory intubation and mechanical ventilation, Arthroplasty of the knee, Cesarean section, Other vascular catheterization, not heart, Diagnostic cardiac catheterization, Coronary Arteriography, Cholecystectomy and common duct exploration, Hysterectomy, abdominal and vaginal, Percutaneous coronary angioplasty (PTCA), Upper GI endoscopy, biopsy, Blood transfusion, other OR upper GI therapeutic procedures, Debridement of wound, infection or burn, Hip replacement (total and partial), Other hernia repair, Diagnostic ultrasound of heart (echocardiography), Other procedures to assist delivery, Spinal fusion, Coronary artery bypass graft (CABG), Hemodylisis, Colorectal resection, Psychological and psychiatric evaluation and therapy, Excision, Lysis, Peritoneal adhesions, Other gastrointestinal diagnostic procedures, Gastrectomy, partial and total, Other OR lower GI therapeutic procedures, Blood transfusion, Other vascular catheterization, not heart, Other OR GI therapeutic procedures, Other OR procedures on vessels other than head and neck, Incision and drainage, skin and subcutaneous tissue, are all associated with morbid obesity. Overweight is associated with same procedures and also Insertion, revision, replacement, removal of cardiac pacemaker or cardioverter/defibrillator, Other vascular catheterization, not heart, Diagnostic ultrasound of heart (echocardiogram), Colorectal resection, Psychological and psychiatric evaluation and therapy, Other OR procedures on vessels other than head and neck.

TABLE 1
2006 National statistics—related diagnoses or procedures
OBESITY COMORBIDITIES

Principal diagnosis = 278.01 Morbid Obesity

ICD-9-CM secondary diagnosis code and name	Total number of discharges	Aggregate charges, $ (the "national bill")	Standard errors	
			Total number of discharges	Aggregate charges, $ (the "national bill")
Principal diagnosis = 278.01 Morbid Obesity	**96,371**	**3,520,016,040**	**7,811**	**307,693,342**
V85.4 Bmi 40 And Over, adult	48,669	1,689,064,505	5,031	178,458,143
401.9 Hypertension Nos	48,465	1,750,750,672	4,016	159,505,577
530.81 Esophageal Reflux	33,247	1,160,643,983	2,995	110,920,479
250.00 Dmii Wo Cmp Nt St Uncntr (after Oct 1, 1997)	26,354	972,219,156	2,237	90,083,078
780.57 Oth Unspcf Sleep Apnea	18,828	668,125,208	1,843	69,534,105
327.23 Obstructive Sleep Apnea	17,136	643,271,473	1,927	73,577,311
311 Depressive Disorder Nec	16,603	557,141,160	1,563	52,861,082
493.90 Asth W/O Stat Asthm Nos (after Oct 1, 2001)	15,231	531,733,326	1,364	51,518,804
272.0 Pure Hypercholesterolemia	15,175	545,980,325	1,714	64,772,531
272.4 Hyperlipidemia Nec/Nos	13,522	457,744,495	1,409	48,589,442
715.90 Osteoarthros Nos-Unspecified	11,902	407,362,437	1,697	51,788,563
244.9 Hypothyroidism Nos	9,148	326,374,614	847	33,270,629
625.6 Fem Stress Incontinence	9,110	306,929,922	1,292	42,351,026
571.8 Chronic Liver Dis Nec	8,404	258,973,892	1,908	55,533,039
V15.82 History Of Tobacco Use	7,908	264,499,810	987	31,604,376
568.0 Peritoneal Adhesions	7,422	314,944,619	891	39,650,817
553.3 Diaphragmatic Hernia	4,703	171,204,380	546	22,939,407
716.90 Arthropathy Nos-Unspec	4,323	154,353,965	676	27,508,341
724.2 Lumbago	4,238	152,047,145	701	26,592,247
724.5 Backache Nos	3,990	126,545,818	673	20,014,185

TABLE 2

OBESITY COMORBIDITIES

Principal diagnosis = 278.01 Morbid Obesity

	CCS secondary diagnosis category and name	Total number of discharges	Aggregate charges, $ (the "national bill")	Standard errors	
				Total number of discharges	Aggregate charges, $ (the "national bill")
Principal diagnosis = 278.01 Morbid Obesity		**130,267**	**5,004,726,591**	**11,824**	**488,216,866**
58	Other nutritional, endocrine, and metabolic disorders	109,631	4,145,894,506	10,879	442,221,423
98	Essential hypertension	71,770	2,724,584,934	6,645	272,530,950
259	Residual codes, unclassified	66,121	2,540,827,498	6,492	260,800,206
138	Esophageal disorders	50,021	1,877,017,703	4,963	203,673,669
53	Hyperlipidemia	48,801	1,837,273,251	4,808	193,166,182
49	Diabetes mellitus without complication	42,293	1,658,811,822	4,026	173,970,855
657	Mood disorders	31,433	1,142,837,022	3,242	117,503,903
203	Osteoarthritis	26,127	919,024,925	3,288	111,802,541
204	Other non-traumatic joint disorders	21,793	881,747,186	3,172	150,855,752
128	Asthma	21,278	824,430,949	2,067	86,238,555
205	Spondylosis, intervertebral disc disorders, other back problems	19,742	753,704,638	2,629	101,885,554
143	Abdominal hernia	18,043	737,312,520	2,379	102,008,317
663	Screening and history of mental health and substance abuse codes	17,845	673,424,299	1,851	71,706,147
48	Thyroid disorders	16,046	614,008,116	1,587	62,341,755
151	Other liver diseases	14,466	531,986,452	2,664	89,483,268
175	Other female genital disorders	13,095	486,572,661	2,100	84,501,025
155	Other gastrointestinal disorders	11,862	541,312,920	1,214	63,956,284
133	Other lower respiratory disease	10,392	417,237,741	2,162	93,383,022
211	Other connective tissue disease	8,353	333,515,169	1,061	40,307,803
257	Other aftercare	8,122	305,766,995	1,005	33,602,543

Morbid Obesity Comorbidities

- Other nutritional, endocrine, and metabolic disorders
- Essential hypertension
- Esophageal reflux
- Type II diabetes
- Obstructive sleep apnea
- Depressive disorder
- Asthma without status Asthmaticus
- Pure hypercholesterolemia/hyperlipidemia
- Osteoarthritis
- Hypothyroidism
- Female stress incontinence
- Chronic liver disease
- History of tobacco use
- Peritoneal adhesions
- Diaphragmatic hernia
- Arthropathy nos—unspecified
- Lumbago
- Backache NOS

Tables 3 and 4 present the obesity associated procedures

TABLE 3

Secondary diagnosis = 278.01 Morbid Obesity

CCS principal procedure category and name	Total number of discharges	LOS (length of stay), days (median)	Charges, $ (median)	Aggregate charges, $ ("the "national bill")
Secondary diagnosis = 278.01 Morbid Obesity	**776,569**	**4.0**	**19,773**	**24,455,547,538**
216	Respiratory intubation and mechanical ventilation	30,962	6.0	32,221	1,600,788,810
152	Arthroplasty knee	29,598	3.0	36,963	1,290,077,708
134	Cesarean section	25,974	3.0	14,071	459,222,541
54	Other vascular catheterization, not heart	25,589	6.0	27,716	994,768,108
47	Diagnostic cardiac catheterization, coronary arteriography	22,262	3.0	26,253	731,486,077
84	Cholecystectomy and common duct exploration	16,026	3.0	27,172	562,927,371
124	Hysterectomy, abdominal and vaginal	15,600	3.0	21,205	424,747,257
45	Percutaneous coronary angioplasty (PTCA)	14,600	2.0	44,004	761,876,401
70	Upper gastrointestinal endoscopy, biopsy	13,987	4.0	20,771	391,504,392
222	Blood transfusion	11,521	5.0	19,808	329,033,544
231	Other therapeutic procedures	10,150	4.0	15,676	246,934,084
169	Debridement of wound, infection or burn	9,617	7.0	27,663	451,470,341
153	Hip replacement, total and partial	8,982	3.0	42,802	448,405,750
86	Other hernia repair	8,982	3.0	24,438	295,919,549
193	Diagnostic ultrasound of heart (echocardiogram)	7,747	4.0	19,745	203,414,627
137	Other procedures to assist delivery	7,652	2.0	8,175	79,850,415
158	Spinal fusion	7,591	3.0	61,778	577,249,497
44	Coronary artery bypass graft (CABG)	7,460	8.0	88,281	803,598,765
58	Hemodialysis	7,268	4.0	18,756	213,544,002
168	Incision and drainage, skin and subcutaneous tissue	6,403	5.0	18,282	163,792,699

TABLE 4

OVERWEIGHT COMORBIDITIES

Secondary diagnosis = 278.02 Overweight

	CCS principal procedure category and name	Total number of discharges	LOS (length of stay), days (median)	Charges, $ (median)	Aggregate charges, $ (the "national bill")
	Secondary diagnosis = 278.02 Overweight	**45,811**	**3.0**	**17,276**	**1,250,971,995**
152	Arthroplasty knee	2,276	3.0	35,644	93,517,817
45	Percutaneous coronary angioplasty (PTCA)	2,160	1.0	42,477	106,380,838
47	Diagnostic cardiac catheterization, coronary arteriography	1,728	2.0	22,821	44,785,014
153	Hip replacement, total and partial	1,091	3.0	38,469	47,952,310
158	Spinal fusion	929	3.0	62,645	66,938,517
84	Cholecystectomy and common duct exploration	876	3.0	23,063	25,700,198
124	Hysterectomy, abdominal and vaginal	867	2.0	14,730	16,607,033
70	Upper gastrointestinal endoscopy, biopsy	793	3.0	17,859	18,669,220
231	Other therapeutic procedures	723	2.0	10,215	12,136,186
3	Laminectomy, excision intervertebral disc	659	1.0	21,236	17,434,421
44	Coronary artery bypass graft (CABG)	527	6.0	96,333	58,152,377
222	Blood transfusion	503	4.0	23,212	14,675,718
216	Respiratory intubation and mechanical ventilation	462	5.0	28,204	19,333,790
48	Insertion, revision, replacement, removal of cardiac pacemaker or cardioverter/defibrillator	419	2.0	47,070	28,063,816
54	Other vascular catheterization, not heart	403	5.0	22,903	12,133,727
193	Diagnostic ultrasound of heart (echocardiogram)	337	3.0	16,201	8,414,383
78	Colorectal resection	317	6.0	23,983	12,622,173
218	Psychological and psychiatric evaluation and therapy	301	8.0	18,823	8,381,037
61	Other OR procedures on vessels other than head and neck	296	5.0	42,701	19,267,285

Summary of obesity associated procedures

- Respiratory intubation and mechanical ventilation
- Arthroplasty of the knee
- Cesarean section
- Other vascular catheterization, not heart
- Diagnostic cardiac catheterization, coronary arteriography
- Cholecystectomy and common duct exploration
- Hysterectomy, abdominal and vaginal
- Percutaneous coronary angioplasty (PTCA)
- Upper GI endoscopy, biopsy
- Blood transfusion
- Other OR upper GI therapeutic procedures
- Debridement of wound, infection or burn
- Hip replacement, total and partial
- Other hernia repair
- Diagnostic ultrasound of heart (echocardiography)
- Other procedures to assist delivery
- Spinal fusion
- Coronary artery bypass graft (CABG)
- Hemodylisis
- Colorectal resection
- Psychological and psychiatric evaluation and therapy
- Excision, Lysis, peritoneal adhesions
- Other gastrointestinal diagnostic procedures
- Gastrectomy, partial and total
- Other OR lower GI therapeutic procedures
- Blood transfusion
- Other vascular catheterization, not heart
- Other OR GI therapeutic procedures
- Other OR procedures on vessels other than head and neck
- Incision and drainage, skin and subcutaneous tissue

Toll of Obesity, Comorbidities, and Associated Procedures

Human misery due to:

- Cardiovascular diseases
- Respiratory diseases
- Gastrointestinal diseases
- Hypertension
- Diabetes
- Hormone imbalance and associated comorbidities
- Hyperlipidemia and consequences
- Cancer and other tumors
- Arthritis
- Allergic diseases that are on the rise
- Monetary and income loss for individuals and for the whole country

These obesity and overweight comorbidities and associated procedures are intrinsically related to death in the United States as depicted by the mortality experience in 2007.

Mortality experience in 2007

In 2007, a total of 2,423,712 resident deaths were registered in the United States. The age-adjusted death rate, which takes the aging of the population into account, was 760.2 deaths per 100,000 (US standard population).

- Life expectancy at birth was 77.9 years.
- The fifteen leading causes of death in 2007 were:
  - Diseases of heart (heart disease)
  - Malignant neoplasms (cancer)
  - Cerebrovascular diseases (stroke)
  - Chronic lower respiratory diseases

- Accidents (unintentional injuries)
- Alzheimer's disease
- Diabetes mellitus (diabetes)
- Influenza and pneumonia
- Nephritis, nephrotic syndrome and nephrosis (kidney disease)
- Septicemia
- Intentional self-harm (suicide)
- Chronic liver disease and cirrhosis
- Essential hypertension and hypertensive renal disease (hypertension)
- Parkinson's disease
- Assault (homicide)

Obesity-associated comorbidities ranked at the top in the American mortality experience in 2007. The obesity comorbidities and associated procedures clearly show that obesity is the number one killer in America today and carries the highest healthcare cost burden and should therefore be treated as the most important disease in America today. Physicians have a casual attitude about obesity and prescribe the same diet and exercise regimens for patients that do not work. I suggest that obesity be aggressively treated so as to avoid all the comorbidities that lead to death and economic burden in our society. The reason for declaring war on obesity and it is comorbidities is that they are on the rise. Table 5 presents a snapshot of the 2009 and 2010 obesity rates in each of the states of the US. The difference between the 2010 and 2009 rates is also reported.

TABLE 5

2009 State Obesity Rates

State	%	State	%	State	%	State	%
Alabama	31.0	Illinois	26.5	Montana	23.2	Rhode Island	24.6
Alaska	24.8	Indiana	29.5	Nebraska	27.2	South Carolina	29.4
Arizona	25.5	Iowa	27.9	Nevada	25.8	South Dakota	29.6
Arkansas	30.5	Kansas	28.1	New Hampshire	25.7	Tennessee	32.3
California	24.8	Kentucky	31.5	New Jersey	23.3	Texas	28.7
Colorado	18.6	Louisiana	33.0	New Mexico	25.1	Utah	23.5
Connecticut	20.6	Maine	25.8	New York	24.2	Vermont	22.8
Delaware	27.0	Maryland	26.2	North Carolina	29.3	Virginia	25.0
Washington DC	19.7	Massachusetts	21.4	North Dakota	27.9	Washington	26.4
Florida	25.2	Michigan	29.6	Ohio	28.8	West Virginia	31.1
Georgia	27.2	Minnesota	24.6	Oklahoma	31.4	Wisconsin	28.7
Hawaii	22.3	Mississippi	34.4	Oregon	23.0	Wyoming	24.6
Idaho	24.5	Missouri	30.0	Pennsylvania	27.4		

2010 State Obesity Rates

State	%	State	%	State	%	State	%
Alabama	32.2	Illinois	28.2	Montana	23.0	Rhode Island	25.5
Alaska	24.5	Indiana	29.6	Nebraska	26.9	South Carolina	31.5
Arizona	24.3	Iowa	28.4	Nevada	22.4	South Dakota	27.3
Arkansas	30.1	Kansas	29.4	New Hampshire	25.0	Tennessee	30.8
California	24.0	Kentucky	31.3	New Jersey	23.8	Texas	31.0
Colorado	21.0	Louisiana	31.0	New Mexico	25.1	Utah	22.5
Connecticut	22.5	Maine	26.8	New York	23.9	Vermont	23.2
Delaware	28.0	Maryland	27.1	North Carolina	27.8	Virginia	26.0
Washington DC	22.2	Massachusetts	23.0	North Dakota	27.2	Washington	25.5
Florida	26.6	Michigan	30.9	Ohio	29.2	West Virginia	32.5
Georgia	29.6	Minnesota	24.8	Oklahoma	30.4	Wisconsin	26.3
Hawaii	22.7	Mississippi	34.0	Oregon	26.8	Wyoming	25.1
Idaho	26.5	Missouri	30.5	Pennsylvania	28.6		

2009–2010 State Obesity Rates

State	2009	2010	State	2009	2010	State	2009	2010	State	2009	2010
AL	31.0	32.2	IL	26.5	28.2	MT	23.2	23.0	RI	24.6	25.5
AK	24.8	24.5	IN	29.5	29.6	NE	27.2	26.9	SC	29.4	31.5
AZ	25.5	24.3	IA	27.9	28.4	NV	25.8	22.4	SD	29.6	27.3
AR	30.5	30.1	KS	28.1	29.4	NH	25.7	25.0	TN	32.3	30.8
CA	24.8	24.0	KY	31.5	31.3	NJ	23.3	23.8	TX	28.7	31.0
CO	18.6	21.0	LA	33.0	31.0	NM	25.1	25.1	UT	23.5	22.5
CT	20.6	22.5	ME	25.8	26.8	NY	24.2	23.9	VT	22.8	23.2
DE	27.0	28.0	MD	26.2	27.1	NC	29.3	27.8	VA	25.0	26.0
DC	19.7	22.2	MA	21.4	23.0	ND	27.9	27.2	WA	26.4	25.5
FL	25.2	26.6	MI	29.6	30.9	OH	28.8	29.2	WV	31.1	32.5
GA	27.2	29.6	MN	24.6	24.8	OK	31.4	30.4	WI	28.7	26.3
HI	22.3	22.7	MS	34.4	34.0	OR	23.0	26.8	WY	24.6	25.1
ID	24.5	26.5	MO	30.0	30.5	PA	27.4	28.6			

The 2009 and 2010 state obesity rates are compared in this table.

Rate Change (2010 Rate–2009 Rate)

State	Change	State	Change	State	Change	State	Change
AL	1.2	IL	1.7	MT	−0.2	RI	0.9
AK	−.3	IN	0.1	NE	−0.3	SC	1.1
AZ	−1.2	IA	0.5	NV	−3.4	SD	−2.3
AR	−0.4	KS	1.3	NH	−0.7	TN	−2.5
CA	−0.8	KY	−0.2	NJ	0.5	TX	2.3
CO	2.4	LA	−2.0	NM	0.0	UT	−1.0
CT	1.9	ME	1.0	NY	−0.3	VT	0.4
DE	1.0	MD	0.9	NC	−2.5	VA	1.0
DC	2.5	MA	1.6	ND	−0.7	WA	−0.9
FL	1.4	MI	1.3	OH	0.4	WV	1.4
GA	2.4	MN	0.2	OK	−1.0	WI	−2.4
HI	0.4	MS	−0.4	OR	3.8	WY	1.5
ID	2.0	MO	0.5	PA	1.2		

The rates presented in Table 5 are estimates from data collected through the CDC's Behavioral Risk Factor Surveillance System (BRFSS). Each year, state health departments use standard procedures to collect data through a series of monthly telephone interviews with US adults. Prevalence estimates generated for obesity maps reported in Chapter 3, may vary slightly from those generated for the states by the BRFSS as slightly different analytic methods are used.

In 2010, no state had a prevalence of obesity less than 20%. Thirty-six states had prevalence equal to or greater than 25%; twelve of these states (Alabama, Arkansas, Kentucky, Louisiana, Michigan, Mississippi, Missouri, Oklahoma, South Carolina, Tennessee, Texas, and West Virginia) had prevalence equal to or greater than 30%. Taking the rate difference between 2010 and 2009, shows that the Mississippi embayment states have had a mild decrease in their obesity rates with the largest decrease occurring in Louisiana and Tennessee (–2.0 and –2.5, respectively). Overall twenty states saw a decrease in their obesity rates with the highest decrease in Nevada at 3.4%. Thirty states and the District of Columbia had an increase in their rates. Five states (Colorado, Georgia, Idaho, Oregon, Texas, and the District of Columbia) had rate increase greater than 2%. The largest increase was in Oregon with 3.8%. The biggest surprise is Colorado that has jumped to 21% from 18.6% a year ago. The mild decrease in the obesity rates in the South may be due to Southern state policies for weight control, but it is too soon to draw conclusions. However, with the Mississippi river flooding this year, we will see what impact that will have on the obesity rates of the Mississippi embayment states in 2011 and the years to come.

These statistics undeniably demonstrate that obesity has quickly gained ground in the past twenty five years. The fast rise of the obesity and hence its comorbidities forces us to wonder why this "obesitization or leptinization" of America now? And why this seemingly geometric progression? The following chapters will attempt to shed light on this obesity enigma.

CHAPTER 3

FARMING AND OBESITY IN THE UNITED STATES

Evidence from the CDC Obesity maps, USGS Pesticides Maps, and Healthcare Cost and Utilization Project Data Analysis

The US obesity epidemic started in the South and the Midwest and has now spread to the whole United States. The CDC has kept track of US obesity since 1985 through the BRFSS surveys. In that time, the leading states have been in the South and Midwest. What these states have in common are agriculture and pesticides/herbicides usage. The South, especially the Mississippi Embayment States (Mississippi, Louisiana, Arkansas, Tennessee, Kentucky, Missouri, and contiguous states such as Alabama and Texas), seem to start the obesity trends that progressively spread northward through the Midwest, then to the Northeast and finally to the West. Even though obesity is often attributed to overeating and lack of exercise, the CDC BRFSS survey maps, coupled with the USGS (US Geological Survey) pesticides/herbicides spray maps, tell a different story. The BRFSS survey also indicates that African-Americans and Hispanic-Americans lead in the obesity rates followed by whites. The evidence based on the HCUP (HealthCare Cost and Utilization Project) database seems to point to whites and the well-to-do as having higher rates of obesity than blacks and the poor.

The pesticides/herbicides used in agriculture lead to hyper-estrogenism, hypothyroidism and hypoandrogenism that lead to multiple pathological syndromes that manifest as symptoms in patients. The CDC obesity maps correlate strikingly with the USGS pesticides/herbicides maps, suggesting that the pesticides and herbicides used in farming have a major impact on the increasing obesity epidemic in the US. The South uses three times more chemicals in farming than other regions in the US because of cotton farming that requires more herbicides and pesticides. The Mississippi River drains many important rivers in the US and therefore all the chemicals sprayed in farmlands in the Upper Midwest and Midwest are carried downward into the Mississippi Embayment states which, hence, have higher obesity rates than all other states.

Controlling for population, it appears that obesity and its comorbidities (hypertension, diabetes, heart disease, etc.), are more prevalent in the South and the Midwest than the Northeast and the West. Allergic diseases such as asthma, allergic rhinitis, chronic sinusitis, food allergy... are on the rise and are also more prevalent in the South and the Midwest.

The next section presents the CDC obesity maps and correlates these maps with the 1997 and 2002 USGS pesticides/herbicides maps. This gives the reader a visual representation of what is happening to the country in terms of obesity. Follow the obesity rates and maps and notice how they are increasing quickly, year after year since 1985.

CDC Obesity Maps 1985–2009

Obesity Trends* Among US Adults
BRFSS, 1985
(*BMI ≥30, or ~ 30 lbs. overweight for 5' 4" person)

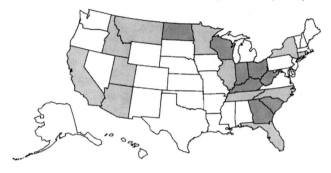

No Data   <10%   10%–14%

Source: Behavioral Risk Factor Surveillance System, CDC.

Obesity Trends* Among US Adults
BRFSS, 1986
(*BMI ≥30, or ~ 30 lbs. overweight for 5' 4" person)

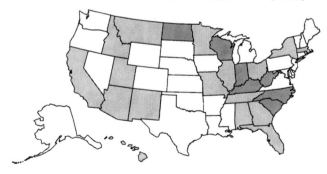

No Data   <10%   10%–14%

Source: Behavioral Risk Factor Surveillance System, CDC.

Obesity Trends* Among US Adults
BRFSS, 1987
(*BMI ≥30, or ~ 30 lbs. overweight for 5' 4" person)

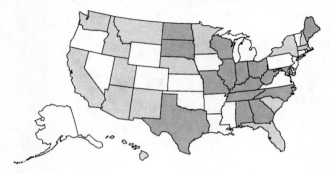

No Data   <10%   10%–14%

Source: Behavioral Risk Factor Surveillance System, CDC.

Obesity Trends* Among US Adults
BRFSS, 1988
(*BMI ≥30, or ~ 30 lbs. overweight for 5' 4" person)

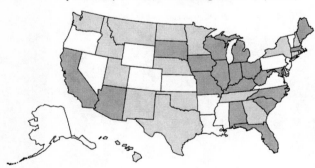

No Data   <10%   10%–14%

Source: Behavioral Risk Factor Surveillance System, CDC.

Obesity Trends* Among US Adults
BRFSS, 1989
(*BMI ≥30, or ~ 30 lbs. overweight for 5′ 4″ person)

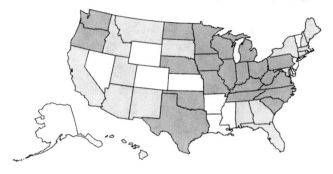

| No Data | <10% | 10%–14% |

Source: Behavioral Risk Factor Surveillance System, CDC.

Obesity Trends* Among US Adults
BRFSS, 1990
(*BMI ≥30, or ~ 30 lbs. overweight for 5′ 4″ person)

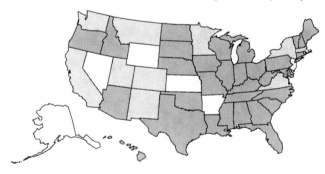

| No Data | <10% | 10%–14% |

Source: Behavioral Risk Factor Surveillance System, CDC.

Obesity Trends* Among US Adults
BRFSS, 1991
(*BMI ≥30, or ~ 30 lbs. overweight for 5' 4" person)

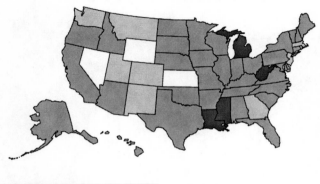

No Data   <10%   10%–14%   15%–19%

Source: Behavioral Risk Factor Surveillance System, CDC.

Obesity Trends* Among US Adults
BRFSS, 1992
(*BMI ≥30, or ~ 30 lbs. overweight for 5' 4" person)

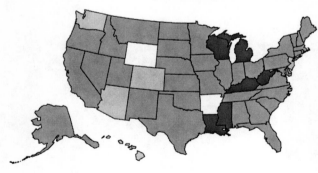

No Data   <10%   10%–14%   15%–19%

Source: Behavioral Risk Factor Surveillance System, CDC.

Obesity Trends* Among US Adults
BRFSS, 1993
(*BMI ≥30, or ~ 30 lbs. overweight for 5' 4" person)

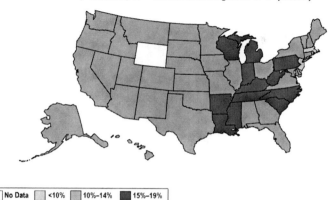

No Data   <10%   10%–14%   15%–19%

Source: Behavioral Risk Factor Surveillance System, CDC.

Obesity Trends* Among US Adults
BRFSS, 1994
(*BMI ≥30, or ~ 30 lbs. overweight for 5' 4" person)

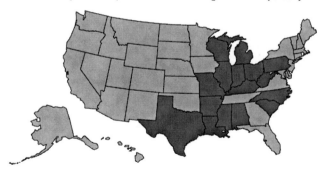

No Data   <10%   10%–14%   15%–19%

Source: Behavioral Risk Factor Surveillance System, CDC.

Obesity Trends* Among US Adults
BRFSS, 1995
(*BMI ≥30, or ~ 30 lbs. overweight for 5' 4" person)

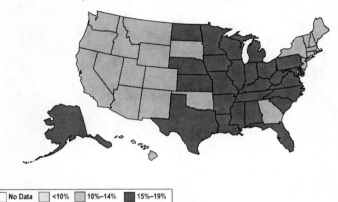

No Data ☐   <10% ☐   10%–14% ☐   15%–19% ■

Source: Behavioral Risk Factor Surveillance System, CDC.

Obesity Trends* Among US Adults
BRFSS, 1996
(*BMI ≥30, or ~ 30 lbs. overweight for 5' 4" person)

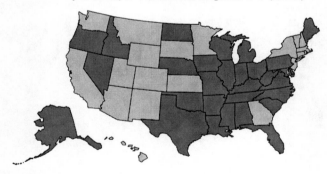

No Data ☐   <10% ☐   10%–14% ☐   15%–19% ■

Source: Behavioral Risk Factor Surveillance System, CDC.

Obesity Trends* Among US Adults
BRFSS, 1997
(*BMI ≥30, or ~ 30 lbs. overweight for 5' 4" person)

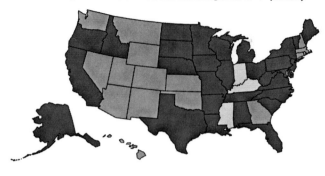

| No Data | <10% | 10%–14% | 15%–19% | ≥20% |

Source: Behavioral Risk Factor Surveillance System, CDC.

Atrazine Pesticide Spray in the US in 1997—See how the Spray Area seems to Exactly Correspond to the 1997 CDC Map of Highest Obesity Rates

ATRAZINE - herbicide
1997 estimated annual agricultural use

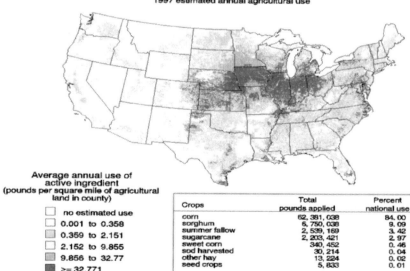

Average annual use of
active ingredient
(pounds per square mile of agricultural
land in county)

☐ no estimated use
☐ 0.001 to 0.358
☐ 0.359 to 2.151
☐ 2.152 to 9.855
☐ 9.856 to 32.77
■ >= 32.771

Crops	Total pounds applied	Percent national use
corn	62, 381, 038	84. 00
sorghum	6, 750, 038	9. 09
summer fallow	2, 539, 169	3. 42
sugarcane	2, 203, 421	2. 97
sweet corn	340, 452	0. 46
sod harvested	30, 214	0. 04
other hay	13, 224	0. 02
seed crops	5, 833	0. 01

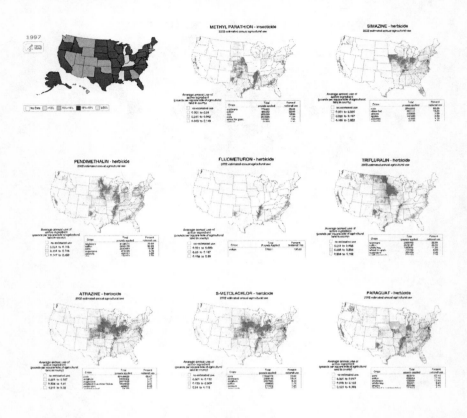

The areas with the highest obesity rates reported by the CDC in 1997 correspond to the areas that see the greatest use of herbicides and pesticides, as reported by the USGS in the same year. Coincidence or not?

TABLE 6

Outcomes by patient and hospital characteristics for ICD-9-CM principal diagnosis code 244.9 Hypothyroidism Nos

		Total number of discharges	LOS (length of stay), days (median)	Charges, $ (median)	Standard errors Total number of discharges
All discharges		4,438 (100.00%)	4.0	6,807	216
Age group	<1	*	*	*	*
	1–17	*	3.0	3,659	*
	18–44	556 (12.52%)	3.0	5,740	65
	45–64	927 (20.88%)	3.0	6,770	82
	65–84	2,139 (48.19%)	4.0	7,246	132
	85+	748 (16.85%)	5.0	6,807	63
	Missing	*	*	*	*
Sex	Male	1,204 (27.14%)	4.0	6,852	84
	Female	3,234 (72.86%)	4.0	6,807	178
Region	Northeast	875 (19.72%)	5.0	8,693	78
	Midwest	1,111 (25.04%)	4.0	6,196	107
	South	1,580 (35.61%)	4.0	6,048	136
	West	871 (19.62%)	3.0	7,225	103

Most physicians agree that hypothyroidism causes weight gain. The 1997 hypothyroidism hospital discharges were more prevalent in women at 73% and increases with age starting at 12.5% for ages (18–44), 21% for ages (45–64), and 48% for ages (65–84). Hypothyroidism discharges in 1997 were more prevalent in the South at 35.6% and the Midwest at 25% followed by the Northeast at 19.7% and the West at 19.6%.

TABLE 7

Outcomes by patient and hospital characteristics for ICD-9-CM principal diagnosis code 278.01 Morbid Obesity

		Total number of discharges	Aggregate charges, $ (the "national bill")	Standard errors	
				Total number of discharges	Aggregate charges, $ (the "national bill")
All discharges		12,353 (100.00%)	226,923,613	3,156	60,589,817
Age group	1–17	*	2,016,664	*	866,099
	18–44	8,143 (65.92%)	145,853,191	2,072	39,179,047
	45–64	3,862 (31.26%)	75,076,257	1,051	20,565,783
	65–84	209 (1.69%)	3,977,501	43	1,142,425
Sex	Male	2,207 (17.87%)	52,068,245	550	15,709,118
	Female	10,146 (82.13%)	174,855,369	2,615	45,549,748
Region	Northeast	*	55,835,488	*	16,897,400
	Midwest	1,293 (10.46%)	21,294,322	360	6,146,648
	South	*	64,684,248	*	23,198,974
	West	*	85,109,555	*	53,005,945

TABLE 8

Outcomes by patient and hospital characteristics for ICD-9-CM principal diagnosis code 278.1 Localized Adiposity

		Total number of discharges	Aggregate charges, $ (the "national bill")	Standard errors	
				Total number of discharges	Aggregate charges, $ (the "national bill")
All discharges		3,514 (100.00%)	37,797,720	537	4,479,287
Age group	1–17	*	*	*	*
	18–44	1,657 (47.16%)	18,057,482	252	2,523,361
	45–64	1,578 (44.89%)	16,872,820	277	2,068,048
	65–84	245 (6.97%)	2,531,262	45	557,000
	85+	*	*	*	*
Sex	Male	386 (10.97%)	4,497,675	60	727,492
	Female	3,129 (89.03%)	33,300,046	495	4,134,637
Region	Northeast	1,124 (31.97%)	10,584,832	296	2,923,380
	Midwest	492 (14.00%)	5,556,382	70	779,053
	South	1,477 (42.03%)	16,270,084	438	3,165,226
	West	421 (11.99%)	5,386,422	67	944,607

The morbid obesity discharges in 1997 were also more prevalent in women and were 82.1% for females and 17.9% for males. Morbid obesity was more prevalent in the young ("prime") ages (18–44) at 66%, followed by old adults ages (45–64) at 31.3%. The data by region were not reported. Localized adiposity followed the same pattern and was higher in the South followed by the Northeast, then the Midwest and the West.

Obesity Trends* Among US Adults
BRFSS, 1998
(*BMI ≥30, or ~ 30 lbs. overweight for 5' 4" person)

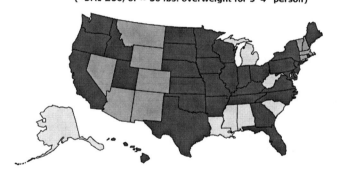

| No Data | <10% | 10%–14% | 15%–19% | ≥20% |

Source: Behavioral Risk Factor Surveillance System, CDC.

This obesity map clearly shows that the Southern states lead in the obesity rates and that Mississippi, Louisiana, and Alabama start the trend that progresses upward and spreads by contiguity to the Midwest and Upper Midwest states and then to the Northeast and to the West. This progression will be clear in the 1999 map and will continue through the years without much change.

TABLE 9

1998 National statistics—principal diagnosis only

Outcomes by patient and hospital characteristics for
ICD-9-CM principal diagnosis code
244.9 Hypothyroidism Nos

		Total number of discharges	Aggregate charges, $ (the "national bill")	Standard errors	
				Total number of discharges	Aggregate charges, $ (the "national bill")
All discharges		4,526 (100.00%)	48,360,757	234	3,633,341
Age group	<1	*	*	*	*
	1–17	*	*	*	*
	18–44	488 (10.79%)	3,079,464	53	412,889
	45–64	1,009 (22.30%)	11,467,373	97	1,894,836
	65–84	2,256 (49.84%)	26,088,794	137	2,080,296
	85+	698 (15.43%)	7,311,133	65	907,964
Sex	Male	1,086 (23.99%)	11,662,537	92	1,531,950
	Female	3,440 (76.01%)	36,698,219	182	3,106,639
Region	Northeast	786 (17.36%)	12,960,506	82	2,573,884
	Midwest	998 (22.04%)	9,675,519	81	1,228,279
	South	1,805 (39.88%)	16,115,327	176	1,733,265
	West	938 (20.72%)	9,609,405	103	1,436,459

The 1998 hypothyroidism hospital discharges were more prevalent in women at 76% and increased with age starting at 10.8% for ages 18–44, 22.3% for ages 45–64, 49.8% for ages 65–84, and 15.4% for ages greater than 85. Hypothyroidism discharges in 1998 were more prevalent in the South at 39.9% and the Midwest at 22% followed by the West at 20.7% and the Northeast at 17.4%. The hypothyroidism trend also follows the trend observed in the obesity rate maps.

TABLE 10

Outcomes by patient and hospital characteristics for
ICD-9-CM principal diagnosis code
278.01 Morbid Obesity

| | | Total number of discharges | Aggregate charges, $ (the "national bill") | Standard errors | |
				Total number of discharges	Aggregate charges, $ (the "national bill")
All discharges		13,904 (100.00%)	318,617,244	1,986	49,602,369
Age group	1–17	*	1,722,776	*	529,434
	18–44	9,315 (66.99%)	198,734,499	1,382	32,039,831
	45–64	4,309 (31.00%)	114,245,943	614	18,609,393
	65–84	144 (1.03%)	*	32	*
Sex	Male	2,706 (19.46%)	74,121,089	374	11,665,960
	Female	11,198 (80.54%)	244,496,154	1,655	39,695,450
Region	Northeast	*	55,144,231	*	21,422,936
	Midwest	*	51,588,276	*	16,990,934
	South	3,998 (28.75%)	84,440,369	877	18,815,655
	West	4,156 (29.89%)	127,444,367	1,125	36,860,984

TABLE 11

Outcomes by patient and hospital characteristics for
ICD-9-CM principal diagnosis code
278.1 Localized Adiposity

| | | Total number of discharges | Aggregate charges, $ (the "national bill") | Standard errors | |
				Total number of discharges	Aggregate charges, $ (the "national bill")
All discharges		3,795 (100.00%)	44,176,600	549	5,969,565
Age group	1–17	*	*	*	*
	18–44	1,759 (46.37%)	19,265,386	278	3,142,467
	45–64	1,786 (47.06%)	21,741,708	264	3,068,180
	65–84	240 (6.34%)	3,144,615	42	685,950
	85+	*	*	*	*
Sex	Male	403 (10.63%)	6,580,724	61	1,695,827
	Female	3,386 (89.23%)	37,495,822	511	5,077,477
	Missing	*	*	*	*
Region	Northeast	947 (24.97%)	6,710,923	266	1,718,998
	Midwest	796 (20.99%)	12,218,389	141	2,482,325
	South	1,274 (33.56%)	13,283,971	368	2,510,765
	West	*	11,963,317	*	4,496,096

Women made up 80.5% of morbid obesity discharges in 1998. The same discharges are seen more among the young (prime) (18–44) years of age at 67%, followed by the older adults ages (45–64) at 31%. The data by region were not completely reported. This pattern is the same for all years of obesity trends reported by the CDC. Morbid obesity is a disease of women in their prime in the South and Midwest states of the US.

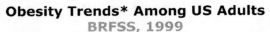

Obesity Trends* Among US Adults
BRFSS, 1999

(*BMI ≥30, or ~ 30 lbs. overweight for 5′ 4″ person)

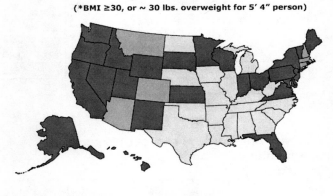

| No Data | <10% | 10%–14% | 15%–19% | ≥20% |

Source: Behavioral Risk Factor Surveillance System, CDC.

In 1998, an obesity rate ≥ 20% was observed in Mississippi, Alabama, South Carolina, West Virginia, and Michigan. Since 1999, this rate has spread contiguously to most Southern and Midwestern states as previously mentioned.

TABLE 12

1999 National statistics—principal diagnosis only

Outcomes by patient and hospital characteristics for
ICD-9-CM principal diagnosis code
244.9 Hypothyroidism Nos

		Total number of discharges	LOS (length of stay), days (median)	Charges, $ (median)	Aggregate charges, $ (the "national bill")
All discharges		3,976 (100.00%)	4.0	7,009	45,182,792
Age group	<1	*	*	*	*
	1–17	*	*	*	*
	18–44	547 (13.75%)	2.0	5,086	4,762,263
	45–64	798 (20.06%)	3.0	6,622	10,022,332
	65–84	1,902 (47.84%)	4.0	7,213	22,017,771
	85+	680 (17.11%)	6.0	7,541	8,112,843
	Missing	*	*	*	*
Sex	Male	945 (23.76%)	4.0	7,166	11,156,071
	Female	3,032 (76.24%)	4.0	6,978	34,026,720
Region	Northeast	797 (20.04%)	4.0	8,511	11,289,405
	Midwest	986 (24.80%)	4.0	7,003	10,658,385
	South	1,460 (36.72%)	4.0	6,113	12,571,017
	West	733 (18.44%)	4.0	7,992	10,663,984

TABLE 13

Outcomes by patient and hospital characteristics for
ICD-9-CM principal diagnosis code
278.01 Morbid Obesity

		Total number of discharges	LOS (length of stay), days (median)	Charges, $ (median)	Aggregate charges, $ (the "national bill")
All discharges		23,577 (100.00%)	4.0	18,006	585,060,642
Age group	1–17	176 (0.75%)	*	*	*
	18–44	14,222 (60.32%)	4.0	17,783	329,584,319
	45–64	8,924 (37.85%)	4.0	18,356	244,153,531
	65–84	251 (1.06%)	4.0	18,472	5,606,133
	Missing	*	*	*	*
Sex	Male	4,410 (18.71%)	4.0	19,894	131,438,471
	Female	19,158 (81.26%)	4.0	17,609	453,394,899
	Missing	*	*	*	*
Region	Northeast	*	4.0	15,581	88,316,634
	Midwest	4,207 (17.84%)	4.0	21,587	106,935,016
	South	7,023 (29.79%)	4.0	19,413	163,100,600
	West	*	3.0	16,149	226,708,392

The hypothyroidism and morbid obesity rates followed the same pattern in 1999 as in previous years and reflected the obesity rate patterns in the four major US regions.

Obesity Trends* Among US Adults
BRFSS, 2000
(*BMI ≥30, or ~ 30 lbs. overweight for 5′ 4″ person)

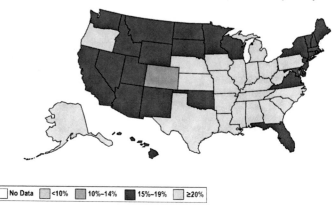

| No Data | <10% | 10%–14% | 15%–19% | ≥20% |

Source: Behavioral Risk Factor Surveillance System, CDC.

In 2000, the increased obesity rate has spread to most of the Midwest states and in the Northeast to Pennsylvania and in the West to Oregon.

TABLE 14

2000 National statistics—principal diagnosis only

Outcomes by patient and hospital characteristics for
ICD-9-CM principal diagnosis code
244.9 Hypothyroidism Nos

		Total number of discharges	LOS (length of stay), days (median)	Charges, $ (median)	Aggregate charges, $ (the "national bill")
All discharges		4,409 (100.00%)	4.0	7,210	53,393,023
Age group	1–17	*	*	*	*
	18–44	626 (14.19%)	2.0	5,739	5,974,899
	45–64	1,043 (23.66%)	3.0	6,773	10,205,423
	65–84	1,945 (44.12%)	4.0	8,108	28,160,564
	85+	764 (17.33%)	5.0	7,191	8,417,499
Sex	Male	1,101 (24.97%)	*	7,711	14,761,870
	Female	3,308 (75.03%)	4.0	6,987	38,631,153
Region	Northeast	859 (19.49%)	4.0	9,065	14,190,842
	Midwest	1,038 (23.54%)	4.0	7,572	10,805,482
	South	1,586 (35.98%)	4.0	6,245	15,434,988
	West	926 (20.99%)	*	8,464	12,961,711

TABLE 15

Outcomes by patient and hospital characteristics for
ICD-9-CM principal diagnosis code
278.01 Morbid Obesity

		Total number of discharges	LOS (length of stay), days (median)	Charges, $ (median)	Aggregate charges, $ (the "national bill")
All discharges		32,023 (100.00%)	3.0	17,973	803,527,608
Age group	1–17	158 (0.49%)	4.0	14,364	3,053,828
	18–44	19,997 (62.44%)	3.0	17,579	483,669,021
	45–64	11,597 (36.21%)	4.0	18,800	308,703,121
	65–84	257 (0.80%)	5.0	21,878	7,913,248
	85+	*	*	*	*
	Missing	*	*	*	*
Sex	Male	4,895 (15.29%)	4.0	19,472	140,017,845
	Female	27,123 (84.70%)	3.0	17,771	663,442,337
	Missing	*	*	*	*
Region	Northeast	10,239 (31.97%)	3.0	21,289	282,247,671
	Midwest	4,479 (13.99%)	4.0	19,429	99,950,090
	South	11,617 (36.28%)	3.0	10,993	217,719,428
	West	5,688 (17.76%)	4.0	32,818	203,610,420

Hypothyroidism and morbid obesity patterns were the same
in 2000.

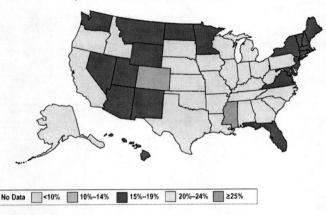

Obesity Trends* Among US Adults
BRFSS, 2001
(*BMI ≥30, or ~ 30 lbs. overweight for 5' 4" person)

No Data   <10%   10%–14%   15%–19%   20%–24%   ≥25%

Source: Behavioral Risk Factor Surveillance System, CDC.

In 2001, Mississippi started a new obesity rate, and you will notice that the new rate will spread contiguously to all the Southern states and then upward to the Midwest states and then to the Northeast and to the West.

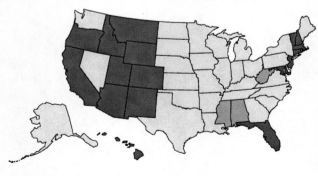

Obesity Trends* Among US Adults
BRFSS, 2002
(*BMI ≥30, or ~ 30 lbs. overweight for 5' 4" person)

No Data   <10%   10%–14%   15%–19%   20%–24%   ≥25%

Source: Behavioral Risk Factor Surveillance System, CDC.

Since 2002, Alabama and West Virginia have joined Mississippi in the new rate trend, and you will notice that the new rate also spreads contiguously to all the Southern states and then upward to the Midwest states and then to the Northeast and to the West.

The following section presents the spatial association between pesticide use and levels of obesity and its comorbidities in the US. Recent studies are pointing to endocrine disrupting chemicals as possible culprits. The CDC obesity maps compiled from data collected through CDC's Behavioral Risk Factor Surveillance System (BRFSS), which each year reports state health departments data obtained through a series of telephone interviews with US adults, and the USGS pesticide use estimate summarized by county, were used to correlate hypothyroidism, obesity and selected comorbidities to pesticide use density. Thyroid disrupting chemicals such as alachlor, acetochlor, paraquat, malathion, and glyphosate and estrogen and androgen disrupting chemicals such as carbaryl, endosulfan, and atrazine, are shown here in relation to the obesity maps. Hospital discharges for hypothyroidism, morbid obesity and selected comorbidities, and pesticide use density, were analyzed for all US regions. The following figures and tables 16 and 17 focused on year 2002 that encompassed all three databases.

TABLE 16

2002 National statistics—principal diagnosis only

Outcomes by patient and hospital characteristics for
ICD-9-CM principal diagnosis code
244.9 Hypothyroidism Nos

		Total number of discharges	LOS (length of stay), days (median)	Charges, $ (median)	Aggregate charges, $ (the "national bill")
All discharges		5,051 (100.00%)	4.0	9,832	75,844,783
Age group	<1	*	*	*	*
	1–17	*	*	*	*
	18–44	684 (13.54%)	2.0	6,709	7,782,867
	45–64	1,200 (23.76%)	3.0	9,513	17,847,895
	65–84	2,086 (41.29%)	4.0	10,648	35,565,710
	85+	1,023 (20.26%)	*	10,341	13,773,683
Sex	Male	1,324 (26.21%)	4.0	9,832	22,772,197
	Female	3,727 (73.79%)	4.0	9,802	53,072,586
Region	Northeast	909 (17.99%)	4.0	11,135	17,029,025
	Midwest	1,115 (22.08%)	3.0	8,603	14,864,053
	South	1,952 (38.64%)	4.0	8,857	25,154,482
	West	1,075 (21.29%)	*	11,766	18,797,224

The 2002 hypothyroidism rate in women was 73.8% and
26.2 % in men. The South had 38.6%, the Midwest 22.1%, the
West 21.3%, and the Northeast 18%.

TABLE 17

Outcomes by patient and hospital characteristics for
ICD-9-CM principal diagnosis code
278.01 Morbid Obesity

		Total number of discharges	LOS (length of stay), days (median)	Charges, $ (median)	Aggregate charges, $ (the "national bill")
All discharges		74,179 (100.00%)	3.0	23,122	2,234,317,964
Age group	1–17	272 (0.37%)	4.0	20,791	6,105,743
	18–44	44,049 (59.38%)	3.0	22,479	1,251,511,915
	45–64	29,121 (39.26%)	3.0	24,008	950,543,694
	65–84	737 (0.99%)	4.0	26,740	26,156,611
Sex	Male	11,955 (16.12%)	3.0	24,773	404,492,142
	Female	62,224 (83.88%)	3.0	22,830	1,829,825,821
Region	Northeast	22,844 (30.80%)	3.0	23,469	655,276,724
	Midwest	13,026 (17.56%)	3.0	21,792	332,013,440
	South	20,502 (27.64%)	3.0	23,188	576,720,704
	West	17,808 (24.01%)	3.0	23,863	670,307,096

In 2002, morbid obesity discharges were also more prevalent among women at 83.9%. Males had a rate of 16.1%. Discharges were more prevalent among prime-age women, ages 18–44 at 59.4% followed by older adults at 39.3%.

In all tables drawn from the HCUP database, descriptive statistics employed [means and standard error (SE), and proportions], as appropriate. A two-tailed p-value < 0.05 denotes statistical significance. When the three databases were analyzed concomitantly for 2002, it was found that the thyroid, estrogen and androgen disrupting chemicals used in this analysis had highest average annual use of active ingredient (pounds per square mile) and cumulative effects in the South, especially in the Mississippi delta and the Midwest Corn Belt areas. Hypothyroidism discharges for 2002 were also more prevalent in females [3,727 (248), 73%] and in the South [1,952 (150), 38.6%] and the Midwest [1,115 (102), 22%]. The Northeast had [909 (78), 17.99%] and the West had [1,075 (199), 21.3%] for 2002. Statistics for 1997 painted the same picture. Morbid obesity hospital discharges in 2002 were 74,179(8,601) total and were also more prevalent in females [62,224 (7,107), 83.9%] and consistent with the high hypothyroidism rate in this group. The regional obesity rates were [20,502 (3,605), 27.6%] for the South, [13,026 (2,965), 17.6%], for the Midwest, [22,844 (5,840), 30.8%] for the Northeast and [17,808 (4,251), 24%] for the West in 2002. The regional rates were not reported by the HCUP in 1997.

These results indicate that endocrine disrupting chemicals should be scrutinized and regarded with greatest suspicion for contributing to the American obesity epidemic. Although the areas with highest pesticide use density also seem to have the highest hypothyroidism and obesity rates, this book is not focusing on a causality analysis and therefore no cause and effect conclusions are drawn. However, you the reader, may connect the dots yourself.

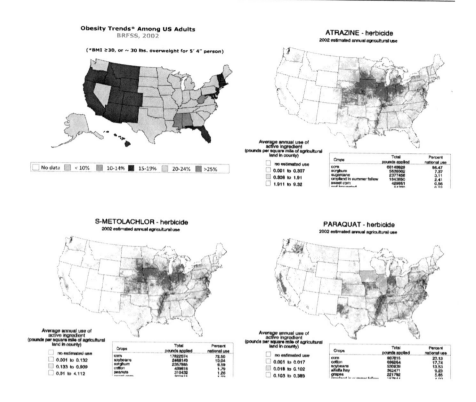

This figure shows the obesity map by the CDC and selected herbicide maps by the USGS (US Geological Survey). Notice that the 2002 herbicide spray areas depicted in the USGS maps seem to coincide with the CDC 2002 map of high obesity rates.

Darker areas in these pesticides maps are red in the color maps and depict the highest pesticides spray intensity.

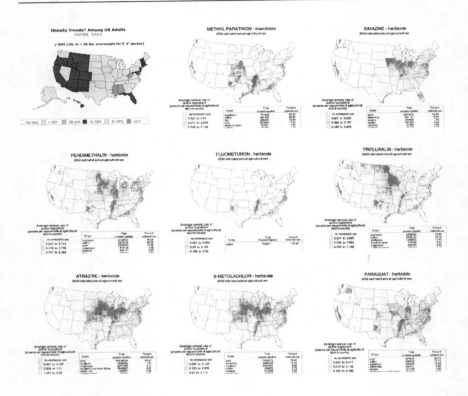

This figure shows the obesity maps by the CDC and selected herbicide maps by USGS (US Geological Survey). Notice that the 2002 herbicide spray areas depicted in the USGS maps seem to coincide with the CDC 2002 obesity map area of high obesity rates. The areas with herbicides spray intensity are in red and shown in darker color in the black and white maps. Note that the Mississippi Delta is red as is the Corn Belt. The cumulative effects of these chemicals over the years are the major problems. The consequences of the interaction of these chemicals are not even known.

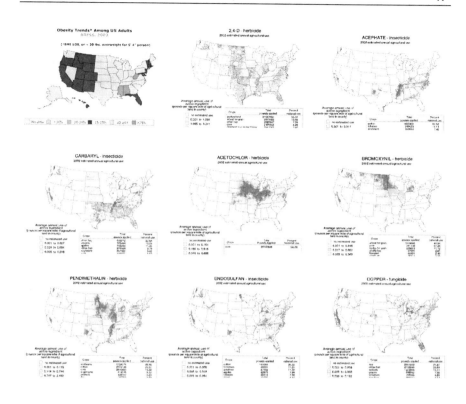

The same pattern is seen for various herbicides and pesticides spray maps and the obesity maps.

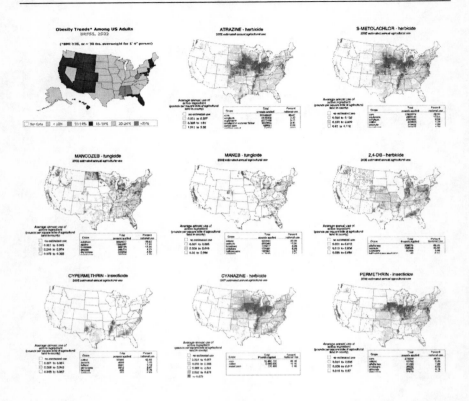

The same pattern is seen for various herbicides and pesticides spray maps and the obesity maps.

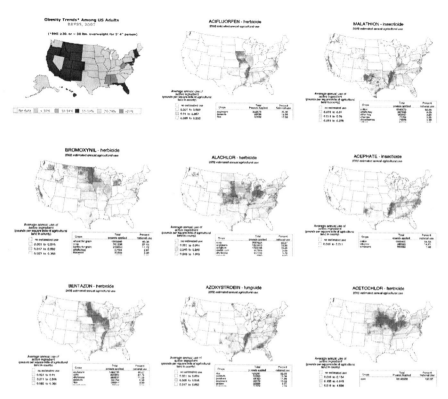

Spatial Association between Pesticide Use and Levels of Obesity and its Comorbidities in the US Case of thyroid disputing chemicals

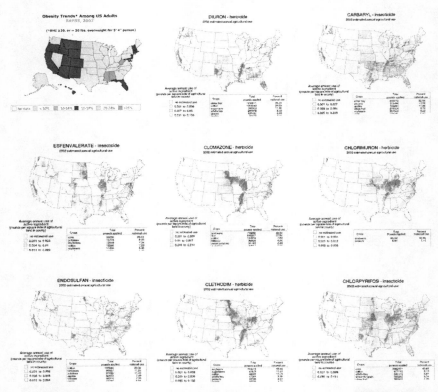

Spatial Association between Pesticide Use and Levels of Obesity and its Comorbidities in the US Case of thyroid disputing chemicals

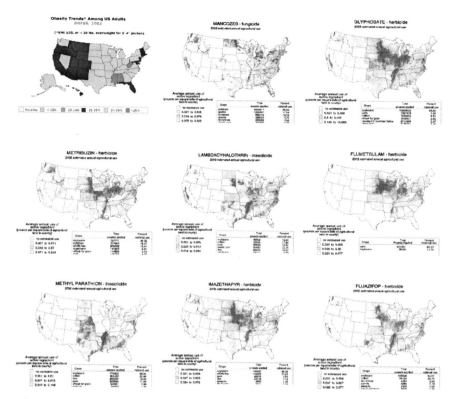

Spatial Association between Pesticide Use and Levels of Obesity and its Comorbidities in the U.S. Case of thyroid disputing chemicals

**Atrazine water contamination map
published by the USGS in 2002**

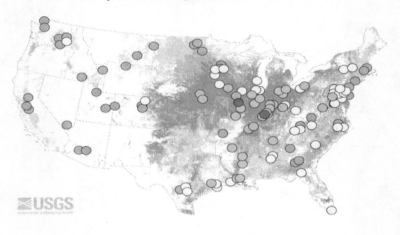

Measured Atrazine in Streams

Concentrations of atrazine measured in agricultural streams correlated with the distribution of its use on crops—primarily corn—with some of the highest concentrations (shown by red and orange) occurring in the corn-growing areas of Illinois, Indiana, Iowa, Nebraska, and Ohio.

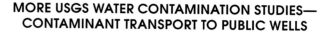

MORE USGS WATER CONTAMINATION STUDIES— CONTAMINANT TRANSPORT TO PUBLIC WELLS

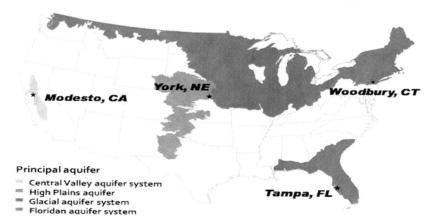

Principal aquifer

 Central Valley aquifer system
 High Plains aquifer
 Glacial aquifer system
 Floridan aquifer system

Contaminant transport to public wells

New USGS groundwater studies explain what, when, and how contaminants may reach public-supply wells. All wells are not equally vulnerable to contamination because of differences in three factors: the general chemistry of the aquifer, groundwater age, and direct paths within aquifer systems that allow water and contaminants to reach a well. The USGS tracked the movement of contaminants in groundwater and in public-supply wells in four aquifers in California, Connecticut, Nebraska, and Florida. The importance of each factor differs among the various aquifer settings, depending upon natural geology and local aquifer conditions, as well as human activities related to land use and well construction and operation. Findings in the four different aquifer systems can be applied to similar aquifer settings and wells throughout the nation.

Obesity Trends* Among US Adults
BRFSS, 2003
(*BMI ≥30, or ~ 30 lbs. overweight for 5' 4" person)

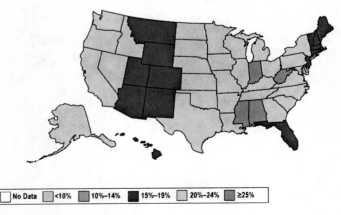

| No Data | <10% | 10%–14% | 15%–19% | 20%–24% | ≥25% |

Source: Behavioral Risk Factor Surveillance System, CDC.

In 2003, the new obesity rate ≥ 25% set in Mississippi, Alabama, and West Virginia in 2002, had extended to Indiana. Keep an eye on this new trend and see how it spreads by contiguity to all the states in the Mississippi Delta, the South, and the Midwest within only four years. Follow the progressive obesity spread in years 2004, 2005, 2006, and 2007. By 2007, Southern states, and most of the Midwest states except for Illinois and Wisconsin, had attained the rates ≥ 25%.

Obesity Trends* Among US Adults
BRFSS, 2004
(*BMI ≥30, or ~ 30 lbs. overweight for 5' 4" person)

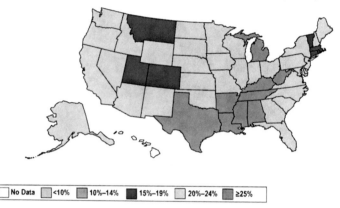

| | No Data | | <10% | | 10%–14% | | 15%–19% | | 20%–24% | | ≥25% |

Source: Behavioral Risk Factor Surveillance System, CDC.

Obesity Trends* Among US Adults
BRFSS, 2005
(*BMI ≥30, or ~ 30 lbs. overweight for 5' 4" person)

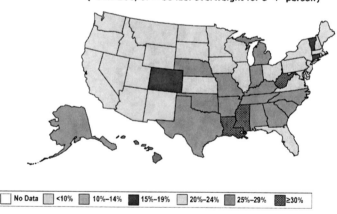

| | No Data | | <10% | | 10%–14% | | 15%–19% | | 20%–24% | | 25%–29% | | ≥30% |

Source: Behavioral Risk Factor Surveillance System, CDC.

Notice the new obesity rate ≥ 30% in Mississippi, Alabama, and West Virginia in 2005

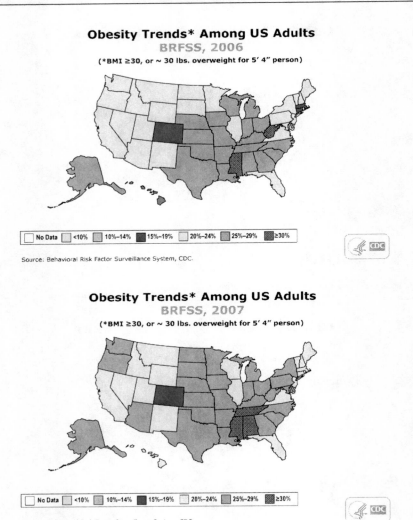

In 2007, Tennessee had joined in the new rate ≥ 30% set in 2005.

Obesity Trends* Among US Adults
BRFSS, 2008
(*BMI ≥30, or ~ 30 lbs. overweight for 5' 4" person)

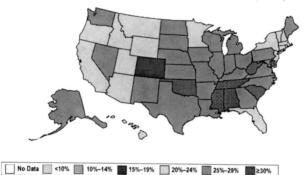

No Data | <10% | 10%–14% | 15%–19% | 20%–24% | 25%–29% | ≥30%

Source: Behavioral Risk Factor Surveillance System, CDC.

Obesity Trends* Among US Adults
BRFSS, 2009
(*BMI ≥30, or ~ 30 lbs. overweight for 5' 4" person)

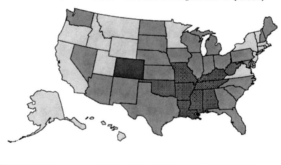

No Data | <10% | 10%–14% | 15%–19% | 20%–24% | 25%–29% | ≥30%

Source: Behavioral Risk Factor Surveillance System, CDC.

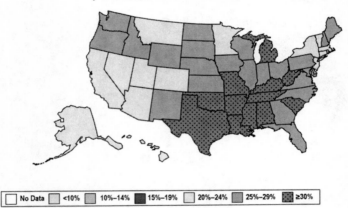

Obesity Trends* Among U.S. Adults
BRFSS, 2010
(*BMI ≥30, or ~ 30 lbs. overweight for 5' 4" person)

| No Data | <10% | 10%–14% | 15%–19% | 20%–24% | 25%–29% | ≥30% |

Source: Behavioral Risk Factor Surveillance System, CDC.

In 2009, all the states in the Mississippi embayment had achieved the obesity rate of ≥ 30%. Notice the contiguity effect of the spread. The rate started in Mississippi, Alabama, and West Virginia and progressively spread to Tennessee, Louisiana, Arkansas, Missouri, Kentucky, and Oklahoma. In 2010 Texas, South Carolina and Michigan have joined this group. This is not pure coincidence, and the population in the Mississippi Delta does not consume any more "junk food" than the rest of America. What goes through the Mississippi Delta may account for the higher obesity rate in that area.

TABLE 18

2008 National statistics—principal diagnosis only

Outcomes by patient and hospital characteristics for
ICD-9-CM principal diagnosis code
244.9 Hypothyroidism Nos

		Total number of discharges	LOS (length of stay), days (median)	Charges, $ (median)	Costs, $ (median)	Aggregate costs
All discharges		5,474 (100.00%)	3.0	15,797	5,524	41,499,598
Age group	<1	*	*	*	*	*
	1–17	*	*	*	*	*
	18–44	712 (13.01%)	3.0	13,120	4,327	4,487,846
	45–64	1,561 (28.52%)	3.0	15,444	5,653	12,556,615
	65–84	2,158 (39.42%)	4.0	17,274	5,767	16,674,937
	85+	977 (17.85%)	4.0	15,256	5,652	7,150,845
Sex	Male	1,428 (26.09%)	3.0	16,593	5,732	11,191,637
	Female	4,040 (73.82%)	3.0	15,406	5,378	30,276,904
	Missing	*	*	*	*	*
Median income for zip code	Low	1,688 (30.83%)	3.0	13,358	5,145	11,426,805
	Not low	3,676 (67.15%)	3.0	17,206	5,687	29,134,340
	Missing	111 (2.02%)	*	*	4,330	938,454
Region	Northeast	1,058 (19.33%)	4.0	15,985	5,465	8,428,620
	Midwest	1,156 (21.11%)	*	14,785	6,006	9,537,699
	South	2,235 (40.84%)	3.0	13,727	4,755	14,086,522
	West	1,024 (18.71%)	3.0	23,070	6,338	9,446,756

Hypothyroidism discharges in 2008 followed the same pattern as those of previous years. The highest rate was in women; the South and the Midwest had the highest prevalence.

TABLE 19

Outcomes by patient and hospital characteristics for
ICD-9-CM principal diagnosis code
278.01 Morbid Obesity

		Total number of discharges	LOS (length of stay), days (median)	Charges, $ (median)	Costs, $ (median)	Aggregate costs
All discharges		130,267 (100.00%)	2.0	32,743	10,276	1,548,060,384
Age group	1–17	254 (0.20%)	*	33,426	9,064	3,238,210
	18–44	62,627 (48.08%)	2.0	32,060	10,220	728,569,432
	45–64	61,539 (47.24%)	2.0	33,138	10,456	751,433,641
	65–84	5,713 (4.39%)	1.0	34,479	9,222	63,369,167
	85+	*	*	*	*	*
	Missing	129 (0.10%)	2.0	45,275	10,517	1,439,250
Sex	Male	27,453 (21.07%)	2.0	34,297	10,397	344,474,306
	Female	102,443 (78.64%)	2.0	32,261	10,242	1,199,675,406
	Missing	*	2.0	45,275	9,965	3,910,672
Median income for zip code	Low	24,525 (18.83%)	2.0	30,924	10,094	284,746,824
	Not low	101,365 (77.81%)	2.0	33,426	10,443	1,221,950,836
	Missing	*	2.0	24,220	7,966	41,362,723
Region	Northeast	35,041 (26.90%)	2.0	25,936	8,528	363,972,046
	Midwest	21,448 (16.46%)	2.0	31,363	12,275	296,318,826
	South	38,448 (29.52%)	2.0	32,387	10,990	473,230,415
	West	35,329 (27.12%)	2.0	41,925	10,342	414,539,097

Obesity discharges in 2008 also followed the same pattern as those of previous years. The highest rate was in women, and the South and the Midwest had the highest prevalence. However, the obesity rate decreased slightly in 2008.

Following the CDC obesity maps from 1985 to 2010, a pattern emerges. It is clear that the Southern states start the trend that spread by contiguity to all the other states going through the Midwest, then the Northeast, and finally the West. The states in the Mississippi Delta are hardest hit as shown in the latest obesity maps. This trend may be due to the Mississippi River draining most of the Midwest and Southern rivers that carry with them the endocrine-disrupting pesticides and herbicides sprayed in the farmlands. The 2008 HCUP discharges for hypothyroidism correlate well with this picture. The South had 41%, followed by the Midwest with 21%, the Northeast with 19%, and the West with 18%. The hypothyroidism discharge rate patterns continued the same through all the years of the published obesity maps and rates.

The obesity pattern held constant from 1985 to 2010. From 1997 to 2009, women continued to have the highest discharge rates. Prime age women, 18 to 44, had the highest discharges, followed by older adults, ages 45 to 64. In 2008, the cost associated with morbid obesity related hospitalization was $1.5 billion. The low income group accounted for 19% of the discharges whereas the high income group contributed 78%. The 2008 discharge data showed regional obesity rates of 29.5% for the South, 27% for the West, 26.9% for the Northeast, and 16.5% for the Midwest. This regional report does not seem to correlate with the trend observed from 1985 to 2009.

These observations raise several questions: Why are the Mississippi Delta states so much more vulnerable? Why do women, especially those of prime-age, have so much more obesity discharges than all other groups? Why is hypothyroidism so much more prevalent in women? The following chapters will shed some light on these questions.

The South is more populous than the rest of the US regions. Some may argue that it is therefore logical that the South has more obesity, more hypothyroidism, and more of the obesity related comorbidities. Looking at the population distribution in the South, Texas and Florida have more population than the other Southern states. Hence, it is only logical to see if Texas and Florida have more obesity and hypothyroidism discharges than the rest of the Southern states. Examination of the obesity and hypothyroidism discharges in Texas and Florida in 2008, showed that the two states have low discharges for these two conditions. Thus, the high hypothyroidism and high obesity rates and associated comorbidities in the South and especially in the Mississippi Delta are due to something more sinister.

TABLE 20

2009 National statistics — principal diagnosis only

Outcomes by patient and hospital characteristics for
ICD-9-CM principal diagnosis code 278.01 Morbid Obesity

		Total number of discharges	LOS (length of stay), days (mean)	LOS (length of stay), days (median)	Charges, $ (mean)	Costs, $ (mean)	Aggregate costs	Aggregate charges, $ (the "national bill")
All discharges		132,448 (100.00%)	2.2	2.0	41,931	12,405	1,642,293,490	5,551,321,702
Age group	<1	*	*	*	*	*	*	*
	1-17	239 (0.18%)	1.8	1.0	45,263	12,517	2,990,436	10,813,997
	18-44	62,928 (47.51%)	2.0	2.0	40,730	12,065	759,046,843	2,562,558,773
	45-64	61,559 (46.48%)	2.3	2.0	42,800	12,742	783,801,225	2,632,831,033
	65-84	7,600 (5.74%)	2.4	2.0	44,406	12,475	94,831,997	337,486,654
	85+	*	*	*	*	*	*	*
	Missing	*	1.6	2.0	65,329	13,650	1,519,210	7,270,703
Sex	Male	29,663 (22.40%)	2.3	2.0	44,923	13,264	393,248,481	1,331,855,347
	Female	102,535 (77.42%)	2.1	2.0	41,017	12,155	1,245,838,173	4,204,354,124
	Missing	*	1.6	1.0	60,983	12,881	3,206,836	15,112,232
Payer	Medicare	19,590 (14.79%)	2.6	2.0	45,293	13,062	255,856,502	887,061,485
	Medicaid	8,749 (6.61%)	2.3	2.0	37,053	11,252	98,372,490	323,921,588
	Private insurance	90,385 (68.24%)	2.1	2.0	41,190	12,154	1,098,041,647	3,721,456,035
	Uninsured	9,051 (6.83%)	1.9	2.0	47,455	14,530	131,432,107	429,311,292
	Other	4,409 (3.33%)	2.3	2.0	40,134	12,389	54,629,047	176,964,840
	Missing	*	1.8	2.0	47,737	15,002	3,961,697	12,606,462
Median income for zipcode	Low	27,210 (20.54%)	2.3	2.0	41,430	12,555	341,407,106	1,126,810,038
	Not low	101,560 (76.68%)	2.1	2.0	42,385	12,457	1,264,542,474	4,302,598,180
	Missing	3,679 (2.78%)	2.6	2.0	33,117	9,874	36,343,910	121,913,484
Region	Northeast	26,254 (19.82%)	2.0	2.0	37,725	10,056	263,996,863	990,412,895
	Midwest	37,669 (28.44%)	2.5	2.0	37,384	13,466	507,079,579	1,408,037,599
	South	41,671 (31.46%)	2.0	2.0	44,221	13,138	547,126,914	1,841,671,575
	West	26,855 (20.28%)	2.1	2.0	49,016	12,076	324,090,133	1,311,199,633

* Denotes missing values

The morbid obesity discharges in 2009, showed that women
continue to bear the bulk of this disease and had a rate of 77.4%
compared to men with only 22.4%. The 18-44 age groups still

have the highest rate followed by the 45-64 age groups. In 2009, the South clearly had the highest morbid obesity discharges at 31.5%, followed by the Midwest at 28.4%, then the West at 20.3% and the Northeast at 19.8%. The well to do had the highest rate at 76.7% and the low income group had only 20.5%.

TABLE 21

Outcomes by patient and hospital characteristics for ICD-9-CM principal diagnosis code 244.9 Hypothyroidism Nos

		Total number of discharges	LOS (length of stay), days (mean)	LOS (length of stay), days (median)	Charges, $ (mean)	Costs, $ (mean)	Aggregate costs	Aggregate charges, $ (the "national bill")
All discharges		5,336 (100.00%)	4.3	3.0	25,124	7,173	38,275,928	134,045,978
Age group	<1	*	*	*	*	*	*	*
	1-17	57 (1.07%)	1.7	2.0	7,627	2,569	147,083	436,701
	18-44	831 (15.58%)	3.3	3.0	19,451	5,561	4,623,007	16,171,424
	45-64	1,622 (30.40%)	4.6	3.0	29,209	7,999	12,955,114	47,290,026
	65-84	1,869 (35.02%)	4.3	3.0	24,994	7,131	13,335,248	46,731,174
	85+	936 (17.54%)	5.0	4.0	24,165	7,402	6,925,671	22,613,412
Sex	Male	1,490 (27.92%)	4.6	3.0	24,542	7,614	11,348,032	36,594,163
	Female	3,847 (72.08%)	4.3	3.0	25,349	7,003	26,927,896	97,451,815
Payer	Medicare	3,040 (56.97%)	4.5	3.0	23,744	7,053	21,442,891	72,194,891
	Medicaid	655 (12.27%)	4.9	3.0	*	8,974	5,875,459	*
	Private insurance	949 (17.78%)	3.8	3.0	22,301	6,581	6,245,193	21,161,391
	Uninsured	527 (9.87%)	3.8	3.0	20,820	6,804	3,582,666	10,963,172
	Other	136 (2.54%)	4.2	3.0	21,866	7,060	958,388	2,968,342
	Missing	*	*	*	*	*	*	*
Median income for zipcode	Low	1,648 (30.89%)	4.4	3.0	27,287	7,214	11,878,592	44,919,490
	Not low	3,547 (66.47%)	4.2	3.0	23,989	7,133	25,311,396	85,127,288
	Missing	*	6.0	4.0	28,321	7,690	1,085,940	3,999,200
Region	Northeast	975 (18.28%)	4.8	4.0	*	8,126	7,926,115	*
	Midwest	1,193 (22.35%)	4.4	3.0	19,963	7,358	8,777,218	23,812,965
	South	2,096 (39.28%)	4.3	3.0	19,830	6,055	12,689,878	41,560,358
	West	1,072 (20.09%)	4.0	3.0	34,401	8,312	8,882,717	36,632,264

* Denotes missing values

The 2009 hypothyroidism hospital discharges were more prevalent in women at 72.1% and increased with age starting at 1.1 for the young, then 15.6% for ages (18-44), 30.4% for ages (45-64), 35% for ages (65-84), and slightly less for ages 85+ at 17.5%. Hypothyroidism discharges in 2009 were more prevalent in the South at 39.3% and the Midwest at 22.4% followed by the West at 20.1% and the Northeast at 18.3%. Notice that the regional hypothyroidism rate mirrors the regional obesity rate in 2010.

TABLE 22

STATE STATISTICS—2008 TEXAS-PRINCIPAL DIAGNOSIS ONLY

Outcomes by patient and hospital characteristics for ICD-9-CM principal diagnosis code 244.9 Hypothyroidism Nos

		Total number of discharges	LOS (length of stay), days (median)	Charges, $ (median)
All discharges		323 (100.00%)	3.0	17,115
Age group	<1	*	*	*
	1–17	*	*	*
	18–44	49 (15.17%)	3.0	12,981
	45–64	116 (35.91%)	3.0	19,135
	65–84	118 (36.53%)	4.0	17,956
	85+	35 (10.84%)	4.0	20,174
Sex	Male	96 (29.72%)	3.0	16,250
	Female	227 (70.28%)	4.0	17,368
Race/ethnicity	White	164 (50.77%)	3.5	17,008
	Black	52 (16.10%)	4.0	16,773
	Hispanic	81 (25.08%)	3.0	19,577
	Asian/Pacific Islander	*	*	*
	Native American	*	*	*
	Other	11 (3.41%)	2.0	11,948
	Missing	*	*	*

The hypothyroidism rate in Texas, one of the states with large population, does not account for the high hypothyroidism rate in the South.

TABLE 23

STATE STATISTICS—2008 TEXAS-PRINCIPAL DIAGNOSIS ONLY

Outcomes by patient and hospital characteristics for
ICD-9-CM principal diagnosis code
278.01 Morbid Obesity

		Total number of discharges	LOS (length of stay), days (median)	Charges, $ (median)
All discharges		9,486 (100.00%)	2.0	40,432
Age group	<1	*	*	*
	1–17	58 (0.61%)	2.0	45,273
	18–44	4,678 (49.31%)	2.0	41,339
	45–64	4,163 (43.89%)	2.0	40,198
	65–84	581 (6.12%)	1.0	36,275
	85+	*	*	*
	Missing	*	*	*
Sex	Male	2,017 (21.26%)	2.0	42,063
	Female	7,465 (78.69%)	2.0	40,099
	Missing	*	*	*
Race/ethnicity	White	5,398 (56.90%)	2.0	39,003
	Black	1,355 (14.28%)	2.0	44,741
	Hispanic	1,395 (14.71%)	2.0	47,483
	Asian/Pacific Islander	47 (0.50%)	1.0	81,304
	Native American	334 (3.52%)	2.0	29,469
	Other	684 (7.21%)	2.0	32,769
	Missing	273 (2.88%)	1.0	43,031

The obesity rate in Texas does not explain the high obesity rate in the south.

TABLE 24

STATE STATISTICS—2008 FLORIDA-PRINCIPAL DIAGNOSIS ONLY

Outcomes by patient and hospital characteristics for
ICD-9-CM principal diagnosis code
244.9 Hypothyroidism Nos

		Total number of discharges	LOS (length of stay), days (median)	Charges, $ (median)	Costs, $ (median)	Aggregate costs
All discharges		345 (100.00%)	3.0	19,053	4,422	2,123,947
Age group	1–17	*	*	*	*	*
	18–44	86 (24.93%)	3.0	15,908	3,595	443,224
	45–64	101 (29.28%)	3.0	18,577	4,692	554,445
	65–84	107 (31.01%)	4.0	20,479	4,865	784,818
	85+	50 (14.49%)	4.0	18,571	4,982	339,933
Sex	Male	85 (24.64%)	4.0	19,223	4,857	593,603
	Female	260 (75.36%)	3.0	18,565	4,368	1,530,344
Race/ ethnicity	White	236 (68.41%)	3.0	18,321	4,384	1,377,620
	Black	40 (11.59%)	3.0	17,661	4,479	249,655
	Hispanic	48 (13.91%)	3.0	21,670	4,939	353,995
	Asian/Pacific Islander	*	*	*	*	*
	Other	16 (4.64%)	3.0	26,809	4,722	109,237
	Missing	*	*	*	*	*

The hypothyroidism rate in Florida, one of the states with the largest population, does not account for the high hypothyroidism rate in the South. Controlling for the population in both Texas and Florida, the hypothyroidism rate is still higher in the South than in other regions.

TABLE 25

STATE STATISTICS—2008 FLORIDA-PRINCIPAL DIAGNOSIS ONLY

Outcomes by patient and hospital characteristics for
ICD-9-CM principal diagnosis code
278.01 Morbid Obesity

		Total number of discharges	LOS (length of stay), days (median)	Charges, $ (median)	Costs, $ (median)	Aggregate costs
All discharges		5,629 (100.00%)	2.0	39,488	8,372	57,517,771
Age group	1–17	18 (0.32%)	2.0	38,128	8,006	136,206
	18–44	2,478 (44.02%)	2.0	39,162	8,213	24,516,225
	45–64	2,704 (48.04%)	2.0	39,815	8,571	28,794,711
	65–84	429 (7.62%)	1.0	38,505	8,015	4,070,630
Sex	Male	1,412 (25.08%)	2.0	41,513	8,733	15,677,313
	Female	4,217 (74.92%)	2.0	38,794	8,274	41,840,458
Race/ ethnicity	White	4,135 (73.46%)	2.0	38,948	8,326	40,845,811
	Black	745 (13.24%)	2.0	38,881	8,458	7,728,327
	Hispanic	479 (8.51%)	2.0	42,942	9,902	6,456,866
	Asian/Pacific Islander	12 (0.21%)	2.0	42,262	7,505	98,795
	Native American	*	*	*	*	*
	Other	174 (3.09%)	1.0	45,731	7,656	1,606,457
	Missing	79 (1.40%)	1.0	35,377	7,410	679,933

The obesity rates in these two large states in terms of population do not account for the large proportion of obesity in the South.

Why Does the Obesity Trend Start in the Mississippi Embayment States?

- The Mississippi Embayment states grow cotton.
- Cotton requires more pesticides and herbicides than any other crops in the US.
- The Mississippi River drains most of Upper Midwest and Midwest rivers that carry with them the pesticides and herbicides sprayed in farmlands in these regions.

Mississippi Embayment States and Estimated harvested Cotton in the US in 1967.
This map is only provided as reference.

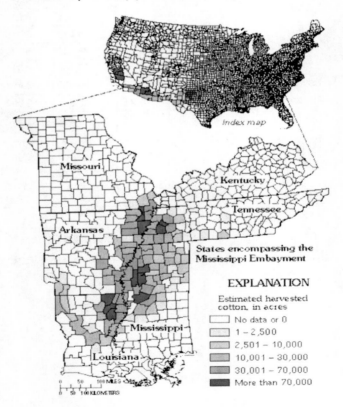

Figure 1. Estimated harvested cotton in the United States, 1967 (data from Battaglin and Goolsby, 1995).

Pesticides and Herbicides used in the US 1990–1993

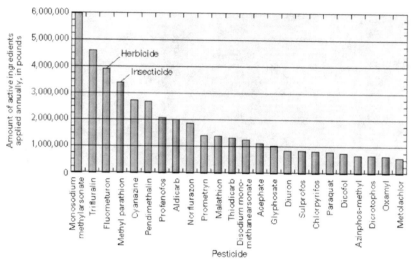

Figure 3. Cotton pesticide usage in the United States, 1990—93 (data from Gianessi and Anderson, 1995).

Concentrations of Insecticides detected in Surface—Water Samples of the Mississippi Embayment for January–December 1996

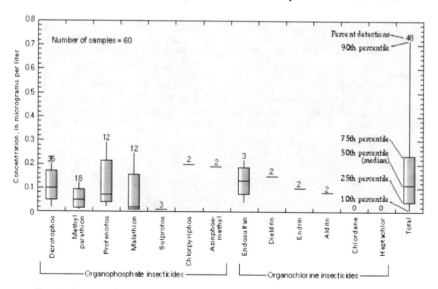

Figure 8. Concentrations of insecticides detected in surface-water samples from the Mississippi Embayment, January—December 1996.

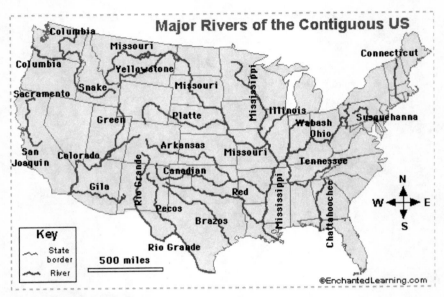

Major Rivers of the Contiguous US

Key
~ State border
~ River

500 miles

©EnchantedLearning.com

River, Length in miles (flows into)

1. Missouri, 2,540 miles (flows into Mississippi River)
2. Mississippi, 2,340 miles (flows into Gulf of Mexico)
3. Yukon, 1,980 miles (flows into Bering Sea)
4. Rio Grande, 1,900 miles (flows into Gulf of Mexico)
5. St. Lawrence, 1,900 miles (flows into Gulf of St. Lawrence)
6. Arkansas, 1,460 miles (flows into Mississippi River)
7. Colorado, 1,450 miles (flows into Gulf of California)
8. Red, 1,290 miles (flows into Mississippi River)
9. Brazos, 1,280 miles (flows into Gulf of Mexico)
10. Columbia, 1,240 miles (flows into Pacific Ocean)
11. Snake, 1,040 miles (flows into Columbia River)
12. Platte, 990 miles (flows into Missouri River)
13. Ohio, 981 miles (flows into Mississippi River)
14. Pecos, 926 miles (flows into Gulf of Mexico)
15. Canadian, 906 miles (flows into Arkansas River)
16. Tennessee, 886 miles (flows into Ohio River)
17. Colorado, 862 miles (flows into Matagordo Bay)
18. North Canadian, 800 miles (flows into Canadian River)
19. Mobile, 774 miles (flows into Gulf of Mexico)
20. Kansas, 743 miles (flows into Missouri River)
21. Kuskokwim, 724 miles (flows into Bering Sea)
22. Green, 730 miles (flows into Colorado River)
23. James, 710 miles (flows into Missouri River)
24. Yellowstone, 692 miles (flows into Missouri River)
25. Tanana, 659 miles (flows into Yukon River)
26. Gila, 630 miles (flows into Colorado River)
27. Milk, 625 miles (flows into Missouri River)
28. Quachita, 605 miles (flows into Red River)

Refs. Encyclopedia Britannica and Kammerer, J.C., May, 1990, *Largest Rivers in United States*, US Geological Survey Fact Sheet, Open File Report 87-242.
Note: Measuring the exact length of a river is difficult, and the length can change over time. Many references cite different lengths for the same river. Average have to be taken in these cases.

This map clearly shows that the most important rivers in the Midwest and the South drain into the Mississippi River that carries with it all the pesticides and herbicides from farm lands in the upper Midwest and Midwest into the Mississippi Embayment states (Mississippi, Louisiana, Arkansas, Missouri, Kentucky, Tennessee, and the contiguous neighboring states of Alabama, Texas, Oklahoma, etc.).

TABLE 26

2009 State Obesity Rates—
Mississippi Embayment States are indicated by **

State	%	State	%	State	%	State	%
**Alabama	31.0	Illinois	26.5	Montana	23.2	Rhode Island	24.6
Alaska	24.8	Indiana	29.5	Nebraska	27.2	South Carolina	29.4
Arizona	25.5	Iowa	27.9	Nevada	25.8	South Dakota	29.6
**Arkansas	30.5	Kansas	28.1	New Hampshire	25.7	**Tennessee	32.3
California	24.8	**Kentucky	31.5	New Jersey	23.3	Texas	28.7
Colorado	18.6	**Louisiana	33.0	New Mexico	25.1	Utah	23.5
Connecticut	20.6	Maine	25.8	New York	24.2	Vermont	22.8
Delaware	27.0	Maryland	26.2	North Carolina	29.3	Virginia	25.0
Washington DC	19.7	Massachusetts	21.4	North Dakota	27.9	Washington	26.4
Florida	25.2	Michigan	29.6	Ohio	28.8	West Virginia	31.1
Georgia	27.2	Minnesota	24.6	Oklahoma	31.4	Wisconsin	28.7
Hawaii	22.3	**Mississippi	34.4	Oregon	23.0	Wyoming	24.6
Idaho	24.5	**Missouri	30.0	Pennsylvania	27.4		

Based on all the evidence presented above, it is therefore not surprising that the Mississippi Embayment states and their contiguous neighbors represented here by ** carry the highest obesity rates in the US. West Virginia, one of the most polluted states in the US, also carries an obesity rate similar to the states in the Mississippi Delta. The states in the Midwest follow the Southern states as indicated above.

Do Herbicides and Pesticides Cause Any Harm to Humans?

From the evidence shown above, it seems appropriate to look with increased suspicion at herbicides and pesticides sprayed in farmlands. There are studies that point to the concentration of these chemicals in the US water supply and in foods. Endocrine disrupting effects of these herbicides and pesticides have been reported and heavily debated. Looking at the USGS reports and comparing the USGS herbicides/pesticides maps with the CDC obesity maps and the HCUP discharges for hypothyroidism and morbid obesity by region, you may draw the conclusions yourself.

While awaiting a definitive verdict, many are recommending solutions to avoid mass casualties. Organic foods are highly recommended by the experts and therefore are high in demand. The high demand and the low supply leads to higher prices for these organic food items, and not all Americans can afford to go organic. Organic farms are still limited in numbers, despite the organic food production act of 1990. The nation should therefore transition into organic farming from synthetic chemical farming. This will be a challenge since synthetic chemical farming has high yields and the ability to feed not only the US population but the rest of the world.

We are, therefore, in a situation I call conflicting responsibilities. On one hand we need to produce more to feed a growing population and that can be achieved with agrichemicals. However, agrichemicals are making us sick and organic farming that is safe, has low yield. How do we get out of this bad situation? Some solutions to reduce pesticide use such as creating genetically modified plants that can sustain a heavy dosage of only one pesticide such as Roundup (glyphosate), have become controversial. Safer farming, therefore, calls for a more intensive research and the government should start putting more resources and encourage scientists to engage in this type of research for a better America and world tomorrow. The following sections provide evidence on the destructive effects of agrichemicals.

EFFECTS OF ENDOCRINE DISRUPTING CHEMICALS

TABLE 27

Pesticide	CAS number	Pesticide class	Type of pesticide	Maximum LT-MDL (µg/L)
Atrazine	1912-24-9	Triazine	Herbicide	0.004
Acetochlor	34256-82-1	Acetanilide	Herbicide	0.003
Metolachlor	51218-45-2	Acetanilide	Herbicide	0.006
Alachlor	15972-60-8	Acetanilide	Herbicide	0.002
Cyanazine	21725-46-2	Triazine	Herbicide	0.009
EPTC	759-94-4	Thiocarbamate	Herbicide	0.002
Simazine	122-34-9	Triazine	Herbicide	0.006
Metribuzin	21087-64-9	Triazine	Herbicide	0.014
Prometon	1610-18-0	Triazine	Herbicide	0.007
Chlorpyrifos	2921-88-2	Organothiophosphate	Insecticide	0.003
Diazinon	333-41-5	Organothiophosphate	Insecticide	0.003

Trends in Pesticide Concentrations in Corn-Belt Streams, 1996–2006

Two related concepts—statistical significance and p-value are used to discuss and compare the trends results from the various methods. The less likely the obtained value of a particular trend statistic (such as the SEAKEN test statistic or the estimated trend slope from the SEAWAVE model) could have occurred by chance (that is, even if there was no trend), the more confidence we have that the trend is real and not an artifact of random variation. The p-value is the probability that the trend statistic could have been as extreme, or more extreme, than the value obtained simply by chance. All p-values in this report are two-sided p-values, which means they do not distinguish between negative values (downtrends) or positive values (uptrends). Thus, the p-value is the probability that the absolute value of the trend statistic could have been as large, or larger than, the obtained value simply by chance. A significance level often is specified, which is the p-value below which a trend is deemed to be "statistically significant." For this report, two significance levels—1 % and 10 %—are used. A trend is significant at the 1-% level if the p-value is less than or equal to 0.01 and significant at the 10-% level if the p-value is less than or equal to 0.10. The p-value sometimes is referred to as the "attained significance level," because it is the smallest significance level for which the trend can be deemed significant.

Effect of Endocrine Disrupting Chemicals

- *Our Stolen Future* published data on endocrine disrupting chemicals that I am using in this book for illustration.
- Most pesticides and herbicides used in the US have major effects on:
  - The thyroid gland
  - Estrogen and
  - The reproductive system
- Hypothyroidism, hyperestrogenism and hypoandrogenism in men and women are the most important direct effects of these chemicals.
- Please note the effects of the pesticides and herbicides in the following tables to corroborate the statements above.

TABLE 28

Persistent organohalogens

Compound(s)	Hormone system affected	Mechanism if known	References
Benzenehexachloride (BHC)	Thyroid		Akhtar et al. 1996
1,2-dibromoethane	Reproductive		Brittebo et al. 1987
Chloroform	Reproductive		Brittebo et al. 1987
Dioxins and furans (in order of antiestrogenic potency: 2,3,7,8-tetrachlorodibenzo-p-dioxin > 2,3,7,8-tetrachlorodibenzofuran > 2,3,4,7,8-pentachlorodibenzofuran > 1,2,3,7,9-pentachlorodibenzofuran > 1,3,6,8-tetrachlo-rodibenzofuran)	Estrogen	work as anti-estrogen through binding with Ah receptor, which then inhibits estrogen receptor binding to estrogen response elements, thereby inhibiting estrogen action.	Krishnan and Safe 1993 Klinge et al. 1999
Octachlorostyrene	Thyroid		Sandan et al. 2000
PBBs	Estrogen/Thyroid		Bahn et al. 1980 Hendreson et al. 1995
PCBs (in order of antiestrogenic potency: 3,3' – pentachlorobiphenyl > 3,3,4,4,5,5' – hexachlorobiphenyl 3,3', 4,4– tetrachlorobiphenyl > 2,3,3',4,4',5'–hexa, 2,3,3',4,4' – and 2,3,4,4',5– pentachlorobiphyenyl > Aroclors 1221, 1232. 1248, 1254, and 1260 were inactive as antiestrogens at the highest concentrations used in this study (10–6 NI)	Estrogen/androgen/Thyroid Adverse outcomes in reproductive systems.	Inhibits estrogen binding to the receptor; works as anti-estrogen. anti-androgenic via Ah receptor interaction	Korach et al. 1988 Zoeller et al. 2000 Grey et al. 1999
PCB, hydroxylated	Thyroid	Binds to thyroid hormone binding protein, but not to the thyroid hormone receptor.	Cheek et al. 1999
PBDEs	Thyroid	Interfere with thyroxine (T4) binding with transthryetin	Ilonka et al. 2000
Pentachlorophenol	Thyroid	Reduces thyroid hormone possibly through a direct effect on the thyroid gland.	Bear et al. 1999 Gerhard et al. 1999

Food Antioxidant

Compound	Hormone system affected	Mechanism if known	References
Butylated hydroxyanisole (BHA)	Estrogen	Inhibits binding to the estrogen receptor.	Jobling et al. 1995

Pesticide (for information organized by pesticide class)

Compound	Hormone system affected	Mechanism if known	References
Acetochlor	Thyroid (decrease of thyroid hormone levels, increase in TSH)		Hurley et al. 1998
Alachlor	Thyroid (decrease of thyroid hormone levels, increase in TSH)		Wilson et al. 1996
Aldrin	Estrogen	Binds to estrogen receptors; competes with estradiol.	Jorgenson et al. 2001
Allethrin, d-trans	Estrogen		Go et al. 1999
Amitrol	Thyroid	Thyroid peroxidase inhibitors; inhbits thyroid hormone synthesis.	Hurley et al. 1998
Atrazine	Neuroendocrine-pituitary (depression of LH surge), testosterone metabolism	Inhibits ligand binding to androgen and estrogen receptors.	Danzo et al. 1997
Carbaryl	Estrogen and progesterone		Klotz et al. 1997
Chlofentezine	Thyroid	Enhances secretion of thyroid hormone.	Hurley et al. 1998
Chlordane	Testosterone and progesterone		Willingham et al. 2000
Cypermethrin	Disruption of reproductive function		Moore and Waring et al. 2001

DDT	Estrogen	DDT and related compounds act in a number of ways to disrupt endocrine function by binding with the estrogen receptor, including estrogen mimickry and antagonism, altering the pattern of synthesis or metabolism of hormones, and (4) modifying hormone receptor levels.	Soto *et al.* 1994 Lascombe *et al.* 2000 Kupfer *et al.* 1980 Rajapakse *et al.* 2001
DDT Metabolite, p,p'–DDE	Androgen	Inhibits androgen binding to the androgen receptor.	Kelce 1995
Dicofol (Kelthan)	Estrogen		Vinggaard *et al.* 1999
Dieldrin	Estrogen	Binds to estrogen receptor; competes with estradiol.	Soto *et al.* 1994 Jorgenson 2001
Endosulfan	Estrogen		Soto *et al.* 1994 Soto *et al.* 1995
Ethylene thiourea	Thyroid	Thyroid peroxidase inhibitor.	Hurley *et al.* 1998
Fenarimol	Estrogen	Estrogen receptor agonist.	Vinggaard *et al.* 1999
Fenbuconazole	Thyroid	Enhances secretion of thyroid hormone.	Hurley *et al.* 1998
Fenitrothion	Antiandrogen	Competitive androgen receptor antagonist.	Tamura *et al.* 2001
Fenvalerate	Estrogen		Go *et al.* 1999
Fipronil	Thyroid	Enhances secretion of thyroid hormone.	Hurley *et al.* 1998
Heptachlor	Thyroid		Akhtar *et al.* 1996 Reuber 1987
Heptachlor-epoxide	Thyroid/Reproductive	Metabolite of heptachlor.	Reuber 1987
Iprodione	Inhibition of testosterone synthesis		Benhamed 1996
Karate	Thyroid	A decrease of thyroid hormone in serum; direct effect on the thyroid gland?	Akhtar *et al.* 1996
Kepone (Chlordecone)	Estrogen	Displays androgen and estrogen receptor-binding affinities.	Waller *et al.* 1996 Soto *et al.* 1994 McLachlan (ed)
Ketoconazole	Effects on reproductive systems		Marty *et al.* 1999 Marty *et al.* 2001
Lindane (Hexachlorocyclohexane)	Estrogen/Androgen	Inhibits ligand binding to androgen and estrogen receptors.	Danzo 1997
Linuron	Androgen	Androgen receptor antagonist.	Waller *et al.* 1996 Lambright *et al.* 2000 Grey *et al.* 1999
Malathion	Thyroid	Significant decrease of thyroid hormone in serum, with perhaps a direct effect on the thyroid gland.	Akhtar *et al.* 1996
Mancozeb	Thyroid	Thyroid peroxidase inhibitors.	Hurley *et al.* 1998
Maneb	Thyroid	The metabolite ethylenthiourea inhibits thyroid hormone synthesis.	Toppari *et al.* 1995
Methomyl	Thyroid		Porter *et al.* 1993 Klotz *et al.* 1997
Methoxychlor	Estrogen	Through mechanisms other than receptor antagonism. Precise mechanism still unclear.	Pickford and Morris 1999
Metribuzin	Thyroid		Porter *et al.* 1993
Mirex	Antiandrogenic activity; inhibits production of LH. Potentially thyroid		Chen *et al.* 1986 Chernoff *et al.* 1976
Nitrofen	Thyroid	Structural similarities to the thyroid hormones; nitrofen or its metabolite may have thyroid hormone activities.	Stevens and Summer 1991
Nonachlor, trans–	Estrogen	Estrogen receptor agonist?	Willingham *et al.* 2000
Oxychlordane	Reproductive		Guillette *et al.* 1999
Pendimethalin	Thyroid	Enhances secretion of thyroid hormone.	Hurley *et al.* 1998
Pentachloronitrobenzene	Thyroid	Enhances secretion of thyroid hormone.	Hurley *et al.* 1998
Permethrin	Estrogenic		Go *et al.* 1999

Procymidone	Androgen	Androgen receptor antagonist.	Ostby *et al.* 1999 Grey *et al.* 1999
Prodiamine	Thyroid	Enhances secretion of thyroid hormone.	Hurley *et al.* 1998
Pyrimethanil	Thyroid	Enhances secretion of thyroid hormone.	Hurley *et al.* 1998
Sumithrin	Androgen		Go *et al.* 1999
Tarstar	Thyroid	A decrease of thyroid hormone in serum; direct effect on the thyroid gland?	Akhtar *et al.* 1996
Thiazopyr	Thyroid	Enhances secretion of thyroid hormone.	Hurley *et al.* 1998
Thiram	Neuroendocrine-pituitary (depression of LH surge), thyroid (decrease of T4, increase of TSH)		Stoker *et al.* 1993
Toxaphene	Estrogen/Thyroid		Soto *et al.* 1994
Triadimefon	Estrogen	Estrogen receptor agonist.	Vinggaard *et al.* 1999
Triadimenol	Estrogen	Estrogen receptor agonist.	Vinggaard *et al.* 1999
Tributyltin	Reproductive		Horiguchi *et al.* 2000
Trifluralin	Reprodutive/Metabolic		Rawlings *et al.* 1998
Vinclozolin	Androgen	Anti-androgenic. (Competes with androgens for the androgen receptor (AR), inhibits AR-DNA binding, and alters androgen-dependent gene expression.)	Soto *et al.* 1994 Soto *et al.* 1995 Kelce *et al.* 1994 Grey *et al.* 1999
Zineb	Thyroid	The metabolite ethylenthiourea inhibits thyroid hormone synthesis.	Toppari *et al.* 1995
Ziram	Thyroid	Inhibits the iodide peroxidase. Structural similarities between ziram and thiram; ziram can be metabolized to thiram in the environment.	Marinovich *et al.* 1997

Phthalate

Compound	Hormones affected	Mechanism	References
Butyl benzyl phthalate (BBP)	Estrogen	Inhibits binding to the estrogen receptor.	Jobling *et al.* 1995
Di-n-butyl phthalate (DBP)	Estrogen Androgen	Inhibits binding to the estrogen receptor. anti-androgenic	Jobling *et al.* 1995 Harris *et al.* 1997 Grey *et al.* 1999
Di-ethylhexyl phthalate (DEHP)	Estrogen Androgen	Inhibits binding to the estrogen receptor. anti-androgenic	Jobling *et al.* 1995 Harris *et al.* 1997 Moore *et al.* 2001 Grey *et al.* 1999
Diethyl Phthalate (DEP)	Estrogen		Harris *et al.* 1997

Other Compounds

Compound	Hormones affected	Mechanism	References
Benzophenone	Estrogen	Binds weakly to estrogen	Schlupf *et al.*
Bisphenol A	Estrogen	Estrogenic; binds to estrogen receptor	Fisher *et al.* 1999 Anderson *et al.* 1999 Rajapakse *et al.* 2001
Bisphenol F	Estrogen	Estrogenic; binds to estrogen receptor	Perez *et al.* 1998
Benzo(a)pyrene	Androgen	anti-androgenic	Thomas 1990
Carbendazim	Reproductive		Gray *et al.* 1990
Ethane Dimethane Sulphonate	Reproductive		Gray *et al.* 1999
Perfluorooctane sulfonate (PFOS)	Thyroid, reproductive	suppression of T3, T4; mechanism unknown	3M data
Nonylphenol, octylphenol	Estrogen	Estrogen receptor agonists; reduces estradiol binding to the estrogen receptor.	Soto *et al.* 1991 Soto *et al.* 1995 Danzo *et al.* 1997 Lascombe *et al.* 2000 Rajapakse *et al.* 2001

| Resorcinol | Thyroid | | Lindsay *et al.* 1989 |
| Styrene dimers and trimers | Estrogen | Estrogen receptor agonists | Ohyama *et al.* 2001 |

Metals

Compound	Hormones affected	Mechanism	References
Arsenic	Glucocorticoid	Selective inhibition of DNA transcription normally stimulated by the glucocorticoid-GR complex.	Kaltreider *et al.* 2001
Cadmium	Estrogenic	Activates estrogen receptor through an interaction with the hormone-binding domain of the receptor.	Stoica *et al.* 2000 Johnson *et al.* 2003
Lead	Reproductive		Telisman *et al.* 2000 Hanas *et al.* 1999
Mercury	Reproductive/Thyroid		Facemire *et al.*

Source: Colborn, Our Stolen Future: Are we Threatening our Fertility, Intelligence and Survival? A Scientific Detective Story

Again, notice that most of the reported pesticides and herbicides adversely affect the thyroid, increase estrogen, and have a major impact on the reproductive system. This may explain why women have more morbid obesity than men. Women have more endogenous production of estrogen than men. This endogenous estrogen, coupled with the exogenous estrogens may lead to obesity. This connection will be made clearer in later sections of the book.

The USGS in 1992, 1997, and 2002 published the pesticides/herbicides usage maps in farmlands in the US. The maps showed the average annual pesticide and herbicide use intensity expressed as average weight (in pounds) of a pesticide or herbicide applied to each square mile of agricultural land in a county. The area of each map is based on state-level estimates of pesticide/herbicide use rates for individual crops that were compiled by the Crop Life Foundation and Crop Protection Research Institute based on information collected during 1999 through 2004 and on 2002 Census of Agriculture county crop acreage. These pesticides and herbicides are reported in Table 29. Many of these chemicals are present in "Our Stolen Future" tables, and all the reported chemical groups are present in these tables. Some of these chemicals are also banned in the European Union. Until proven otherwise, I will suspect that all these synthetic chemicals are endocrine disruptors even if it is minor. I am concerned about the thyroid, estrogen and androgen disruption potential of these chemicals. Selected maps from this group of chemicals that either had thyroid disruption or estrogen disruption capacity were compared with the obesity maps on pages 47–53, and you saw how the areas in the chemical maps matched perfectly well the areas of the CDC obesity maps.

TABLE 29
Pesticide

Herbicide Name	Tthyroid Disruptors (Potential)	Estrogen Disruptors (Potential)
1,3-D	YES	YES
2,4-D	YES	YES
2,4-DB	YES	YES
abamectin	YES	YES
acephate	YES	YES
acetochlor	YES	YES
acifluorfen	YES	YES
alachlor	YES	YES
aldicarb	YES	YES
ametryn	YES	YES
amitraz	YES	YES
asulam	YES	YES
atrazine	YES	YES
azadirachtin	YES	YES
azinphos-methyl	YES	YES
azoxystrobin	YES	YES
benefin	YES	YES
benomyl	YES	YES
bensulfuron	YES	YES
bensulide	YES	YES
bentazon	YES	YES
benzyladenine	YES	YES
bifenthrin	YES	YES
bispyribac	YES	YES
bromacil	YES	YES

Herbicide Name	Tthyroid Disruptors (Potential)	Estrogen Disruptors (Potential)
bromoxynil	YES	YES
buprofezin	YES	YES
butenoic acid	YES	YES
butralin	YES	YES
cacodylic acid	YES	YES
captan	YES	YES
carbaryl	YES	YES
carbofuran	YES	YES
carfentrazone	YES	YES
chlorethoxyfos	YES	YES
chlorimuron	YES	YES
chloropicrin	YES	YES
chlorothalonil	YES	YES
chlorpyrifos	YES	YES
chlorsulfuron	YES	YES
clethodim	YES	YES
clodinafop	YES	YES
clofentezine	YES	YES
clomazone	YES	YES
clopyralid	YES	YES
cloransulam	YES	YES
copper	YES	YES
cryolite	YES	YES
cyclanilide	YES	YES
cycloate	YES	YES
cyfluthrin	YES	YES
cyhalofop	YES	YES
cymoxanil	YES	YES
cypermethrin	YES	YES
cyprodinil	YES	YES
cyromazine	YES	YES
cytokinins	YES	YES
DCNA	YES	YES
DCPA	YES	YES
deltamethrin	YES	YES
desmedipham	YES	YES
diazinon	YES	YES

Herbicide Name	Tthyroid Disruptors (Potential)	Estrogen Disruptors (Potential)
dicamba	YES	YES
dichlobenil	YES	YES
diclofop	YES	YES
diclosulam	YES	YES
dicofol	YES	YES
dicrotophos	YES	YES
difenzoquat	YES	YES
diflubenzuron	YES	YES
diflufenzopyr	YES	YES
dimethenamid	YES	YES
dimethipin	YES	YES
dimethoate	YES	YES
dimethomorph	YES	YES
diquat	YES	YES
disulfoton	YES	YES
diuron	YES	YES
dodine	YES	YES
DSMA	YES	YES
emamectin	YES	YES
endosulfan	YES	YES
endothall	YES	YES
EPTC	YES	YES
esfenvalerate	YES	YES
ethalfluralin	YES	YES
ethephon	YES	YES
ethofumesate	YES	YES
ethoprop	YES	YES
etridiazole	YES	YES
fenamiphos	YES	YES
fenarimol	YES	YES
fenbuconazole	YES	YES
fenbutatin oxide	YES	YES
fenhexamid	YES	YES
fenoxaprop	YES	YES
fenpropathrin	YES	YES
fenpyroximate	YES	YES
ferbam	YES	YES

Herbicide Name	Tthyroid Disruptors (Potential)	Estrogen Disruptors (Potential)
fipronil	YES	YES
fluazifop	YES	YES
fluazinam	YES	YES
fludioxonil	YES	YES
flufenacet	YES	YES
flumetralin	YES	YES
flumetsulam	YES	YES
flumiclorac	YES	YES
flumioxazin	YES	YES
fluometuron	YES	YES
fluroxypyr	YES	YES
flutolanil	YES	YES
fomesafen	YES	YES
foramsulfuron	YES	YES
formetanate hcl	YES	YES
fosetyl-al	YES	YES
gibberellic acid	YES	YES
glufosinate	YES	YES
glyphosate	YES	YES
halosulfuron	YES	YES
hexazinone	YES	YES
hexythiazox	YES	YES
imazamethabenz	YES	YES
imazamox	YES	YES
imazapic	YES	YES
imazapyr	YES	YES
imazaquin	YES	YES
imazethapyr	YES	YES
imidacloprid	YES	YES
indoxacarb	YES	YES
iprodione	YES	YES
isoxaflutole	YES	YES
kaolin	YES	YES
kresoxim	YES	YES
lactofen	YES	YES
lambdacyhalothrin	YES	YES
linuron	YES	YES

Herbicide Name	Tthyroid Disruptors (Potential)	Estrogen Disruptors (Potential)
malathion	YES	YES
maleic hydrazide	YES	YES
mancozeb	YES	YES
maneb	YES	YES
MCPA	YES	YES
MCPB	YES	YES
mefenoxam	YES	YES
mepiquat chloride	YES	YES
mesotrione	YES	YES
metaldehyde	YES	YES
metam sodium	YES	YES
methamidophos	YES	YES
methidathion	YES	YES
methomyl	YES	YES
methoxyfenozide	YES	YES
methyl bromide	YES	YES
methyl parathion	YES	YES
metiram	YES	YES
metribuzin	YES	YES
metsulfuron	YES	YES
molinate	YES	YES
MSMA	YES	YES
myclobutanil	YES	YES
NAA	YES	YES
NAD	YES	YES
naled	YES	YES
napropamide	YES	YES
naptalam	YES	YES
nicosulfuron	YES	YES
norflurazon	YES	YES
oil	YES	YES
oryzalin	YES	YES
oxamyl	YES	YES
oxydemeton-methyl	YES	YES
oxyfluorfen	YES	YES
oxytetracycline	YES	YES
paraquat	YES	YES

Herbicide Name	Tthyroid Disruptors (Potential)	Estrogen Disruptors (Potential)
PCNB	YES	YES
pebulate	YES	YES
pendimethalin	YES	YES
permethrin	YES	YES
phenmedipham	YES	YES
phorate	YES	YES
phosmet	YES	YES
picloram	YES	YES
primisulfuron	YES	YES
profenofos	YES	YES
prohexadione	YES	YES
prometryn	YES	YES
pronamide	YES	YES
propamocarb	YES	YES
propanil	YES	YES
propargite	YES	YES
propiconazole	YES	YES
prosulfuron	YES	YES
pymetrozine	YES	YES
pyraclostrobin	YES	YES
pyrazon	YES	YES
pyridaben	YES	YES
pyridate	YES	YES
pyriproxyfen	YES	YES
pyrithiobac	YES	YES
quinclorac	YES	YES
quizalofop	YES	YES
rimsulfuron	YES	YES
sethoxydim	YES	YES
simazine	YES	YES
s-metolachlor	YES	YES
sodium chlorate	YES	YES
spinosad	YES	YES
streptomycin	YES	YES
sulfentrazone	YES	YES
sulfosulfuron	YES	YES
sulfur	YES	YES

Herbicide Name	Tthyroid Disruptors (Potential)	Estrogen Disruptors (Potential)
sulfuric acid	YES	YES
tebuconazole	YES	YES
tebufenozide	YES	YES
tebupirimphos	YES	YES
tebuthiuron	YES	YES
tefluthrin	YES	YES
terbacil	YES	YES
terbufos	YES	YES
tetraconazole	YES	YES
thiamethoxam	YES	YES
thidiazuron	YES	YES
thifensulfuron	YES	YES
thiobencarb	YES	YES
thiodicarb	YES	YES
thiophanate methyl	YES	YES
thiram	YES	YES
tralkoxydim	YES	YES
tralomethrin	YES	YES
triadimefon	YES	YES
triallate	YES	YES
triasulfuron	YES	YES
tribenuron	YES	YES
tribufos	YES	YES
triclopyr	YES	YES
trifloxystrobin	YES	YES
triflumizole	YES	YES
trifluralin	YES	YES
triflusulfuron	YES	YES
triforine	YES	YES
triphenyltin hyd	YES	YES
vinclozolin	YES	YES
z-cypermethrin	YES	YES
ziram	YES	YES
zoxamide	YES	YES

Table 29 is not exhaustive and there are thousands of other chemicals that are not reported or mentioned here. In the introduction, I briefly mentioned the CDC report on human exposure to the environmental chemicals. The next section presents the summary of the latest CDC report for your appreciation and here again you may draw your own conclusions.

THE CDC FOURTH REPORT

The *Fourth National Report on Human Exposure to Environmental Chemicals 2009* and the *Updated Tables, February 2011*, together are the most comprehensive assessment of environmental chemical exposure in the US population. Since 1999, CDC has measured 219 chemicals in people's blood or urine. The *Fourth Report, 2009*, includes the findings from national samples for 1999–2000, 2001–2002, and 2003–2004.

The blood and urine samples were collected from participants in CDC's National Health and Nutrition Examination Survey (NHANES), which obtains and releases health-related data from a nationally representative sample in two-year cycles.

The *Updated Tables* add more recent and new data to the *Fourth Report, 2009*. The *Updated Tables* are cumulative and include data reported in earlier updates. Therefore, the *Updated Tables, February 2011* includes data that were reported in the previous *Updated Tables, July 2010*. The *Updated Tables, February 2011* presents data from the 2005–2006 and 2007–2008 NHANES survey periods for fifty four of the chemicals previously reported through 2004 in the *Fourth Report, 2009*, along with nine more recently added chemicals. The data are analyzed separately by age, sex, and racial/ethnic groups. Internet links have been provided for those who want to find more about this report.

Executive Summary
Background

The *National Report on Human Exposure to Environmental Chemicals (National Exposure Report)* is a series of ongoing assessments of the US population's exposure to environmental chemicals by measuring chemicals in people's blood and urine, also called *Biomonitoring*. The *Fourth National Report on Human Exposure to Environmental Chemicals (Fourth Report)* presents exposure data for 212 environmental chemicals for the civilian, noninstitutionalized US population. This *Fourth Report* includes results from 2003–2004, as well as data from 1999–2000 and 2001–2002 as reported in the *Second* and *Third National Report on Human Exposure to Environmental Chemicals.*

To obtain data for this *Fourth Report*, the Centers for Disease Control and Prevention (CDC)'s Environmental Health Laboratory at the National Center for Environmental Health measured chemicals or their metabolites in blood and urine from a random sample of participants from the National Health and Nutrition Examination Survey (NHANES). CDC's National Center for Health Statistics conducts NHANES, which is a series of surveys on the health status, health-related behaviors, and nutrition of the US population. Since 1999, NHANES has been conducted in continuous two-year survey cycles.

For the *National Exposure Report*, an environmental chemical refers to a chemical compound or chemical element present in air, water, food, soil, dust, or other environmental media, such as consumer products. Blood and urine levels reflect the amount of the chemical that actually gets into the body from the environment. Either the chemical or its metabolite is measured. A metabolite is a substance produced when body tissues chemically alter the original compound.

The *Fourth Report* includes results for seventy five chemicals measured for the first time in the US population. These chemicals are in the following groups:

- acrylamide and glycidamide adducts;
- arsenic species and metabolites;
- environmental phenols, including bisphenol A and triclosan;

- perchlorate;
- perfluorinated chemicals;
- polybrominated diphenyl ethers;
- volatile organic compounds; and
- some additions to chemical groups previously measured.

A complete listing of the seventy five new chemicals is given in *What's New*. A full listing of all the chemicals included in the *Fourth Report* is available at *http://www.cdc.gov/exposurereport/pdf/NER_CHEMICAL list*.

Public Health Uses of the *Fourth Report*

The *Fourth Report* provides unique exposure information to scientists, physicians, and health officials to help prevent effects that may result from exposure to environmental chemicals. Specific public health uses of the exposure information in the *Fourth Report* are to:

- determine which chemicals get into Americans' bodies and at what concentrations;

- determine what proportion of the population has levels above those associated with adverse health effects for chemicals with a known toxicity level;

- establish reference values that can be used by physicians and scientists to determine whether a person or group has an unusually high exposure;

- assess the effectiveness of public health efforts to reduce exposure of Americans to specific chemicals and track levels over time;

- determine whether exposure levels are higher among minorities, children, women of childbearing age, or other special groups; and

• direct priorities for research on human health effects from exposure.

Interpreting the Data

The presence of an environmental chemical in people's blood or urine does not mean that it will cause effects or disease. The toxicity of a chemical is related to its dose or concentration, in addition to a person's individual susceptibility. Small amounts may be of no health consequence, whereas larger amounts may cause adverse health effects. Research studies, separate from the *National Exposure Report*, are required to determine the levels of a chemical that may cause health effects and the levels that are not a significant health concern. For some chemicals, such as lead, research studies provide a good understanding of health risks associated with various blood levels. For most of the environmental chemicals included in the *Fourth Report*, more research is needed to determine whether exposure at the levels reported is a cause for health concern. CDC conducts and provides biomonitoring measurements for this type of research in collaboration with other agencies and institutions.

The *Fourth Report* presents data that provides estimates of exposure for the civilian, non-institutionalized US population. The current survey design does not permit CDC to estimate exposure on a state-by-state or city-by-city basis. For example, CDC cannot extract a subset of data and examine levels of blood lead that represent a state population.

Key Highlights and Findings

First-Time Exposure Information for the US Population Provided for Seventy Five Chemicals

The *Fourth Report*, for the first time, provides population reference values in blood and urine, including ninety fifth percentile levels, for seventy five chemicals. The ninety fifth percentile level means that 95% of the population has concentrations below that level. Public health officials use such reference values to determine whether groups of people are experiencing an exposure that is unusual compared with an exposure experienced by the rest of the population.

To provide scientists and public health officials these new data quickly, CDC published much of this exposure information on new chemicals in separate, scientific, peer-reviewed publications before the *Fourth Report* was released. Abstracts and links to full-text articles are available at *http://www.cdc.gov/exposurereport/*.

Widespread Exposure to Some Industrial Chemicals

Findings in the *Fourth Report* indicate widespread exposure to some commonly used industrial chemicals.

- Polybrominated diphenyl ethers are fire retardants used in certain manufactured products. These accumulate in the environment and in human fat tissue. One type of polybrominated diphenyl ether, BDE-47, was found in the serum of nearly all of the NHANES participants.
- Bisphenol A (BPA), a component of epoxy resins and polycarbonates, may have potential reproductive toxicity. General population exposure to BPA may occur through ingestion of foods in contact with BPA-containing materials. CDC scientists found bisphenol A in more than 90% of the urine samples representative of the US population.
- Another example of widespread human exposure included several of the perfluorinated chemicals. One of these chemicals, perfluorooctanoic acid (PFOA), was a byproduct of the synthesis of other perfluorinated chemicals and was a synthesis aid in the manufacture of a commonly used polymer, polytetrafluoroethylene, which is used to create heat-resistant non-stick coatings in cookware. Most

participants had measurable levels of this environmental contaminant.

Ongoing Progress in Reducing Blood Lead Levels in Children

Progress is being made in reducing children's blood lead levels. New data on blood lead levels in children aged one to five years enable estimates of the number of children with elevated levels (that is, levels greater than or equal to 10 micrograms per deciliter [µg/dL]). Figure 1 shows how the percentage of blood lead levels in children has declined since the late 1970s. For example, for the period 1999–2004, 1.4% of children aged one to five years had elevated blood lead levels, the smallest percentage of any of the prior survey periods.

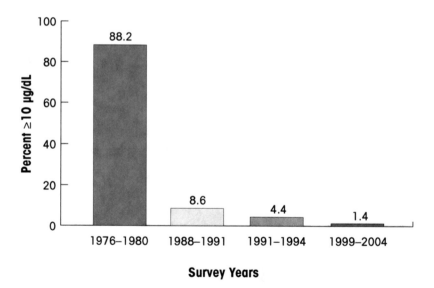

Survey Years

Figure 1. Percentage of children 1–5 years old in the US population with elevated blood lead levels (≥ 10µg/dL).[1]

[1] Jones RL, Homa DM, Meyer PA, Brody DJ, Caldwell KL, Pirkle JL, Brown MJ. Trends in blood lead levels and blood lead testing among US children aged 1 to 5 Years, 1988–2004. *Pediatrics* 2009 Mar;123(3):e376–e385.

These data document that public health efforts to reduce the number of children with elevated blood lead levels in the general population continue to be successful. However, the *Fourth Report* also notes that other data sources show that special populations of children at high risk for lead exposure (for example, children living in homes containing lead-based paint or lead-contaminated dust) have higher rates of elevated blood lead levels and remain a major public health concern.

First Available Exposure Data on Mercury in the US Population

For the first time, the *Fourth Report* characterizes mercury exposure of the US population aged one year and older. Previous *National Exposure Reports* presented mercury levels for children 1–5 years old and women 16–49 years old. Total blood mercury levels are primarily composed of one type of mercury, methyl mercury, which enters the body mainly from dietary seafood sources. Findings in the *Fourth Report* show that total blood mercury levels increase with age for all groups and begin to decline after the fifth decade of life. Compared to older women of childbearing age, younger women have higher birth rates and lower mercury levels (see Figure 2).

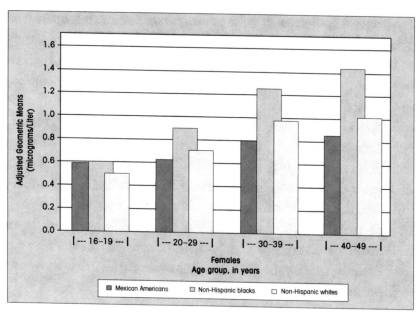

Figure 2. Age-related changes in total blood mercury levels for females aged 16–49 years by race/ethnicity, 1999–2006.[2]

Eight Different Species and Metabolites of Arsenic Measured

By using special laboratory methods, CDC researchers measured total arsenic and seven other forms of arsenic in the urine of NHANES participants for the first time. Some of the forms of arsenic measured are metabolites of inorganic arsenic and others are less toxic species that are formed in the environment. By differentiating these types of arsenic exposure, the *Fourth Report* helps scientists understand which forms of arsenic are important to human health.

---

[2]   Caldwell KL, Mortensen ME, Jones RL, Caudill SP, Osterloh JD. Total blood mercury concentrations in the US population: 1999–2006. *Int J Hyg Environ Health* 2009.

First-Time Assessment of Acrylamide Exposure in the US Population

Acrylamide is formed when foods containing carbohydrates are cooked at high temperatures (e.g., French fries) and as a byproduct of tobacco smoke. Most people are exposed to acrylamide through the diet and from smoking. Because acrylamide is a reactive chemical, it can bind to proteins. These reaction products are called *adducts*. CDC's Environmental Health Laboratory developed a new method to measure acrylamide and its metabolite, glycidamide, as adducts of hemoglobin, a major blood protein. This measure reflects the dose of acrylamide and glycidamide over the previous several months of intake. The data in the *Fourth Report* show that acrylamide exposure is extremely common in the US population.

Perchlorate and Thyroid Function

The chemical perchlorate is both naturally occurring and manmade and is used to manufacture fireworks, explosives, flares, and rocket propellant. For decades, scientists have known that large medical doses of perchlorate affect thyroid function. Low-level exposure to perchlorate from the environment has been under investigation by many scientists in recent years. The *Fourth Report* shows that all NHANES participants have detectable perchlorate in their urine and provides reference values for urinary perchlorate levels (see Table 1). This knowledge helps scientists target the levels of human exposure for future study.

Urinary Perchlorate

Geometric mean and selected percentiles of urine concentrations (in mg/L) for the U.S. population from the National Health and Nutrition Examination Survey.

	Survey years	Geometric mean (95% conf. interval)	Selected percentiles (95% confidence interval)				Sample size
			50th	75th	90th	95th	
Total	01-02	**3.54** (3.29-3.81)	**3.70** (3.50-4.00)	**6.30** (5.80-6.90)	**10.0** (9.10-11.0)	**14.0** (11.0-17.0)	2820
	03-04	**3.22** (2.93-3.55)	**3.30** (2.90-3.80)	**5.50** (5.00-6.40)	**9.50** (8.40-11.0)	**13.0** (12.0-15.0)	2522
Age Group							
6-11 years	01-02	**4.93** (4.22-5.76)	**5.20** (4.40-6.40)	**8.10** (6.90-9.80)	**12.0** (9.30-19.0)	**19.0** (12.0-23.0)	374
	03-04	**4.32** (3.67-5.09)	**4.60** (4.00-5.20)	**7.90** (5.70-9.50)	**13.0** (8.81-16.0)	**16.0** (11.0-29.0)	314
12-15 years	01-02	**3.80** (3.44-4.20)	**4.40** (3.80-4.80)	**6.80** (6.30-7.30)	**10.0** (8.90-11.0)	**13.0** (11.0-17.0)	828
	03-04	**3.62** (3.19-4.12)	**3.80** (3.20-4.40)	**6.40** (5.50-7.10)	**9.80** (7.90-12.0)	**13.0** (10.0-18.0)	721
20 years and older	01-02	**3.35** (3.08-3.65)	**3.50** (3.20-3.70)	**5.90** (5.30-6.60)	**10.0** (8.70-11.0)	**13.0** (11.0-17.0)	1618
	03-04	**3.05** (2.75-3.38)	**3.20** (2.70-3.60)	**5.20** (4.70-6.10)	**9.10** (7.90-10.0)	**12.0** (11.0-14.0)	1487
Gender							
Males	01-02	**4.19** (3.93-4.46)	**4.40** (4.20-4.60)	**7.10** (6.40-7.90)	**11.0** (9.70-12.0)	**14.0** (11.0-19.0)	1335
	03-04	**3.75** (3.39-4.16)	**3.90** (3.40-4.40)	**6.40** (5.60-7.50)	**11.0** (9.20-12.0)	**14.0** (13.0-17.0)	1229
Females	01-02	**3.01** (2.74-3.31)	**3.10** (2.70-3.40)	**5.40** (5.00-6.00)	**9.20** (8.20-11.0)	**13.0** (11.0-17.0)	1485
	03-04	**2.79** (2.49-3.11)	**2.90** (2.50-3.20)	**4.90** (4.40-5.50)	**8.20** (6.90-9.84)	**11.0** (8.80-15.0)	1293
Race/ethnicity							
Mexican Americans	01-02	**4.02** (3.47-4.66)	**4.40** (3.70-5.00)	**7.10** (5.80-8.40)	**12.0** (9.40-13.0)	**14.0** (12.0-18.0)	708
	03-04	**3.76** (3.45-4.11)	**3.96** (3.50-4.40)	**6.20** (5.30-7.50)	**11.0** (9.10-12.0)	**15.0** (12.0-17.0)	617
Non-Hispanic blacks	01-02	**3.51** (3.07-4.03)	**3.70** (3.10-4.10)	**5.90** (5.10-7.00)	**9.20** (7.80-12.0)	**15.0** (11.0-20.0)	681
	03-04	**3.21** (2.90-3.56)	**3.20** (2.87-3.50)	**5.40** (4.60-6.30)	**8.60** (7.50-11.0)	**13.0** (9.30-17.0)	652
Non-Hispanic whites	01-02	**3.51** (3.18-3.88)	**3.70** (3.40-4.10)	**6.30** (5.70-7.10)	**10.0** (8.90-11.0)	**14.0** (11.0-18.0)	1228
	03-04	**3.26** (2.89-3.68)	**3.30** (2.80-4.00)	**5.60** (4.90-6.80)	**9.40** (8.10-11.0)	**13.0** (11.0-15.0)	1092

Limit of detection (LOD, see Data Analysis section) for Survey years 01-02 and 03-04 are 0.05 and 0.05. For the 2001-2002 Survey period, surplus samples were used, and data are unavailable at NHANES website.

Table 1. Perchlorate table as provided in the *Fourth Report*.

Exposure to Cadmium

Recent research studies show that urine cadmium levels as low as 1 microgram per gram of creatinine in people may be associated with subtle markers of effects on the kidney and with an increased risk for low bone-mineral density. The *Fourth Report* shows that about 5% of the US population aged 20 years and older has urinary cadmium levels at or near these levels. Cigarette smoking is the most likely source for these higher cadmium levels. These findings should promote further research on the public health consequences of cadmium in people.

Reduced Exposure to Environmental Tobacco Smoke

Environmental tobacco smoke (ETS) has significant health effects on cardiovascular and respiratory disease. Cotinine is a metabolite of nicotine, and for nonsmokers, levels of Cotinine in people's blood tracks exposure to ETS. In the past fifteen years, data show that blood Cotinine levels for nonsmokers in the US population have decreased about 70%, indicating that public health interventions to reduce ETS exposure have been successful.

US Population's Exposure to Volatile Organic Compounds

People are exposed every day to volatile chemicals in the air we breathe. The *Fourth Report* provides measurements on thirty three of these hydrocarbon and halohydrocarbon-type chemicals. One example is the gasoline additive methyl *tert*-butyl ether (MTBE). Exposure to this chemical can occur through the air we breathe or from contaminated water sources. A high percentage of the NHANES participants representing the US population showed detectable levels of MTBE.

Selection of Chemicals for the *Fourth Report*

Chemicals presented in the *Fourth Report* were selected on the basis of scientific data that suggested exposure in the US population; the seriousness of health effects known or suspected to result from exposure; the need to assess the efficacy of public health actions to reduce exposure to a chemical; the availability of a Biomonitoring analytical method with adequate accuracy, precision, sensitivity, specificity, and speed; the availability of sufficient quantity of blood or urine samples; and the incremental analytical cost to perform the analyses. More information is available at *http://www.cdc.gov/exposurereport/chemical_ selection.html.*

Plans for Future *National Exposure Reports*

CDC's goal is to make new Biomonitoring exposure information available as soon as possible to the public and scientific community. To meet this goal, CDC periodically releases the *National Exposure Report* and also publishes Biomonitoring exposure information in peer-reviewed publications. The *National Exposure Report* is cumulative, providing Biomonitoring exposure data starting in 1999 through the latest available data at the time of the report release. Future plans include releasing data on additional chemicals and providing more information on exposure in population groups defined by age, sex, and race or ethnicity. Peer-reviewed journal articles published since the latest release of the *National Exposure Report* provide more recent and supplementary Biomonitoring data for the U.S. population. These peer-reviewed publications typically also contain more extensive data analysis than that provided in the *National Exposure Report.*

For the most up-to-date Biomonitoring information, users can view the *National Exposure Report* Web site (*http://www.cdc.gov/exposurereport/*), a one-stop source that contains the most recent version of the *Report* as well as the Biomonitoring publications.

About CDC's Environmental Health Laboratory

By using advanced laboratory science and innovative techniques, CDC's Environmental Health Laboratory at the National Center for Environmental Health has been at the forefront of efforts to assess people's exposure to environmental chemicals. CDC's laboratory scientists have built on more than three decades of experience in measuring chemicals directly in people's blood or urine, a process known as Biomonitoring. Biomonitoring measurements are the most health-relevant assessments of exposure because they measure the total amount of the chemical that actually gets into people from all environmental sources (e.g., air, soil, water, dust, or food). With a few exceptions, the concentration of the chemical in people provides the best exposure information for public health officials to evaluate the potential for adverse health effects.

TABLE 30
Chemicals in the *Fourth Report:* Updated Tables, February 2011

CDC's Fourth National Report on Human Exposure to Environmental Chemicals: Updated Tables provides exposure data on the following chemicals or classes of chemicals. The updated tables contain cumulative data from national samples collected in 1999–2000, 2001–2002, 2003–2004, 2005–2006, and 2007–2008. Not all chemicals were measured in each national sample. The data tables are available at *http://www.cdc.gov/exposurereport*. An asterisk (*) denotes a chemical presented for the first time in the 2007–2008 national sample.

Tobacco Smoke	Parabens
Cotinine	Butyl paraben
NNAL (4-(methylnitrosamino)-1-(3-pyridyl)-1-butanol) *	Ethyl paraben
	Methyl paraben
	Propyl paraben
Environmental Phenols	**Perfluorochemicals**
Benzophenone-3 (2-Hydroxy-4-methoxybenzophenone) Bisphenol A (2,2-bis[4-Hydroxyphenyl] propane) 4-tert-Octylphenol (4-[1,1,3,3-Tetramethylbutyl] phenol) Triclosan (2,4,4'-Trichloro-2'-hydroxyphenyl ether)	Perfluorobutane sulfonic acid (PFBuS) Perfluorodecanoic acid (PFDeA) Perfluorododecanoic acid (PFDoA) Perfluoroheptanoic acid (PFHpA) Perfluorohexane sulfonic acid (PFHxS) Perfluorononanoic acid (PFNA) Perfluorooctanoic acid (PFOA) Perfluorooctane sulfonic acid (PFOS) Perfluorooctane sulfonamide (PFOSA) 2-(N-Ethyl-perfluorooctane sulfonamido) acetic acid (Et-PFOSA-AcOH) 2-(N-Methyl-perfluorooctane sulfonamido) acetic acid (Me-PFOSA-AcOH) Perfluoroundecanoic acid (PFUA)

Fungicides	Phthalates	
ortho-Phenylphenol	Mono-benzyl phthalate (MBzP)Mono-isobutyl phthalate (MiBP)Mono-n-butyl phthalate (MnBP)Mono-cyclohexyl phthalate (MCHP)Mono-ethyl phthalate (MEP) Mono-2-ethylhexyl phthalate (MEHP)Mono-(2-ethyl-5-hydroxyhexyl) phthalate (MEHHP)Mono-(2-ethyl-5-oxohexyl) phthalate (MEOHP)Mono-(2-ethyl-5-carboxypentyl) phthalate (MECPP)Mono-(carboxynonyl) phthalate (MCNP) Mono-isononyl phthalate (MiNP) Mono-(carboxyoctyl) phthalate (MCOP) Mono-methyl phthalate (MMP)Mono-(3-carboxypropyl) phthalate (MCPP)Mono-n-octyl phthalate (MOP)	
2,4-Dichlorophenol		
Organochlorine Pesticides 2,4,5-Trichlorophenol 2,4,6-Trichlorophenol		
Other Pesticides 2,5-Dichlorophenol		
Metals		
Antimony	Monomethylarsonic acid	Lead
Arsenic, Total	Trimethylarsine oxide	Mercury
Arsenic (V) acid	Barium	Molybdenum
Arsenobetaine	Beryllium	Platinum
Arsenocholine	Cadmium	Thallium
Arsenous (III) acid	Cesium	Tungsten
Dimethylarsinic acid	Cobalt	Uranium

The Dirty Dozen

In May 1995, the Environmental Program Governing Council (GC) decided to begin investigating POPs (persistent organic pollutants), initially beginning with a short list of the following twelve POPs, known as the "dirty dozen": aldrin, chlordane, DDT, dieldrin, endrin, heptachlor, hexachlorobenzene, mirex, polychlorinated biphenyls, polychlorinated dibenzo-p-dioxins, polychlorinated dibenzofurans, and toxaphene. Since then, this list has generally been understood to include such substances as carcinogenic polycyclic aromatic hydrocarbons (PAHs) and certain brominated flame-retardants, as well as some organo-metallic compounds such as tributyltin (TBT). The groups of compounds that make up POPs are also classified as PBTs (Persistent, Bioaccumulative and Toxic) or TOMPs (Toxic Organic Micro Pollutants).

The 12 Dirty Dozen POPs, as identified by The Stockholm Convention, are:

Aldrin – A pesticide applied to soils to kill termites, grasshoppers, corn rootworm, and other insect pests.

Chlordane – Used extensively to control termites and as a broad-spectrum insecticide on a range of agricultural crops.

DDT – Perhaps the best known of the POPs, DDT was widely used during World War II to protect soldiers and civilians from malaria, typhus, and other diseases spread by insects. It continues to be applied against mosquitoes in several countries to control malaria.

Dieldrin – Used principally to control termites and textile pests, dieldrin has also been used to control insect-borne diseases and insects living in agricultural soils.

Dioxins – These chemicals are produced unintentionally due to incomplete combustion, as well as during the manufacture of certain pesticides and other chemicals. In addition, certain kinds of metal recycling and pulp and paper bleaching can release dioxins. Dioxins have also been found in automobile exhaust, tobacco smoke and wood and coal smoke.

Endrin – This insecticide is sprayed on the leaves of crops such as cotton and grains. It is also used to control mice and other rodents.

Furans – These compounds are produced unintentionally from the same processes that release dioxins, and they are also found in commercial mixtures of PCBs.

Heptachlor – Primarily employed to kill soil insects and termites, heptachlor has also been used more widely to kill cotton insects, grasshoppers, other crop pests, and malaria-carrying mosquitoes.

Hexachlorobenzene (HCB) – HCB kills fungi that affect food crops. It is also released as a byproduct during the manufacture of certain chemicals and as a result of the processes that give rise to dioxins and furans.

Mirex – This insecticide is applied mainly to combat fire ants and other types of ants and termites. It has also been used as a fire retardant in plastics, rubber, and electrical goods.

Polychlorinated Biphenyls (PCBs) – These compounds are employed in industry as heat exchange fluids, in electric transformers and capacitors, and as additives in paint, carbonless copy paper, sealants, and plastics.

Toxaphene – This insecticide, also called camphechlor, is applied to cotton, cereal grains, fruits, nuts, and vegetables. It has also been used to control ticks and mites in livestock.

For more information on The Stockholm Convention, visit *http://www.pops.int/documents/pops/default.htm*

From Our Stolen Future tables, you may have noticed that these chemicals cause hypothyroidism or increased estrogen or affect the reproductive system. The estrogen disruption and consequences follow in the next chapter.

CHAPTER 4

THE ESTROGEN EPIDEMIC AND ASSOCIATED DISEASES

A 2008 review has concluded that obesity may be increased as a function of Bisphenol A (BPA) exposure. Bisphenol A is drawing the attention of the scientific community. A 2009 review of available studies has concluded that perinatal BPA exposure acts to exert persistent effects on body weight and adiposity. Another 2009 review has concluded that eliminating exposures to (BPA) and improving nutrition during development offer the potential for reducing obesity and associated diseases. Other reviews have come with similar conclusions. Bisphenol A is also linked to hyperestrogenism in women, and girls as young as seven are getting menstrual periods. The other chemicals listed in Table 29, the CDC report and the Dirty Dozen that cause an increase in estrogen may have similar effects on humans. These effects are not reported at this time but will be in the near future, as research uncovers these effects.

Medical providers are not keeping up with the new developments and, therefore, measures are not taken to diagnose these endocrine disruptions in patients. Those who are aware and try to diagnose and treat the endocrine related conditions are labeled as quacks or voodoo doctors. The attitudes of most practicing health professionals have not changed in centuries. The path-breakers are sacrificed in the name of standard of care.

Estrogen Induced Cancers

There is evidence that Bisphenol A functions as a xen-oestrogen by binding strongly to estrogen-related receptor γ (ERR-γ). This orphan receptor (endogenous ligand unknown) behaves as a constitutive activator of transcription. BPA seems to bind strongly to ERR-γ (dissociation constant = 5.5 nM) but not to the estrogen receptor (ER). BPA binding to ERR-γ preserves its basal constitutive activity. It can also protect it from deactivation from the selective estrogen receptor modulator 4-hydroxytamoxifen.

Different expressions of ERR-γ in different parts of the body may account for variations in Bisphenol-A effects. For instance, ERR-γ has been found in high concentration in the placenta, explaining reports of high Bisphenol A accumulation in this tissue.

A 2008 review has concluded that perinatal exposure to low doses of BPA alters breast development and increases breast cancer risk. Another 2008 review concluded that animal experiments and epidemiological data strengthen the hypothesis that fetal exposure to xenoestrogens may be an underlying cause of the increased incidence of breast cancer observed over the last fifty years.

A 2009 in vitro study has concluded that BPA is able to induce neoplastic transformation in human breast epithelial cells. Another 2009 study concluded that maternal oral exposure to low concentrations of BPA during lactation increases mammary carcinogenesis in a rodent model.

A 2010 study with the mammary glands of the offspring of pregnant rats treated orally with 0, 25, or 250 µg BPA/kg body weight has found that key proteins involved in signaling pathways such as cellular proliferation were regulated at the protein level by BPA.

A 2010 study has found that BPA may reduce sensitivity to chemotherapy treatment of specific tumors.

All other chemicals in "Our Stolen Future" list that increase the estrogen level in humans are responsible for the increasing cancer rates. The South and the Midwest have an increased prevalence of the estrogen related cancers such as breast, uterine, ovarian, cervical, vaginal, colon, and prostate cancers and benign tumors such as fibroid tumors, benign prostatic hypertrophy, ovarian cysts, fibrocystic breast disease, and cervical dysplasia.

Estrogenic Chemicals and Allergic Diseases: The Case of BPA

A 2010 study on mice has concluded that perinatal exposure to 10 micrograms/mL of BPA in drinking water enhances allergic sensitization and bronchial inflammation and responsiveness in an animal model of asthma (adult-onset allergies due to estrogen dominance will be covered in Chapter 6).

There were striking dose-response relations between serum concentrations of several selected POPs and the prevalence of diabetes. The strong graded association could offer a compelling challenge to future epidemiologic and toxicological research.

- DDE, p, p′-dichlorodiphenyltrichloroethane
- HCB, hexachlorobenzene
- HpCDD, 1,2,3,4,6,7,8-heptachlorodibenzo-p-dioxin
- OCDD, 1,2,3,4,6,7,8,9-octachlorodibenzo-p-dioxin
- PCB, polychlorinated biphenyl
- PCB153, 2,2′,4,4′,5,5′-hexachlorobiphenyl
- PCDD, polychlorinated dibenzo-p-dioxin
- PCDF, polychlorinated dibenzofuran
- TCDD, 2,3,7,8-tetrachlorodibenzo-p-dioxin

Endocrine Disrupting Chemicals, Hormone Imbalance, and Diseases in Humans

Bisphenol A and all the other chemicals reported in the tables, the dirty dozen and the rest of the POPs as well as organophosphates seem to have two major effects. They act as thyroid disruptors or estrogen disruptors. It is, therefore, not surprising that women seem to be most affected by the obesity epidemic and its comorbidities. Women tend to produce more estrogens from their late twenties on. Most women become estrogen dominant because their endogenous production of estrogens increases when they lose their progesterone due to anovulatory menstrual cycles. Women who go on birth control pills tend to develop their hormone disruption sooner. Increased endogenous estrogens, coupled with environmental estrogens (xenoestrogens and phytoestrogens), lead to multiple symptoms that women present with to their doctors. Unfortunately, since there is no true training in hormone disruption and correction of its ill effects in medical schools or residency programs, and since most endocrinologists are busy dealing with diabetes, thyroid diseases and more familiar endocrine conditions, there are few physicians who will touch these symptoms. The few physicians who try to investigate these conditions do well by helping these patients. However, since most medical professionals are not well versed in the literature regarding the effects of endocrine disruptors, they pose as judges of the few who try to find solutions. Names such as voodoo doctor or quack are often used to characterize the few who try.

Most physicians want evidence-based proofs that bio-identical hormone therapy works, but many of them are not willing to engage in research that will demonstrate the efficacy of these hormones. Most physicians are too busy with their daily practices and, therefore, do not have time to read and catch up with progress in the medical field.

Although there are groups of physicians who are making an effort and participate in organizations such as the American Academy of Anti-Aging and Regenerative Medicine (A4M) (please go to *www.A4m.com* for more information about this group and the fellowship in Anti-Aging and Regenerative Medicine), there is still no consensus or unified treatment protocols. This situation makes things more complicated.

Medicine today has practices that I still do not understand. For example, most obstetricians know that fibroid tumors, the number one cause of hysterectomy in the US and the rest of the world, feed on estrogens. There is no measure of the estrogen level in women suffering from fibroid tumors that cause menorrhagia and dysmenorrhea. After hysterectomy, many of these women are placed on more estrogen. The majority of breast cancer is estrogen receptor positive; however, estrogen is hardly ever measured in women who present with this type of cancer, and when they are placed on hormone therapy such as Tamoxifen, the estrogen level is hardly ever measured. Uterine cancer is due to too much estrogen, and yet after a total abdominal hysterectomy and bilateral salpingo-oophorectomy, most patients end up on more synthetic estrogens.

Despite the Women's Health Initiative Trial results, some physicians still start women on synthetic estrogens and progestins such as Premarin or Prempro for hot flashes, not knowing that many of these women have hot flashes because of a lack of progesterone. These physicians, lacking knowledge about hormones, will be quick to criticize the ones who will measure the hormones in an attempt to correct them.

During yearly physical exams, lab work is ordered and most physicians will also order a TSH as a thyroid function test. Some physicians will add free T4. No other hormone levels are ordered even if the patients show signs of gross hormone disruption such as obesity. Many useless laboratory studies are done daily except for the ones that will be truly preventive. Insurance companies may be reluctant to pay for labs ordered for preventive care. In effect, they refuse to pay for preventive care when they ask physicians to prove that the conditions being investigated are not pre-existing conditions.

I suggest that most steroid hormone levels be ordered at age thirty to thirty five. (The hormones in question are progesterone, testosterone, dihydrotestosterone, androstenedione, DHEA, estradiol and estrone.) Other important labs include fasting insulin and glucose, leptin, lipid panel, TSH, free T4, free T3, thyroid antibodies, complete metabolic panel, and vitamin D level. Periodic recheck should be done every three to five years. This will help prevent many pathological conditions that drive up healthcare costs. For example, if a woman is found to have estrogen dominance, starting her on progesterone to balance her estrogen, and giving her supplements that also may help reduce the ill-effects of estrogens, may help avert many types of benign tumors and even cancers and hence prevent human misery and reduce healthcare costs. We all know that there is no free lunch. It may cost the healthcare system a few more dollars in order to save billions in healthcare costs.

The analysis of the HCUP database and the study of the CDC maps in conjunction with the USGS pesticides/herbicides maps, which reveal the role of endocrine disrupting chemicals in obesity through thyroid, estrogen and androgen disruption, show that there is a hyperestrogenism, hypothyroidism and hypo-androgenism epidemic in the US. To address these issues, the symptoms associated with these conditions should be known by all physicians. The next section will present some of the symptoms that the so-called alternative physicians look to determining estrogen dominance issues.

The Estrogen Epidemics and Manifestation in Humans

Often, patients present with multiple complaints which may seem unrelated. However, a careful grouping of these symptoms may reveal a pattern consistent with hormone imbalance syndrome (HIS). The following symptoms may be frequent complaints in both women and men suffering from HIS.

- Acceleration of the aging process (increased wrinkles that is not consistent with chronological age)
- Adrenal exhaustion
- Allergy symptoms (asthma, hives, rashes, sinus congestion, adult-onset allergies including food allergies)
- Autoimmune disorders (systemic lupus erythematosus, thyroiditis, possibly Sjögren's disease, gritty, dry eyes)
- Breast cancer
- Breast tenderness
- Cervical dysplasia
- Cold hands and feet as a symptom of thyroid dysfunction
- Decreased sex drive
- Depression with anxiety or agitation
- Dry eyes
- Early onset of menstruation
- Endometrial (uterine) cancer
- Endometriosis
- Weight gain, especially around the abdomen, hips, and thighs
- Fatigue

- Fertility problems
- Fibrocystic breasts
- Fibromyalgia
- Foggy thinking
- Gallbladder disease
- Hair loss
- Headaches
- Hypoglycemia
- Hysterectomy and salpingo-oophorectomy
- Increased blood clotting (increasing risk of strokes)
- Infertility
- Irregular menstrual periods
- Irritability
- Insomnia
- Magnesium deficiency
- Memory loss
- Mood swings
- Osteoporosis
- PMS (Premenstrual syndrome or premenstrual dysphoric disorder—PMDD)
- PCOS (Polycystic Ovarian Syndrome)
- Post-partum depression
- Premenopausal bone loss
- Premature birth
- Prostate cancer
- Protection against reproductive cancer

- Sluggish metabolism
- Thyroid dysfunction mimicking hypothyroidism
- Rheumatoid arthritis
- Pins and needles
- Sciatica
- Mid-menstrual cycle pain (mittelschmerz)
- Obsessive, irrational thought and behavior patterns: difficulty finding a lost item
- Trying to think of someone's name
- Lack of lateral thinking and ability to multi-task
- Fragmented physically, emotionally, and spiritually
- Headaches and migraines
- Overwhelming panic attacks
- Unfounded fear
- Social phobia, sense of loss of social skills, withdrawal
- Grief and sadness with no apparent cause
- Sluggish liver (aggravated by hormonal overload, overuse of synthetic HRT, medications, xenoestrogens)
- Vocabulary/speech difficulty
- Uterine cancer
- Uterine fibroids
- Water retention, bloating
- Zinc deficiency
- Blurred vision and/or watery eyes, difficulty focusing
- Tender heels and/or feet, from sensitive to burning
- Restless legs syndrome

- Itchy, burning, sore ears
- Sensation of foreign object in ear such as bees or insects, tinnitus
- Vertigo, particularly around ovulation time onward (more profound lying down in bed)
- Palpitations
- Heartburn
- Low resistance to infection
- Sinusitis, head congestion, flu-like headaches
- Pre-menstrual asthma
- Painful, throbbing face, one side more than the other, often reported
- Aching teeth, dental checkup negative for infection
- Constant sore throats every month, tonsillitis
- Upper respiratory problems
- Acne or pimples, particularly just prior to menses, also in older women
- Chronic recurrence of thrush, cystitis, vaginitis,
- Recurrent yeast infections
- Interstitial cystitis
- Reports of acne on the vulva that flares at menses
- Bouts of diarrhea prior to the menses, some alternating constipation, especially with women who have cysts and endometriosis
- Irritable bowel syndrome

- Leaky gut syndrome
- Inability to lose weight and shift fluid
- Stress incontinence
- Extreme dream agitation and anxiety
- Inability to focus
- Inability to concentrate
- Loss of short term memory
- Alienation and loss of confidence
- Androgen side effects: facial hair, increased body hair
- Increased thickening and blacking of limb hair
- Prolonged menstrual periods
- Frequent menstruations
- Irregular menses

Evidence of Endogenous Hormone imbalance

Endogenous estrogen dominance coupled with the xenoestrogens and phytoestrogens generate multiple symptoms in women as described above. Women bear the bulk of the estrogenic effects because of their high endogenous production of this hormone. Progesterone deficiency leads to the endogenous estrogen dominance and thyroid deficiency. Women, therefore, have higher rates of hypothyroidism than men, as demonstrated in previous chapters. The hypothyroidism rate increases with age. Women also have more obesity and its associated comorbidities more often than men due to the high estrogen levels and high rate of hypothyroidism. Some women are born with low progesterone gene, and many others acquire low progesterone starting from the late twenties secondary to anovulatory menstrual cycles (this could also be induced by birth control pills). This progesterone deficiency leads to endogenous estrogen dominance, which in addition to environmental estrogens leads to obesity and its comorbidities. Hence, women between the ages of eighteen and forty four, with increased estrogen surges have more obesity than the rest of the population. Increased estrogen should also produce more menstrual disturbances in women between the ages of eighteen and forty four due to benign tumors and other related comorbidities. Fibroid tumors, ovarian cysts, fibrocystic breast disease, endometriosis, heavy menstrual bleeding, and irregular menstrual periods will prevail in these age groups. Obesity-associated comorbidities such as hypertension, diabetes, and hyperlipidemia should also prevail in women. Obesity causes leptin resistance and leptin resistance causes serotonin production to decrease. If women have more obesity and hence more leptin resistance, then they should have more depressive episodes, anxiety, and panic attacks, than men. In the era of statistics and clinical trials, statements made in vacuum are quickly dismissed.

The following tables (31–98) present more evidence of the devastating effects of estrogen dominance in both men and women.

TABLE 31

Patient and hospital characteristics for ICD-9-CM first-listed diagnosis code 296.20 Depress Psychosis-Unspec

		All ED visits (those that resulted in admission to the hospital and those that did not)	Only hospital visits that originated in the ED	Only ED visits that ended in discharge (no hospital admission)	Standard errors		
					All ED Visits	Admitted to the hospital from the ED	Discharged from the ED
All discharges		101,884 (100.00%)	33,662 (100.00%)	68,222 (100.00%)	7,182	3,318	5,129
Age (mean)		37.73	40.02	36.60	0.27	0.27	0.27
Age group	1–17	11,484 (11.27%)	3,445 (29.99%)	8,040 (70.01%)	1,233	789 (4.53%)	718 (4.53%)
	18–44	55,709 (54.68%)	16,913 (30.36%)	38,796 (69.64%)	4,014	1,633 (2.11%)	3,107 (2.11%)
	45–64	28,402 (27.88%)	10,026 (35.30%)	18,377 (64.70%)	1,988	956 (2.23%)	1,420 (2.23%)
	65–84	5,530 (5.43%)	2,827 (51.11%)	2,704 (48.89%)	389	302 (3.19%)	217 (3.19%)
	85+	758 (0.74%)	452 (59.63%)	306 (40.37%)	78	64 (4.59%)	41 (4.59%)
Sex	Male	46,600 (45.74%)	14,952 (32.09%)	31,648 (67.91%)	3,402	1,462 (2.16%)	2,550 (2.16%)
	Female	55,274 (54.25%)	18,710 (33.85%)	36,565 (66.15%)	3,901	1,914 (2.17%)	2,675 (2.17%)
	Missing	*	*	*	*	*	*
Region	Northeast	20,440 (20.06%)	6,624 (32.41%)	13,816 (67.59%)	3,460	1,364 (4.70%)	2,656 (4.70%)
	Midwest	29,006 (28.47%)	10,161 (35.03%)	18,846 (64.97%)	4,481	1,946 (3.72%)	3,059 (3.72%)
	South	41,167 (40.41%)	13,433 (32.63%)	27,734 (67.37%)	4,154	2,089 (3.50%)	2,996 (3.50%)
	West	11,271 (11.06%)	3,444 (30.56%)	7,827 (69.44%)	1,508	999 (6.22%)	958 (6.22%)

* Denotes missing values

Depression in this table was more prevalent in women than men, 54.3% versus 45.7%, and the prime-age group, ages 18–44, had the highest at 54.7% followed by older adults ages 45–64 at 27.9% and then the young, ages 1–17, at 11.3% and finally the very old, 65–84, at 5.4%. The South leads with 40.4% followed by the Midwest at 28.5%, the Northeast at 20%, and the West at 11%.

TABLE 32

Patient and hospital characteristics for ICD-9-CM first-listed diagnosis code 300.4 Neurotic Depression (after Oct 1, 2004)

		All ED visits (those that resulted in admission to the hospital and those that did not)	Only hospital visits that originated in the ED	Only ED visits that ended in discharge (no hospital admission)	Standard errors		
					All ED Visits	Admitted to the hospital from the ED	Discharged from the ED
All discharges		55,395 (100.00%)	7,708 (100.00%)	47,687 (100.00%)	3,064	892	2,677
Age (mean)		38.89	41.26	38.50	0.30	0.30	0.30
Age group	1–17	4,149 (7.49%)	*	3,078 (74.19%)	559	*	269 (7.48%)
	18–44	31,800 (57.41%)	3,411 (10.73%)	28,389 (89.27%)	1,856	374 (1.08%)	1,732 (1.08%)
	45–64	14,973 (27.03%)	2,138 (14.28%)	12,834 (85.72%)	823	226 (1.28%)	731 (1.28%)
	65–84	3,873 (6.99%)	910 (23.50%)	2,963 (76.50%)	203	93 (2.02%)	172 (2.02%)
	85+	600 (1.08%)	177 (29.48%)	423 (70.52%)	60	32 (4.55%)	51 (4.55%)
Sex	Male	20,420 (36.86%)	3,039 (14.88%)	17,381 (85.12%)	1,356	412 (1.68%)	1,177 (1.68%)
	Female	34,975 (63.14%)	4,669 (13.35%)	30,306 (86.65%)	1,775	504 (1.22%)	1,566 (1.22%)
Region	Northeast	11,702 (21.12%)	1,806 (15.43%)	9,897 (84.57%)	1,287	323 (2.60%)	1,194 (2.60%)
	Midwest	13,583 (24.52%)	2,428 (17.88%)	11,155 (82.12%)	1,145	443 (2.62%)	942 (2.62%)
	South	21,285 (38.42%)	2,913 (13.69%)	18,372 (86.31%)	2,404	696 (2.63%)	2,057 (2.63%)
	West	8,825 (15.93%)	561 (6.36%)	8,264 (93.64%)	798	104 (1.22%)	788 (1.22%)

* Denotes missing values

Neurotic depression has similar pattern as depressive psychosis above.

TABLE 33

Patient and hospital characteristics for ICD-9-CM first-listed diagnosis code 296.50 Bipolar Aff, Depr-Unspec (after Oct 1, 2004)

		All ED visits (those that resulted in admission to the hospital and those that did not)	Only hospital visits that originated in the ED	Only ED visits that ended in discharge (no hospital admission)	Standard errors		
					All ED Visits	Admitted to the hospital from the ED	Discharged from the ED
All discharges		46,696 (100.00%)	24,358 (100.00%)	22,338 (100.00%)	3,297	2,183	1,870
Age (mean)		37.40	39.56	35.04	0.36	0.36	0.36
Age group	1–17	3,544 (7.59%)	1,332 (37.57%)	2,212 (62.43%)	558	389 (5.98%)	249 (5.98%)
	18–44	27,909 (59.77%)	13,772 (49.35%)	14,136 (50.65%)	1,896	1,196 (2.66%)	1,214 (2.66%)
	45–64	13,723 (29.39%)	8,168 (59.52%)	5,555 (40.48%)	1,011	748 (2.62%)	500 (2.62%)
	65–84	1,435 (3.07%)	1,022 (71.20%)	413 (28.80%)	133	105 (3.21%)	60 (3.21%)
	85+	86 (0.18%)	65 (75.10%)	*	21	19 (10.08%)	*
Sex	Male	20,039 (42.91%)	10,144 (50.62%)	9,895 (49.38%)	1,530	982 (2.73%)	898 (2.73%)
	Female	26,657 (57.09%)	14,215 (53.32%)	12,443 (46.68%)	1,840	1,253 (2.49%)	1,017 (2.49%)
Region	Northeast	10,637 (22.78%)	5,150 (48.42%)	5,487 (51.58%)	1,950	1,062 (4.65%)	1,124 (4.65%)
	Midwest	12,396 (26.55%)	7,934 (64.00%)	4,463 (36.00%)	1,583	1,269 (5.01%)	774 (5.01%)
	South	17,273 (36.99%)	8,791 (50.89%)	8,482 (49.11%)	1,882	1,270 (4.16%)	1,094 (4.16%)
	West	6,390 (13.68%)	2,483 (38.86%)	3,906 (61.14%)	1,011	643 (6.65%)	662 (6.65%)

* Denotes missing values

Bipolar disorder has similar pattern: females 57.1%, males 42.9%; ages 18–44, 59.8%; ages 45–64, 29.4%; ages 1–17, 7.6%; and ages 65–84, 3.1%. The South leads with 37% followed by the Midwest at 26.6%, the Northeast, 22.8% and the West at 13.7%.

TABLE 34

Patient and hospital characteristics for ICD-9-CM first-listed diagnosis code 799.2 Nervousness

		All ED visits (those that resulted in admission to the hospital and those that did not)	Only hospital visits that originated in the ED	Only ED visits that ended in discharge (no hospital admission)	Standard errors		
					All ED Visits	Admitted to the hospital from the ED	Discharged from the ED
All discharges		5,464 (100.00%)	*	5,418 (100.00%)	374	*	373
Age (mean)		37.08	44.61	37.01	0.97	0.97	0.97
Age group	<1	496 (9.07%)	*	486 (98.07%)	75	*	73 (1.28%)
	1–17	636 (11.64%)	*	628 (98.66%)	71	*	71 (0.96%)
	18–44	2,122 (38.84%)	*	2,118 (99.80%)	198	*	198 (0.20%)
	45–64	1,468 (26.86%)	*	1,468 (100.00%)	128	*	128 (0.00%)
	65–84	637 (11.65%)	*	620 (97.42%)	69	*	68 (1.31%)
	85+	106 (1.94%)	*	98 (92.46%)	23	*	22 (7.14%)
Sex	Male	2,194 (40.15%)	*	2,185 (99.58%)	146	*	145 (0.30%)
	Female	3,270 (59.85%)	*	3,233 (98.85%)	275	*	275 (0.43%)
Region	Northeast	581 (10.62%)	*	581 (100.00%)	83	*	83 (0.00%)
	Midwest	1,610 (29.47%)	*	1,596 (99.11%)	243	*	242 (0.51%)
	South	2,413 (44.17%)	*	2,386 (98.86%)	258	*	258 (0.51%)
	West	860 (15.74%)	*	855 (99.44%)	87	*	86 (0.54%)

* Denotes missing values

Nervousness follows same pattern: females 59.9%, males 40.2%; ages 18–44, 38.9%; ages 45–64, 26.9%; ages 1–17, 11.6%; and ages 65–84, 11.7%. The South leads with 44.2% followed by the Midwest at 29.5%, the West at 15.7%, and the Northeast at 10.6%.

TABLE 35

2008 National statistics—first-listed diagnosis only

Patient and hospital characteristics for ICD-9-CM first-listed diagnosis code 300.00 Anxiety State Nos

		All ED visits (those that resulted in admission to the hospital and those that did not)	Only hospital visits that originated in the ED	Only ED visits that ended in discharge (no hospital admission)	Standard errors		
					All ED Visits	Admitted to the hospital from the ED	Discharged from the ED
All discharges		531,594 (100.00%)	8,980 (100.00%)	522,614 (100.00%)	12,768	641	12,567
Age (mean)		39.67	51.13	39.47	0.13	0.13	0.13
Age group	<1	*	*	*	*	*	*
	1–17	30,350 (5.71%)	643 (2.12%)	29,707 (97.88%)	1,033	158 (0.51%)	1,004 (0.51%)
	18–44	313,288 (58.93%)	2,669 (0.85%)	310,619 (99.15%)	8,195	256 (0.08%)	8,126 (0.08%)
	45–64	131,895 (24.81%)	3,143 (2.38%)	128,752 (97.62%)	3,221	281 (0.20%)	3,123 (0.20%)
	65–84	47,883 (9.01%)	2,085 (4.35%)	45,799 (95.65%)	1,247	155 (0.30%)	1,203 (0.30%)
	85+	8,157 (1.53%)	440 (5.40%)	7,717 (94.60%)	335	52 (0.59%)	321 (0.59%)
Sex	Male	194,072 (36.51%)	3,389 (1.75%)	190,684 (98.25%)	4,797	278 (0.14%)	4,714 (0.14%)
	Female	337,466 (63.48%)	5,591 (1.66%)	331,875 (98.34%)	8,235	398 (0.11%)	8,118 (0.11%)
	Missing	*	*	*	*	*	*
Region	Northeast	101,905 (19.17%)	1,953 (1.92%)	99,952 (98.08%)	5,705	202 (0.17%)	5,601 (0.17%)
	Midwest	123,381 (23.21%)	2,101 (1.70%)	121,280 (98.30%)	6,039	309 (0.24%)	5,965 (0.24%)
	South	184,890 (34.78%)	3,500 (1.89%)	181,390 (98.11%)	7,445	418 (0.21%)	7,305 (0.21%)
	West	121,418 (22.84%)	1,426 (1.17%)	119,992 (98.83%)	6,212	316 (0.25%)	6,134 (0.25%)

* Denotes missing values

Anxiety follows same pattern: females 63.5%, males 36.5%; ages 18–44, 58.9%; ages 45–64, 24.8%; ages 1–17, 5.7%; and ages 65–84, 9%. The South leads with 34.8% followed by the Midwest at 23.2%, the West at 22.8%, and the Northeast at 19.2%.

TABLE 36

**Patient and hospital characteristics for
ICD-9-CM first-listed diagnosis code
300.01 Panic Disorder (after Oct 1, 2004)**

		All ED visits (those that resulted in admission to the hospital and those that did not)	Only hospital visits that originated in the ED	Only ED visits that ended in discharge (no hospital admission)	Standard errors		
					All ED Visits	Admitted to the hospital from the ED	Discharged from the ED
All discharges		121,182 (100.00%)	4,958 (100.00%)	116,224 (100.00%)	3,359	277	3,274
Age (mean)		35.50	50.20	34.88	0.15	0.15	0.15
Age group	1–17	9,669 (7.98%)	122 (1.26%)	9,547 (98.74%)	404	27 (0.27%)	398 (0.27%)
	18–44	79,636 (65.72%)	1,844 (2.32%)	77,792 (97.68%)	2,324	135 (0.16%)	2,289 (0.16%)
	45–64	24,468 (20.19%)	1,721 (7.03%)	22,747 (92.97%)	746	120 (0.48%)	722 (0.48%)
	65–84	6,476 (5.34%)	1,079 (16.66%)	5,397 (83.34%)	278	85 (1.20%)	254 (1.20%)
	85+	933 (0.77%)	192 (20.60%)	741 (79.40%)	86	32 (3.12%)	77 (3.12%)
Sex	Male	40,655 (33.55%)	1,678 (4.13%)	38,977 (95.87%)	1,222	123 (0.29%)	1,193 (0.29%)
	Female	80,501 (66.43%)	3,280 (4.07%)	77,221 (95.93%)	2,261	195 (0.23%)	2,204 (0.23%)
	Missing	*	*	*	*	*	*
Region	Northeast	25,306 (20.88%)	1,062 (4.19%)	24,244 (95.81%)	1,640	142 (0.53%)	1,594 (0.53%)
	Midwest	28,216 (23.28%)	1,200 (4.25%)	27,016 (95.75%)	1,622	127 (0.42%)	1,579 (0.42%)
	South	44,614 (36.82%)	1,995 (4.47%)	42,619 (95.53%)	1,908	186 (0.39%)	1,850 (0.39%)
	West	23,047 (19.02%)	702 (3.04%)	22,346 (96.96%)	1,524	77 (0.34%)	1,503 (0.34%)

* Denotes missing values

Panic disorder follows the same patterns as other estrogen-induced conditions noted above.

TABLE 37

MIGRAINE HEADACHE 2008

Patient and hospital characteristics for ICD-9-CM first-listed diagnosis code 346.10 Comn Migrne Wo Ntrc Mgrn

		All ED visits (those that resulted in admission to the hospital and those that did not)	Only hospital visits that originated in the ED	Only ED visits that ended in discharge (no hospital admission)	Standard errors		
					All ED Visits	Admitted to the hospital from the ED	Discharged from the ED
All discharges		18,439 (100.00%)	991 (100.00%)	17,448 (100.00%)	2,306	91	2,305
Age (mean)		36.69	43.20	36.32	0.32	0.32	0.32
Age group	1–17	924 (5.01%)	*	877 (94.93%)	119	*	115 (1.68%)
	18–44	12,611 (68.39%)	474 (3.76%)	12,137 (96.24%)	1,735	53 (0.66%)	1,735 (0.66%)
	45–64	4,523 (24.53%)	391 (8.65%)	4,132 (91.35%)	517	52 (1.46%)	516 (1.46%)
	65–84	363 (1.97%)	79 (21.84%)	284 (78.16%)	67	19 (5.70%)	65 (5.70%)
	85+	*	*	*	*	*	*
Sex	Male	3,382 (18.34%)	238 (7.04%)	3,144 (92.96%)	433	37 (1.35%)	432 (1.35%)
	Female	15,053 (81.64%)	753 (5.00%)	14,300 (95.00%)	1,900	75 (0.79%)	1,899 (0.79%)
	Missing	*	*	*	*	*	*
Region	Northeast	1,970 (10.68%)	182 (9.24%)	*	545	34 (3.01%)	*
	Midwest	4,204 (22.80%)	235 (5.59%)	3,969 (94.41%)	1,184	46 (1.85%)	1,182 (1.85%)
	South	10,251 (55.60%)	429 (4.19%)	9,822 (95.81%)	1,846	64 (0.98%)	1,847 (0.98%)
	West	2,013 (10.92%)	145 (7.19%)	1,869 (92.81%)	457	29 (2.08%)	455 (2.08%)

* Denotes missing values

Common migraine follows same pattern: females 81.6%, males 18.3%; ages 18–44, 68.4%; ages 45–64, 24.5%; ages 1–17, 5%; and ages 65–84, 2%. The South leads with 55.6% followed by the Midwest at 22.8%, the West at 10.9%, and the Northeast at 10.7%.

Hormone Imbalance Syndrome

TABLE 38
Patient and hospital characteristics for
ICD-9-CM first-listed diagnosis code
346.90 Migraine, unspecified; without mention of status migrainosus

		All ED visits (those that resulted in admission to the hospital and those that did not)	Only hospital visits that originated in the ED	Only ED visits that ended in discharge (no hospital admission)	Standard errors		
					All ED Visits	Admitted to the hospital from the ED	Discharged from the ED
All discharges		696,410 (100.00%)	12,998 (100.00%)	683,412 (100.00%)	17,826	644	17,626
Age (mean)		37.09	42.57	36.98	0.10	0.10	0.10
Age group	<1	*	*	*	*	*	*
	1–17	31,889 (4.58%)	750 (2.35%)	31,139 (97.65%)	1,518	97 (0.26%)	1,467 (0.26%)
	18–44	470,984 (67.63%)	6,549 (1.39%)	464,436 (98.61%)	12,766	370 (0.08%)	12,661 (0.08%)
	45–64	179,183 (25.73%)	4,515 (2.52%)	174,668 (97.48%)	4,911	252 (0.14%)	4,845 (0.14%)
	65–84	13,668 (1.96%)	1,068 (7.82%)	12,599 (92.18%)	559	87 (0.63%)	541 (0.63%)
	85+	636 (0.09%)	115 (18.15%)	520 (81.85%)	70	24 (3.41%)	64 (3.41%)
	Missing	*	*	*	*	*	*
Sex	Male	115,385 (16.57%)	2,762 (2.39%)	112,623 (97.61%)	3,028	162 (0.14%)	2,985 (0.14%)
	Female	580,970 (83.42%)	10,236 (1.76%)	570,734 (98.24%)	15,106	524 (0.09%)	14,954 (0.09%)
	Missing	*	*	*	*	*	*
Region	Northeast	85,066 (12.21%)	2,633 (3.10%)	82,433 (96.90%)	5,426	347 (0.40%)	5,341 (0.40%)
	Midwest	197,181 (28.31%)	2,966 (1.50%)	194,215 (98.50%)	9,795	273 (0.14%)	9,734 (0.14%)
	South	292,258 (41.97%)	5,467 (1.87%)	286,791 (98.13%)	12,178	431 (0.13%)	12,004 (0.13%)
	West	121,905 (17.50%)	1,931 (1.58%)	119,973 (98.42%)	6,638	188 (0.15%)	6,580 (0.15%)

* Denotes missing values

Migraine unspecified follows the same pattern: females 83.4%, males 16.6%; ages 18–44, 67.6%; ages 45–64, 25.7%; ages 1–17, 5%; and ages 65–84, 2%. The South leads with 42% followed by the Midwest at 28.3%, the West at 17.5%, and the Northeast at 12.2%.

TABLE 39

Patient and hospital characteristics for ICD-9-CM first-listed diagnosis code 346.90 Migrne Unsp without mention of status migrainosus (after Oct 1, 2008)

		All ED visits (those that resulted in admission to the hospital and those that did not)	Only hospital visits that originated in the ED	Only ED visits that ended in discharge (no hospital admission)	Standard errors		
					All ED Visits	Admitted to the hospital from the ED	Discharged from the ED
All discharges		225,651 (100.00%)	3,961 (100.00%)	221,690 (100.00%)	5,754	230	5,681
Age (mean)		37.00	42.74	36.89	0.12	0.12	0.12
Age group	1–17	11,516 (5.10%)	262 (2.28%)	11,253 (97.72%)	588	45 (0.37%)	572 (0.37%)
	18–44	151,932 (67.33%)	1,947 (1.28%)	149,985 (98.72%)	4,114	133 (0.08%)	4,074 (0.08%)
	45–64	57,269 (25.38%)	1,372 (2.40%)	55,897 (97.60%)	1,617	105 (0.18%)	1,597 (0.18%)
	65–84	4,744 (2.10%)	346 (7.29%)	4,398 (92.71%)	237	41 (0.84%)	229 (0.84%)
	85+	186 (0.08%)	*	153 (82.29%)	29	*	26 (5.98%)
	Missing	*	*	*	*	*	*
Sex	Male	38,535 (17.08%)	890 (2.31%)	37,646 (97.69%)	1,055	73 (0.19%)	1,042 (0.19%)
	Female	187,116 (82.92%)	3,071 (1.64%)	184,045 (98.36%)	4,872	191 (0.10%)	4,815 (0.10%)
Region	Northeast	27,292 (12.09%)	823 (3.02%)	26,469 (96.98%)	1,806	106 (0.40%)	1,784 (0.40%)
	Midwest	62,014 (27.48%)	772 (1.25%)	61,241 (98.75%)	3,057	90 (0.14%)	3,036 (0.14%)
	South	95,774 (42.44%)	1,762 (1.84%)	94,012 (98.16%)	3,885	170 (0.16%)	3,818 (0.16%)
	West	40,571 (17.98%)	603 (1.49%)	39,968 (98.51%)	2,326	69 (0.16%)	2,302 (0.16%)

* Denotes missing values

Migraine unspecified has same pattern as in the other migraine types.

TABLE 40

2008 National statistics—first-listed diagnosis only

Patient and hospital characteristics for
ICD-9-CM first-listed diagnosis code
784.0 Headache

| | | All ED visits (those that resulted in admission to the hospital and those that did not) | Only hospital visits that originated in the ED | Only ED visits that ended in discharge (no hospital admission) | Standard errors | | |
					All ED Visits	Admitted to the hospital from the ED	Discharged from the ED
All discharges		1,427,462 (100.00%)	15,886 (100.00%)	1,411,576 (100.00%)	39,896	964	39,315
Age (mean)		37.44	48.65	37.31	0.14	0.14	0.14
Age group	<1	*	*	*	*	*	*
	1–17	150,113 (10.52%)	1,047 (0.70%)	149,066 (99.30%)	6,749	151 (0.09%)	6,657 (0.09%)
	18–44	825,188 (57.81%)	5,751 (0.70%)	819,437 (99.30%)	23,911	435 (0.05%)	23,690 (0.05%)
	45–64	340,893 (23.88%)	5,359 (1.57%)	335,534 (98.43%)	9,839	341 (0.08%)	9,629 (0.08%)
	65–84	94,718 (6.64%)	2,992 (3.16%)	91,726 (96.84%)	2,792	195 (0.17%)	2,683 (0.17%)
	85+	16,049 (1.12%)	737 (4.59%)	15,312 (95.41%)	547	69 (0.42%)	533 (0.42%)
	Missing	*	*	*	*	*	*
Sex	Male	447,782 (31.37%)	5,375 (1.20%)	442,406 (98.80%)	12,302	317 (0.06%)	12,137 (0.06%)
	Female	979,566 (68.62%)	10,510 (1.07%)	969,055 (98.93%)	27,957	697 (0.06%)	27,537 (0.06%)
	Missing	*	*	*	*	*	*
Region	Northeast	228,102 (15.98%)	3,633 (1.59%)	224,468 (98.41%)	21,712	457 (0.12%)	21,354 (0.12%)
	Midwest	352,884 (24.72%)	3,448 (0.98%)	349,436 (99.02%)	18,962	275 (0.07%)	18,843 (0.07%)
	South	600,418 (42.06%)	6,313 (1.05%)	594,105 (98.95%)	24,803	770 (0.11%)	24,309 (0.11%)
	West	246,058 (17.24%)	2,491 (1.01%)	243,567 (98.99%)	12,063	227 (0.09%)	11,987 (0.09%)

* Denotes missing values

Headache has same pattern.

TABLE 41

Patient and hospital characteristics for ICD-9-CM first-listed diagnosis code 784.0 Headache (after Oct 1, 2008)

		All ED visits (those that resulted in admission to the hospital and those that did not)	Only hospital visits that originated in the ED	Only ED visits that ended in discharge (no hospital admission)	Standard errors		
					All ED Visits	Admitted to the hospital from the ED	Discharged from the ED
All discharges		463,227 (100.00%)	5,504 (100.00%)	457,723 (100.00%)	12,973	416	12,762
Age (mean)		37.26	47.26	37.14	0.15	0.15	0.15
Age group	<1	122 (0.03%)	*	109 (89.03%)	33	*	29 (7.06%)
	1–17	49,491 (10.68%)	531 (1.07%)	48,960 (98.93%)	2,185	102 (0.18%)	2,124 (0.18%)
	18–44	268,214 (57.90%)	1,963 (0.73%)	266,250 (99.27%)	7,891	175 (0.06%)	7,818 (0.06%)
	45–64	109,919 (23.73%)	1,756 (1.60%)	108,163 (98.40%)	3,266	149 (0.12%)	3,192 (0.12%)
	65–84	30,294 (6.54%)	1,012 (3.34%)	29,283 (96.66%)	923	78 (0.22%)	884 (0.22%)
	85+	5,181 (1.12%)	229 (4.42%)	4,952 (95.58%)	213	33 (0.61%)	207 (0.61%)
	Missing	*	*	*	*	*	*
Sex	Male	145,522 (31.41%)	2,046 (1.41%)	143,476 (98.59%)	4,005	205 (0.13%)	3,913 (0.13%)
	Female	317,667 (68.58%)	3,458 (1.09%)	314,209 (98.91%)	9,166	244 (0.07%)	9,045 (0.07%)
	Missing	*	*	*	*	*	*
Region	Northeast	74,473 (16.08%)	1,182 (1.59%)	73,291 (98.41%)	7,040	141 (0.13%)	6,940 (0.13%)
	Midwest	112,483 (24.28%)	1,107 (0.98%)	111,376 (99.02%)	5,973	111 (0.09%)	5,929 (0.09%)
	South	194,978 (42.09%)	2,326 (1.19%)	192,652 (98.81%)	8,233	361 (0.16%)	8,035 (0.16%)
	West	81,293 (17.55%)	890 (1.10%)	80,403 (98.90%)	3,910	100 (0.11%)	3,869 (0.11%)

* Denotes missing values

Tables without reported statistics are interpreted by following these steps: (1) look at sex in the table, the first numbers associated with male and female give the total proportions (%) of female and male discharges; (2) look at the age group, and the first numbers give the proportions (%) of each age group; (3) look at region, the proportions (%) of each region is given as % in the first column.

Henceforth, all tables without statistics are interpreted in the same fashion.

Hormone Imbalance Syndrome

TABLE 42

Patient and hospital characteristics for ICD-9-CM first-listed diagnosis code 729.1 Myalgia And Myositis Nos

		All ED visits (those that resulted in admission to the hospital and those that did not)	Only hospital visits that originated in the ED	Only ED visits that ended in discharge (no hospital admission)	Standard errors		
					All ED Visits	Admitted to the hospital from the ED	Discharged from the ED
All discharges		191,205 (100.00%)	4,889 (100.00%)	186,316 (100.00%)	8,138	265	8,017
Age (mean)		41.23	50.77	40.98	0.21	0.21	0.21
Age group	<1	105 (0.05%)	*	101 (95.80%)	23	*	23 (4.12%)
	1–17	15,113 (7.90%)	425 (2.81%)	14,688 (97.19%)	943	68 (0.41%)	919 (0.41%)
	18–44	96,733 (50.59%)	1,322 (1.37%)	95,410 (98.63%)	4,468	98 (0.10%)	4,431 (0.10%)
	45–64	58,112 (30.39%)	1,845 (3.17%)	56,267 (96.83%)	2,625	133 (0.21%)	2,571 (0.21%)
	65–84	18,096 (9.46%)	1,089 (6.02%)	17,007 (93.98%)	735	89 (0.45%)	701 (0.45%)
	85+	3,042 (1.59%)	203 (6.68%)	2,839 (93.32%)	176	35 (1.10%)	168 (1.10%)
	Missing	*	*	*	*	*	*
Sex	Male	65,203 (34.10%)	1,644 (2.52%)	63,560 (97.48%)	3,441	123 (0.18%)	3,395 (0.18%)
	Female	125,987 (65.89%)	3,245 (2.58%)	122,741 (97.42%)	4,906	185 (0.14%)	4,832 (0.14%)
	Missing	*	*	*	*	*	*
Region	Northeast	50,989 (26.67%)	1,185 (2.32%)	49,804 (97.68%)	6,685	174 (0.28%)	6,576 (0.28%)
	Midwest	37,846 (19.79%)	1,186 (3.13%)	36,660 (96.87%)	1,897	97 (0.27%)	1,879 (0.27%)
	South	75,199 (39.33%)	1,639 (2.18%)	73,560 (97.82%)	3,883	150 (0.20%)	3,838 (0.20%)
	West	27,171 (14.21%)	879 (3.23%)	26,292 (96.77%)	1,692	91 (0.33%)	1,665 (0.33%)

* Denotes missing values

Fibromyalgia follows same pattern: females 65.9%, males 34.1%; ages 18–44, 50.6%; ages 45–64, 30.4%; ages 1–17, 7.9%; and ages 65–84, 9.5%. The South leads with 39.3% followed by the Northeast at 26.7% , the Midwest at 19.8%, and the West, 14.2%.

TABLE 43

Patient and hospital characteristics for ICD-9-CM first-listed diagnosis code 780.4 Dizziness And Giddiness

		All ED visits (those that resulted in admission to the hospital and those that did not)	Only hospital visits that originated in the ED	Only ED visits that ended in discharge (no hospital admission)	Standard errors		
					All ED Visits	Admitted to the hospital from the ED	Discharged from the ED
All discharges		822,947 (100.00%)	34,911 (100.00%)	788,037 (100.00%)	24,438	1,716	23,234
Age (mean)		53.40	68.25	52.75	0.20	0.20	0.20
Age group	<1	113 (0.01%)	*	113 (100.00%)	25	*	25 (0.00%)
	1–17	24,148 (2.93%)	182 (0.76%)	23,966 (99.24%)	1,063	40 (0.16%)	1,049 (0.16%)
	18–44	265,291 (32.24%)	2,819 (1.06%)	262,472 (98.94%)	8,962	216 (0.07%)	8,841 (0.07%)
	45–64	261,299 (31.75%)	9,845 (3.77%)	251,454 (96.23%)	8,279	583 (0.16%)	7,883 (0.16%)
	65–84	221,262 (26.89%)	16,627 (7.51%)	204,635 (92.49%)	6,418	826 (0.29%)	5,919 (0.29%)
	85+	50,828 (6.18%)	5,438 (10.70%)	45,389 (89.30%)	1,647	278 (0.45%)	1,508 (0.45%)
	Missing	*	*	*	*	*	*
Sex	Male	308,192 (37.45%)	13,308 (4.32%)	294,884 (95.68%)	8,632	700 (0.17%)	8,186 (0.17%)
	Female	514,527 (62.52%)	21,603 (4.20%)	492,924 (95.80%)	16,057	1,068 (0.14%)	15,288 (0.14%)
	Missing	*	*	*	*	*	*
Region	Northeast	176,055 (21.39%)	10,652 (6.05%)	165,403 (93.95%)	15,399	1,186 (0.43%)	14,503 (0.43%)
	Midwest	187,051 (22.73%)	7,228 (3.86%)	179,824 (96.14%)	8,937	536 (0.24%)	8,658 (0.24%)
	South	303,106 (36.83%)	12,457 (4.11%)	290,649 (95.89%)	14,693	1,052 (0.23%)	13,884 (0.23%)
	West	156,735 (19.05%)	4,574 (2.92%)	152,161 (97.08%)	8,021	383 (0.22%)	7,858 (0.22%)

* Denotes missing values

Dizziness and giddiness follows same pattern: females 62.5%, males 37.5%; ages 18–44, 32.2%; ages 45–64, 31.8%; ages 1–17, 3%; and ages 65–84, 26.9%. The South leads with 36.8% followed by the Midwest at 22.7%, the Northeast at 21.4%, and the West, 19.1%.

Hormone Imbalance Syndrome

TABLE 44

Patient and hospital characteristics for ICD-9-CM first-listed diagnosis code 780.79 Malaise And Fatigue Nec

		All ED visits (those that resulted in admission to the hospital and those that did not)	Only hospital visits that originated in the ED	Only ED visits that ended in discharge (no hospital admission)	Standard errors		
					All ED Visits	Admitted to the hospital from the ED	Discharged from the ED
All discharges		426,290 (100.00%)	25,525 (100.00%)	400,765 (100.00%)	16,836	1,593	15,580
Age (mean)		59.72	71.54	58.97	0.79	0.79	0.79
Age group	<1	*	*	*	*	*	*
	1–17	15,186 (3.56%)	*	14,880 (97.98%)	3,091	*	2,919 (0.76%)
	18–44	96,668 (22.68%)	1,708 (1.77%)	94,960 (98.23%)	5,004	274 (0.21%)	4,780 (0.21%)
	45–64	105,886 (24.84%)	4,909 (4.64%)	100,976 (95.36%)	4,088	464 (0.34%)	3,780 (0.34%)
	65–84	144,317 (33.85%)	12,181 (8.44%)	132,135 (91.56%)	4,741	559 (0.32%)	4,439 (0.32%)
	85+	62,145 (14.58%)	6,267 (10.08%)	55,878 (89.92%)	2,399	299 (0.45%)	2,274 (0.45%)
	Missing	*	*	*	*	*	*
Sex	Male	169,252 (39.70%)	10,399 (6.14%)	158,853 (93.86%)	6,906	729 (0.27%)	6,336 (0.27%)
	Female	256,894 (60.26%)	15,122 (5.89%)	241,772 (94.11%)	10,077	900 (0.22%)	9,395 (0.22%)
	Missing	*	*	*	*	*	*
Region	Northeast	76,450 (17.93%)	4,553 (5.96%)	71,898 (94.04%)	7,764	462 (0.38%)	7,396 (0.38%)
	Midwest	99,364 (23.31%)	7,445 (7.49%)	91,919 (92.51%)	4,969	509 (0.50%)	4,790 (0.50%)
	South	164,391 (38.56%)	9,539 (5.80%)	154,851 (94.20%)	13,132	1,406 (0.48%)	11,870 (0.48%)
	West	86,086 (20.19%)	3,988 (4.63%)	82,098 (95.37%)	5,103	297 (0.27%)	4,918 (0.27%)

* Denotes missing values

Malaise and fatigue is more common in women and older adults: females 60.3%, males 39.7%; ages 65–84, 33.9%; ages 45–64, 24.8%; ages 18–44, 22.7%; ages 85+, 14.6%, and ages 1–17, 3.6%. The South leads with 38.6% followed by the Midwest at 23.3%, the West at 20.2%, and the Northeast at 17.9%.

TABLE 45

Patient and hospital characteristics for ICD-9-CM first-listed diagnosis code 625.3 Dysmenorrhea

		All ED visits (those that resulted in admission to the hospital and those that did not)	Only hospital visits that originated in the ED	Only ED visits that ended in discharge (no hospital admission)	Standard errors		
					All ED Visits	Admitted to the hospital from the ED	Discharged from the ED
All discharges		76,288 (100.00%)	324 (100.00%)	75,964 (100.00%)	2,238	38	2,235
Age (mean)		25.18	28.08	25.17	0.10	0.10	0.10
Age group	1–17	13,263 (17.39%)	70 (0.53%)	13,193 (99.47%)	488	19 (0.14%)	486 (0.14%)
	18–44	60,146 (78.84%)	225 (0.37%)	59,921 (99.63%)	1,839	31 (0.05%)	1,836 (0.05%)
	45–64	2,861 (3.75%)	*	2,832 (99.00%)	150	*	149 (0.38%)
	65–84	*	*	*	*	*	*
Sex	Female	76,288 (100.00%)	324 (0.42%)	75,964 (99.58%)	2,238	38 (0.05%)	2,235 (0.05%)
Region	Northeast	13,721 (17.99%)	103 (0.75%)	13,618 (99.25%)	875	22 (0.16%)	870 (0.16%)
	Midwest	17,512 (22.95%)	71 (0.40%)	17,441 (99.60%)	1,054	16 (0.10%)	1,053 (0.10%)
	South	33,530 (43.95%)	81 (0.24%)	33,449 (99.76%)	1,634	19 (0.06%)	1,632 (0.06%)
	West	11,526 (15.11%)	70 (0.61%)	11,456 (99.39%)	681	19 (0.17%)	681 (0.17%)

* Denotes missing values

Dysmenorrhea follows the same patterns as the other estrogen-induced conditions noted above. It is more prevalent in the South and the Midwest and manifests most (78.8%) in menstruating women, ages 18–44.

TABLE 46

Patient and hospital characteristics for ICD-9-CM first-listed diagnosis code 626.2 Excessive Menstruation

		All ED visits (those that resulted in admission to the hospital and those that did not)	Only hospital visits that originated in the ED	Only ED visits that ended in discharge (no hospital admission)	Standard errors		
					All ED Visits	Admitted to the hospital from the ED	Discharged from the ED
All discharges		57,284 (100.00%)	6,416 (100.00%)	50,868 (100.00%)	1,907	304	1,817
Age (mean)		31.31	38.13	30.45	0.15	0.15	0.15
Age group	1–17	4,645 (8.11%)	263 (5.67%)	4,382 (94.33%)	261	42 (0.81%)	244 (0.81%)
	18–44	43,741 (76.36%)	4,064 (9.29%)	39,677 (90.71%)	1,527	213 (0.49%)	1,470 (0.49%)
	45–64	8,835 (15.42%)	2,080 (23.55%)	6,755 (76.45%)	377	124 (1.21%)	328 (1.21%)
	65–84	50 (0.09%)	*	*	15	*	*
	85+	*	*	*	*	*	*
Sex	Female	57,284 (100.00%)	6,416 (11.20%)	50,868 (88.80%)	1,907	304 (0.52%)	1,817 (0.52%)
Region	Northeast	11,543 (20.15%)	1,287 (11.15%)	10,255 (88.85%)	1,123	151 (1.46%)	1,094 (1.46%)
	Midwest	13,972 (24.39%)	1,094 (7.83%)	12,878 (92.17%)	774	92 (0.61%)	739 (0.61%)
	South	18,686 (32.62%)	2,634 (14.09%)	16,053 (85.91%)	938	213 (1.00%)	852 (1.00%)
	West	13,083 (22.84%)	1,401 (10.71%)	11,682 (89.29%)	947	126 (1.02%)	914 (1.02%)

* Denotes missing values

Menorrhagia follows the same patterns as other estrogen-induced conditions noted above. It is more prevalent in the South and the Midwest and manifest most in menstruating women at 76.4% in ages 18–44.

TABLE 47

2008 National statistics—first-listed diagnosis only

Patient and hospital characteristics for
ICD-9-CM first-listed diagnosis code
626.0 Absence Of Menstruation

	All ED visits (those that resulted in admission to the hospital and those that did not)	Only hospital visits that originated in the ED	Only ED visits that ended in discharge (no hospital admission)	Standard errors		
				All ED Visits	Admitted to the hospital from the ED	Discharged from the ED
All discharges	8,450 (100.00%)	*	8,444 (100.00%)	417	*	417
Age (mean)	23.77	24.97	23.77	0.19	0.19	0.19
Age group 1–17	933 (11.04%)	*	930 (99.68%)	76	*	76 (0.32%)
18–44	7,362 (87.12%)	*	7,359 (99.96%)	382	*	382 (0.04%)
45–64	155 (1.83%)	*	155 (100.00%)	32	*	32 (0.00%)
Sex Female	8,450 (100.00%)	*	8,444 (99.93%)	417	*	417 (0.05%)
Region Northeast	2,104 (24.90%)	*	2,104 (100.00%)	274	*	274 (0.00%)
Midwest	2,116 (25.04%)	*	2,116 (100.00%)	206	*	206 (0.00%)
South	3,551 (42.02%)	*	3,545 (99.83%)	222	*	222 (0.12%)
West	679 (8.04%)	*	679 (100.00%)	88	*	88 (0.00%)

* Denotes missing values

Absence of menstruation follows the same patterns as other estrogen-induced conditions noted above. It is more prevalent in the South and the Midwest and manifest most in menstruating women at 87.1% in ages 18–44.

TABLE 48

Patient and hospital characteristics for ICD-9-CM first-listed diagnosis code 626.4 Irregular Menstruation

		All ED visits (those that resulted in admission to the hospital and those that did not)	Only hospital visits that originated in the ED	Only ED visits that ended in discharge (no hospital admission)	Standard errors		
					All ED Visits	Admitted to the hospital from the ED	Discharged from the ED
All discharges		11,952 (100.00%)	*	11,941 (100.00%)	810	*	809
Age (mean)		25.53	44.21	25.51	0.23	0.23	0.23
Age group	<1	*	*	*	*	*	*
	1–17	1,392 (11.65%)	*	1,392 (100.00%)	124	*	124 (0.00%)
	18–44	9,906 (82.88%)	*	9,903 (99.97%)	688	*	688 (0.03%)
	45–64	636 (5.32%)	*	627 (98.67%)	73	*	72 (0.94%)
	65–84	*	*	*	*	*	*
Sex	Female	11,952 (100.00%)	*	11,941 (99.90%)	810	*	809 (0.06%)
Region	Northeast	2,410 (20.16%)	*	2,402 (99.65%)	401	*	400 (0.25%)
	Midwest	2,861 (23.93%)	*	2,861 (100.00%)	368	*	368 (0.00%)
	South	4,716 (39.46%)	*	4,716 (100.00%)	523	*	523 (0.00%)
	West	1,966 (16.44%)	*	1,962 (99.84%)	293	*	293 (0.16%)

* Denotes missing values

Irregular Menstruation follows the same patterns as other estrogen-induced conditions noted above. It is more prevalent in the South and the Midwest and manifest most in menstruating women at 82.9% in ages 18–44.

TABLE 49

Patient and hospital characteristics for ICD-9-CM first-listed diagnosis code 626.8 Menstrual Disorder Nec

		All ED visits (those that resulted in admission to the hospital and those that did not)	Only hospital visits that originated in the ED	Only ED visits that ended in discharge (no hospital admission)	Standard errors		
					All ED Visits	Admitted to the hospital from the ED	Discharged from the ED
All discharges		175,921 (100.00%)	3,593 (100.00%)	172,328 (100.00%)	6,959	222	6,864
Age (mean)		30.94	37.15	30.81	0.10	0.10	0.10
Age group	<1	*	*	*	*	*	*
	1–17	9,147 (5.20%)	301 (3.29%)	8,846 (96.71%)	416	43 (0.45%)	404 (0.45%)
	18–44	141,348 (80.35%)	2,174 (1.54%)	139,174 (98.46%)	5,703	160 (0.11%)	5,641 (0.11%)
	45–64	23,469 (13.34%)	1,021 (4.35%)	22,448 (95.65%)	976	81 (0.32%)	947 (0.32%)
	65–84	1,613 (0.92%)	73 (4.51%)	1,540 (95.49%)	109	19 (1.14%)	106 (1.14%)
	85+	300 (0.17%)	*	276 (91.90%)	40	*	38 (3.79%)
Sex	Female	175,916 (100.00%)	3,593 (2.04%)	172,323 (97.96%)	6,959	222 (0.12%)	6,864 (0.12%)
	Missing	*	*	*	*	*	*
Region	Northeast	34,160 (19.42%)	765 (2.24%)	33,395 (97.76%)	4,012	108 (0.29%)	3,957 (0.29%)
	Midwest	37,058 (21.06%)	505 (1.36%)	36,553 (98.64%)	2,607	53 (0.16%)	2,602 (0.16%)
	South	77,281 (43.93%)	1,570 (2.03%)	75,711 (97.97%)	4,544	167 (0.19%)	4,468 (0.19%)
	West	27,422 (15.59%)	753 (2.75%)	26,669 (97.25%)	2,212	85 (0.29%)	2,175 (0.29%)

* Denotes missing values

Menstrual disorders—dysmenorrhea, excessive menstruation, absence of menstruation, irregular menstruation—are more common in prime-age women ages 18–44, followed by females ages 1–17, then older women ages 45–64, followed by ages 65–84, and even 85+. As usual, these estrogen dominance problems are more common in the South, followed by the Midwest, then the Northeast, and finally the West.

Hormone Imbalance Syndrome

TABLE 50

Patient and hospital characteristics for
ICD-9-CM first-listed diagnosis code
620.2 Ovarian Cyst Nec/Nos

		All ED visits (those that resulted in admission to the hospital and those that did not)	Only hospital visits that originated in the ED	Only ED visits that ended in discharge (no hospital admission)	Standard errors		
					All ED Visits	Admitted to the hospital from the ED	Discharged from the ED
All discharges		234,773 (100.00%)	13,592 (100.00%)	221,181 (100.00%)	8,220	528	7,918
Age (mean)		28.55	30.66	28.42	0.07	0.07	0.07
Age group	<1	*	*	*	*	*	*
	1–17	27,684 (11.79%)	1,875 (6.77%)	25,809 (93.23%)	1,071	156 (0.49%)	1,001 (0.49%)
	18–44	190,433 (81.11%)	10,009 (5.26%)	180,424 (94.74%)	6,894	418 (0.18%)	6,648 (0.18%)
	45–64	15,742 (6.71%)	1,442 (9.16%)	14,301 (90.84%)	608	98 (0.57%)	574 (0.57%)
	65–84	694 (0.30%)	177 (25.54%)	517 (74.46%)	64	29 (3.62%)	56 (3.62%)
	85+	196 (0.08%)	84 (42.90%)	112 (57.10%)	30	20 (7.98%)	23 (7.98%)
Sex	Female	234,773 (100.00%)	13,592 (5.79%)	221,181 (94.21%)	8,220	528 (0.19%)	7,918 (0.19%)
Region	Northeast	44,802 (19.08%)	3,270 (7.30%)	41,532 (92.70%)	2,855	268 (0.57%)	2,746 (0.57%)
	Midwest	45,785 (19.50%)	2,434 (5.32%)	43,351 (94.68%)	2,888	171 (0.41%)	2,836 (0.41%)
	South	104,323 (44.44%)	4,882 (4.68%)	99,441 (95.32%)	6,578	367 (0.25%)	6,318 (0.25%)
	West	39,862 (16.98%)	3,006 (7.54%)	36,856 (92.46%)	2,796	207 (0.48%)	2,682 (0.48%)

* Denotes missing values

Ovarian cyst follows the same patterns as other estrogen-induced conditions noted above. It is more prevalent in the South and the Midwest and manifest most in menstruating women at 81.1% in ages 18–44.

TABLE 51

Patient and hospital characteristics for ICD-9-CM first-listed diagnosis code 623.8 Noninflam Discharge Vagina Nec

		All ED visits (those that resulted in admission to the hospital and those that did not)	Only hospital visits that originated in the ED	Only ED visits that ended in discharge (no hospital admission)	Standard errors		
					All ED Visits	Admitted to the hospital from the ED	Discharged from the ED
All discharges		201,835 (100.00%)	1,742 (100.00%)	200,093 (100.00%)	12,229	111	12,177
Age (mean)		31.46	54.50	31.26	0.13	0.13	0.13
Age group	<1	848 (0.42%)	*	834 (98.34%)	83	*	83 (0.97%)
	1–17	12,213 (6.05%)	*	12,195 (99.85%)	801	*	800 (0.07%)
	18–44	157,664 (78.12%)	664 (0.42%)	157,000 (99.58%)	9,818	61 (0.04%)	9,806 (0.04%)
	45–64	22,283 (11.04%)	404 (1.81%)	21,879 (98.19%)	1,418	48 (0.20%)	1,401 (0.20%)
	65–84	6,435 (3.19%)	423 (6.57%)	6,012 (93.43%)	330	51 (0.68%)	305 (0.68%)
	85+	2,392 (1.19%)	219 (9.16%)	2,173 (90.84%)	146	33 (1.30%)	138 (1.30%)
Sex	Female	201,835 (100.00%)	1,742 (0.86%)	200,093 (99.14%)	12,229	111 (0.05%)	12,177 (0.05%)
Region	Northeast	44,020 (21.81%)	390 (0.89%)	43,630 (99.11%)	10,310	66 (0.14%)	10,262 (0.14%)
	Midwest	44,643 (22.12%)	296 (0.66%)	44,347 (99.34%)	3,543	46 (0.10%)	3,534 (0.10%)
	South	82,005 (40.63%)	717 (0.87%)	81,288 (99.13%)	5,104	60 (0.08%)	5,087 (0.08%)
	West	31,167 (15.44%)	339 (1.09%)	30,828 (98.91%)	2,159	46 (0.15%)	2,147 (0.15%)

* Denotes missing values

Non-inflammatory vaginal discharge follows the same patterns as other estrogen-induced conditions noted above. It is more prevalent in the South and the Midwest and manifest most in menstruating women at 78.1% in ages 18–44.

TABLE 52
2008 National statistics—first-listed diagnosis only

Patient and hospital characteristics for
ICD-9-CM first-listed diagnosis code
183.0 Malign Neopl Ovary

		All ED visits (those that resulted in admission to the hospital and those that did not)	Only hospital visits that originated in the ED	Only ED visits that ended in discharge (no hospital admission)	Standard errors		
					All ED Visits	Admitted to the hospital from the ED	Discharged from the ED
All discharges		7,471 (100.00%)	5,824 (100.00%)	1,647 (100.00%)	333	273	150
Age (mean)		62.91	63.94	59.26	0.45	0.45	0.45
Age group	1–17	*	*	*	*	*	*
	18–44	801 (10.73%)	531 (66.20%)	271 (33.80%)	84	57 (4.16%)	49 (4.16%)
	45–64	2,983 (39.93%)	2,244 (75.21%)	739 (24.79%)	178	139 (2.54%)	96 (2.54%)
	65–84	2,992 (40.05%)	2,440 (81.54%)	552 (18.46%)	170	149 (2.09%)	71 (2.09%)
	85+	637 (8.52%)	557 (87.55%)	79 (12.45%)	58	53 (3.07%)	21 (3.07%)
Sex	Female	7,471 (100.00%)	5,824 (77.95%)	1,647 (22.05%)	333	273 (1.63%)	150 (1.63%)
Region	Northeast	1,695 (22.69%)	1,363 (80.40%)	332 (19.60%)	180	147 (3.17%)	68 (3.17%)
	Midwest	1,485 (19.87%)	985 (66.35%)	500 (33.65%)	155	98 (4.89%)	106 (4.89%)
	South	2,684 (35.93%)	2,155 (80.29%)	529 (19.71%)	180	164 (2.23%)	65 (2.23%)
	West	1,607 (21.51%)	1,321 (82.19%)	286 (17.81%)	148	128 (2.50%)	48 (2.50%)

* Denotes missing values

Endometriosis follows the same patterns as other estrogen-
induced conditions noted above. It is more prevalent in the South
and the Midwest and manifest most in menstruating women at
83.6% in ages 18–44.

TABLE 53

2008 National statistics—first-listed diagnosis only

Patient and hospital characteristics for
ICD-9-CM first-listed diagnosis code
179 Malig Neopl Uterus Nos

		All ED visits (those that resulted in admission to the hospital and those that did not)	Only hospital visits that originated in the ED	Only ED visits that ended in discharge (no hospital admission)	Standard errors		
					All ED Visits	Admitted to the hospital from the ED	Discharged from the ED
All discharges		969 (100.00%)	624 (100.00%)	345 (100.00%)	79	61	46
Age (mean)		64.81	65.60	63.38	1.13	1.13	1.13
Age group	18–44	83 (8.60%)	*	*	24	*	*
	45–64	412 (42.45%)	246 (59.77%)	166 (40.23%)	50	35 (5.45%)	32 (5.45%)
	65–84	371 (38.26%)	266 (71.67%)	105 (28.33%)	46	37 (5.92%)	27 (5.92%)
	85+	104 (10.68%)	67 (64.97%)	*	23	18 (10.45%)	*
Sex	Female	969 (100.00%)	624 (64.40%)	345 (35.60%)	79	61 (3.70%)	46 (3.70%)
Region	Northeast	209 (21.56%)	128 (61.19%)	81 (38.81%)	42	32 (8.64%)	24 (8.64%)
	Midwest	183 (18.92%)	118 (64.41%)	*	35	28 (9.61%)	*
	South	329 (33.93%)	239 (72.73%)	90 (27.27%)	40	33 (5.29%)	21 (5.29%)
	West	248 (25.58%)	139 (56.06%)	109 (43.94%)	41	29 (7.27%)	25 (7.27%)

* Denotes missing values

TABLE 54

Patient and hospital characteristics for ICD-9-CM first-listed diagnosis code 174.8 Malign Neopl Breast Nec

		All ED visits (those that resulted in admission to the hospital and those that did not)	Only hospital visits that originated in the ED	Only ED visits that ended in discharge (no hospital admission)	Standard errors		
					All ED Visits	Admitted to the hospital from the ED	Discharged from the ED
All discharges		2,028 (100.00%)	1,649 (100.00%)	379 (100.00%)	194	162	81
Age (mean)		61.99	62.63	59.23	0.85	0.85	0.85
Age group	18–44	249 (12.26%)	186 (74.77%)	63 (25.23%)	43	35 (5.77%)	18 (5.77%)
	45–64	904 (44.59%)	721 (79.72%)	*	119	94 (5.49%)	*
	65–84	693 (34.15%)	591 (85.36%)	101 (14.64%)	68	63 (3.00%)	22 (3.00%)
	85+	183 (9.01%)	151 (82.69%)	*	31	29 (6.16%)	*
Sex	Female	2,028 (100.00%)	1,649 (81.31%)	379 (18.69%)	194	162 (3.29%)	81 (3.29%)
Region	Northeast	902 (44.48%)	721 (79.87%)	*	160	127 (6.24%)	*
	Midwest	220 (10.82%)	156 (70.89%)	*	36	31 (9.38%)	*
	South	682 (33.61%)	570 (83.57%)	112 (16.43%)	96	88 (3.66%)	27 (3.66%)
	West	225 (11.09%)	203 (90.34%)	*	38	37 (4.22%)	*

* Denotes missing values

TABLE 55

Patient and hospital characteristics for ICD-9-CM first-listed diagnosis code 174.9 Malign Neopl Breast Nos

		All ED visits (those that resulted in admission to the hospital and those that did not)	Only hospital visits that originated in the ED	Only ED visits that ended in discharge (no hospital admission)	Standard errors		
					All ED Visits	Admitted to the hospital from the ED	Discharged from the ED
All discharges		7,465 (100.00%)	3,125 (100.00%)	4,339 (100.00%)	346	178	271
Age (mean)		59.65	62.59	57.54	0.48	0.48	0.48
Age group	18–44	1,112 (14.90%)	307 (27.62%)	805 (72.38%)	98	42 (3.43%)	87 (3.43%)
	45–64	3,675 (49.23%)	1,518 (41.32%)	2,156 (58.68%)	219	112 (2.50%)	176 (2.50%)
	65–84	2,307 (30.90%)	1,075 (46.59%)	1,232 (53.41%)	149	85 (2.77%)	111 (2.77%)
	85+	371 (4.97%)	225 (60.72%)	146 (39.28%)	42	31 (5.97%)	29 (5.97%)
Sex	Female	7,465 (100.00%)	3,125 (41.87%)	4,339 (58.13%)	346	178 (1.90%)	271 (1.90%)
Region	Northeast	1,273 (17.06%)	537 (42.18%)	736 (57.82%)	132	77 (4.41%)	97 (4.41%)
	Midwest	1,866 (25.00%)	587 (31.48%)	1,279 (68.52%)	207	70 (4.04%)	191 (4.04%)
	South	2,823 (37.82%)	1,380 (48.87%)	1,443 (51.13%)	196	127 (2.55%)	115 (2.55%)
	West	1,502 (20.12%)	621 (41.35%)	881 (58.65%)	145	68 (3.94%)	119 (3.94%)

TABLE 56

2008 National statistics—first-listed diagnosis only

Patient and hospital characteristics for
ICD-9-CM first-listed diagnosis code
185 Malign Neopl Prostate

		All ED visits (those that resulted in admission to the hospital and those that did not)	Only hospital visits that originated in the ED	Only ED visits that ended in discharge (no hospital admission)	Standard errors		
					All ED Visits	Admitted to the hospital from the ED	Discharged from the ED
All discharges		8,877 (100.00%)	5,185 (100.00%)	3,692 (100.00%)	477	253	380
Age (mean)		73.89	75.47	71.67	0.37	0.37	0.37
Age group	1–17	*	*	*	*	*	*
	18–44	*	*	*	*	*	*
	45–64	1,805 (20.33%)	947 (52.50%)	857 (47.50%)	140	83 (3.47%)	103 (3.47%)
	65–84	5,365 (60.44%)	3,005 (56.00%)	2,361 (44.00%)	347	173 (3.21%)	287 (3.21%)
	85+	1,634 (18.40%)	1,212 (74.18%)	422 (25.82%)	111	88 (3.34%)	67 (3.34%)
Sex	Male	8,877 (100.00%)	5,185 (58.41%)	3,692 (41.59%)	477	253 (2.66%)	380 (2.66%)
Region	Northeast	2,241 (25.24%)	1,489 (66.42%)	*	326	167 (6.81%)	*
	Midwest	1,752 (19.73%)	826 (47.16%)	926 (52.84%)	157	91 (4.13%)	122 (4.13%)
	South	3,370 (37.96%)	1,961 (58.21%)	1,408 (41.79%)	276	140 (4.99%)	257 (4.99%)
	West	1,515 (17.07%)	909 (59.99%)	606 (40.01%)	142	91 (3.23%)	81 (3.23%)

* Denotes missing values

TABLE 57

Patient and hospital characteristics for ICD-9-CM first-listed diagnosis code 617.1 Ovarian Endometriosis

| | All ED visits (those that resulted in admission to the hospital and those that did not) | Only hospital visits that originated in the ED | Only ED visits that ended in discharge (no hospital admission) | Standard errors | | |
				All ED Visits	Admitted to the hospital from the ED	Discharged from the ED
All discharges	1,239 (100.00%)	998 (100.00%)	241 (100.00%)	93	79	38
Age (mean)	34.39	34.94	32.12	0.60	0.60	0.60
Age group 1–17	*	*	*	*		*
Age group 18–44	1,035 (83.59%)	824 (79.57%)	212 (20.43%)	86	73 (2.90%)	36 (2.90%)
Age group 45–64	199 (16.06%)	174 (87.60%)	*	30	29 (4.87%)	*
Sex Female	1,239 (100.00%)	998 (80.58%)	241 (19.42%)	93	79 (2.64%)	38 (2.64%)
Region Northeast	264 (21.33%)	216 (81.62%)	*	43	40 (5.77%)	*
Region Midwest	305 (24.65%)	231 (75.58%)	*	42	35 (6.35%)	*
Region South	394 (31.78%)	318 (80.87%)	75 (19.13%)	52	45 (3.99%)	18 (3.99%)
Region West	276 (22.25%)	233 (84.71%)	*	48	38 (5.28%)	*

* Denotes missing values

Endometriosis follows the same patterns as other estrogen-induced conditions noted above. It is more prevalent in the South and the Midwest and manifest most in menstruating women at 83.6% in ages 18–44.

TABLE 58

Patient and hospital characteristics for ICD-9-CM first-listed diagnosis code 617.3 Pelv Perit Endometriosis

| | | All ED visits (those that resulted in admission to the hospital and those that did not) | Only hospital visits that originated in the ED | Only ED visits that ended in discharge (no hospital admission) | Standard errors | | |
					All ED Visits	Admitted to the hospital from the ED	Discharged from the ED
All discharges		1,100 (100.00%)	608 (100.00%)	492 (100.00%)	107	56	88
Age (mean)		30.28	31.47	28.81	0.51	0.51	0.51
Age group	1–17	*	*	*	*	*	*
	18–44	1,028 (93.43%)	553 (53.80%)	475 (46.20%)	105	54 (5.01%)	87 (5.01%)
	45–64	*	*	*	*	*	*
Sex	Female	1,100 (100.00%)	608 (55.26%)	492 (44.74%)	107	56 (4.88%)	88 (4.88%)
Region	Northeast	186 (16.90%)	109 (58.61%)	*	32	21 (9.47%)	*
	Midwest	366 (33.22%)	177 (48.50%)	*	74	28 (9.40%)	*
	South	371 (33.74%)	187 (50.40%)	184 (49.60%)	64	37 (8.12%)	50 (8.12%)
	West	178 (16.14%)	135 (75.83%)	*	28	24 (6.86%)	*

* Denotes missing values

Pelvic/Peritoneal Endometriosis follows the same patterns as other estrogen-induced conditions noted above. It is more prevalent in the South and the Midwest and manifest most in menstruating women at 93.4% in ages 18–44.

TABLE 59

Patient and hospital characteristics for
ICD-9-CM first-listed diagnosis code
617.9 Endometriosis Nos

		All ED visits (those that resulted in admission to the hospital and those that did not)	Only hospital visits that originated in the ED	Only ED visits that ended in discharge (no hospital admission)	All ED Visits	Admitted to the hospital from the ED	Discharged from the ED
						Standard errors	
All discharges		11,678 (100.00%)	471 (100.00%)	11,207 (100.00%)	496	56	486
Age (mean)		28.19	29.38	28.14	0.17	0.17	0.17
Age group	1–17	230 (1.97%)	*	210 (90.98%)	35	*	34 (4.36%)
	18–44	11,134 (95.34%)	419 (3.76%)	10,715 (96.24%)	483	55 (0.48%)	472 (0.48%)
	45–64	314 (2.69%)	*	282 (89.89%)	39	*	37 (3.68%)
Sex	Female	11,678 (100.00%)	471 (4.03%)	11,207 (95.97%)	496	56 (0.48%)	486 (0.48%)
Region	Northeast	1,841 (15.77%)	158 (8.60%)	1,683 (91.40%)	188	39 (2.06%)	181 (2.06%)
	Midwest	2,823 (24.18%)	125 (4.41%)	2,699 (95.59%)	214	25 (0.88%)	210 (0.88%)
	South	5,249 (44.95%)	153 (2.92%)	5,096 (97.08%)	362	29 (0.54%)	356 (0.54%)
	West	1,764 (15.10%)	*	1,729 (98.01%)	183	*	183 (0.71%)

* Denotes missing values

Endometriosis Nos follows the same patterns as other estrogen-induced conditions noted above. It is more prevalent in the South and the Midwest and manifest most in menstruating women at 95.3% in ages 18–44.

TABLE 60

2008 National statistics—first-listed diagnosis only

Patient and hospital characteristics for
ICD-9-CM first-listed diagnosis code
595.0 Acute Cystitis

		All ED visits (those that resulted in admission to the hospital and those that did not)	Only hospital visits that originated in the ED	Only ED visits that ended in discharge (no hospital admission)	Standard errors		
					All ED Visits	Admitted to the hospital from the ED	Discharged from the ED
All discharges		89,158 (100.00%)	4,328 (100.00%)	84,831 (100.00%)	5,155	344	5,096
Age (mean)		40.11	69.51	38.61	0.41	0.41	0.41
Age group	<1	176 (0.20%)	*	159 (90.32%)	48	*	47 (5.18%)
	1–17	8,596 (9.64%)	92 (1.07%)	8,504 (98.93%)	669	24 (0.29%)	668 (0.29%)
	18–44	47,601 (53.39%)	424 (0.89%)	47,176 (99.11%)	3,050	60 (0.13%)	3,045 (0.13%)
	45–64	17,006 (19.07%)	794 (4.67%)	16,213 (95.33%)	956	96 (0.59%)	948 (0.59%)
	65–84	12,365 (13.87%)	1,991 (16.10%)	10,374 (83.90%)	630	166 (1.27%)	587 (1.27%)
	85+	3,414 (3.83%)	1,010 (29.58%)	2,404 (70.42%)	213	110 (2.58%)	172 (2.58%)
Sex	Male	10,424 (11.69%)	1,461 (14.02%)	8,963 (85.98%)	567	116 (1.13%)	540 (1.13%)
	Female	78,734 (88.31%)	2,867 (3.64%)	75,867 (96.36%)	4,690	282 (0.38%)	4,648 (0.38%)
Region	Northeast	11,042 (12.39%)	919 (8.33%)	10,123 (91.67%)	1,558	110 (1.37%)	1,537 (1.37%)
	Midwest	16,621 (18.64%)	588 (3.54%)	16,033 (96.46%)	1,766	65 (0.50%)	1,757 (0.50%)
	South	42,869 (48.08%)	1,852 (4.32%)	41,017 (95.68%)	4,319	224 (0.61%)	4,278 (0.61%)
	West	18,626 (20.89%)	968 (5.20%)	17,657 (94.80%)	1,542	228 (1.17%)	1,491 (1.17%)

* Denotes missing values

TABLE 61

Patient and hospital characteristics for ICD-9-CM first-listed diagnosis code 595.9 Cystitis Nos

		All ED visits (those that resulted in admission to the hospital and those that did not)	Only hospital visits that originated in the ED	Only ED visits that ended in discharge (no hospital admission)	Standard errors		
					All ED Visits	Admitted to the hospital from the ED	Discharged from the ED
All discharges		115,440 (100.00%)	7,438 (100.00%)	108,002 (100.00%)	4,860	408	4,763
Age (mean)		41.76	69.05	39.88	0.35	0.35	0.35
Age group	<1	286 (0.25%)	*	267 (93.17%)	47	*	44 (3.82%)
	1–17	11,065 (9.59%)	124 (1.12%)	10,941 (98.88%)	564	24 (0.21%)	560 (0.21%)
	18–44	58,021 (50.26%)	859 (1.48%)	57,163 (98.52%)	2,734	91 (0.15%)	2,713 (0.15%)
	45–64	22,466 (19.46%)	1,359 (6.05%)	21,107 (93.95%)	986	105 (0.48%)	969 (0.48%)
	65–84	17,935 (15.54%)	3,243 (18.08%)	14,692 (81.92%)	798	208 (1.09%)	734 (1.09%)
	85+	5,660 (4.90%)	1,828 (32.29%)	3,832 (67.71%)	306	130 (1.89%)	252 (1.89%)
	Missing	*	*	*	*	*	*
Sex	Male	17,387 (15.06%)	2,635 (15.15%)	14,753 (84.85%)	745	162 (0.86%)	685 (0.86%)
	Female	98,025 (84.91%)	4,803 (4.90%)	93,222 (95.10%)	4,243	289 (0.33%)	4,199 (0.33%)
	Missing	*	*	*	*	*	*
Region	Northeast	19,990 (17.32%)	1,266 (6.33%)	18,724 (93.67%)	2,955	131 (1.01%)	2,926 (1.01%)
	Midwest	25,071 (21.72%)	1,421 (5.67%)	23,650 (94.33%)	1,843	134 (0.55%)	1,801 (0.55%)
	South	45,668 (39.56%)	3,190 (6.99%)	42,478 (93.01%)	2,625	259 (0.54%)	2,529 (0.54%)
	West	24,711 (21.41%)	1,560 (6.31%)	23,150 (93.69%)	2,144	254 (1.08%)	2,118 (1.08%)

* Denotes missing values

Cystitis Nos follows the same patterns as other estrogen-induced conditions noted above. It is more prevalent in the South and the Midwest and manifest most in menstruating women at 83.6% in ages 18–44.

TABLE 62

Patient and hospital characteristics for
ICD-9-CM first-listed diagnosis code
595.1 Chr Interstit Cystitis

		All ED visits (those that resulted in admission to the hospital and those that did not)	Only hospital visits that originated in the ED	Only ED visits that ended in discharge (no hospital admission)	Standard errors		
					All ED Visits	Admitted to the hospital from the ED	Discharged from the ED
All discharges		4,693 (100.00%)	740 (100.00%)	3,953 (100.00%)	320	68	292
Age (mean)		41.07	53.54	38.73	0.75	0.75	0.75
Age group	1–17	104 (2.21%)	*	*	28	*	*
	18–44	3,099 (66.03%)	286 (9.22%)	2,813 (90.78%)	276	45 (1.17%)	251 (1.17%)
	45–64	976 (20.79%)	172 (17.60%)	804 (82.40%)	122	27 (3.06%)	118 (3.06%)
	65–84	428 (9.12%)	195 (45.63%)	233 (54.37%)	50	33 (5.57%)	36 (5.57%)
	85+	87 (1.86%)	*	*	24	*	*
Sex	Male	363 (7.74%)	88 (24.23%)	*	101	22 (7.84%)	*
	Female	4,325 (92.15%)	652 (15.07%)	3,673 (84.93%)	300	63 (1.26%)	272 (1.26%)
	Missing	*	*	*	*	*	*
Region	Northeast	683 (14.55%)	132 (19.39%)	550 (80.61%)	112	29 (3.55%)	99 (3.55%)
	Midwest	1,177 (25.09%)	187 (15.88%)	990 (84.12%)	131	37 (2.83%)	118 (2.83%)
	South	1,680 (35.80%)	248 (14.78%)	1,432 (85.22%)	133	34 (1.94%)	125 (1.94%)
	West	1,153 (24.56%)	172 (14.95%)	981 (85.05%)	235	35 (2.57%)	214 (2.57%)

* Denotes missing values

Chronic interstitial cystitis follows the same patterns as other estrogen-induced conditions. It is more prevalent in the South and the Midwest and manifests most in females at 92.2% with males at only 7.7%. Menstruating women ages 18–44 have the highest rate, 66.0%, followed by the older females 45–64 at 20.8%. The young and the very old have rates of 2.2% and 1.9% respectively.

TABLE 63
2008 National statistics—first-listed diagnosis only

Patient and hospital characteristics for ICD-9-CM first-listed diagnosis code 710.0 Syst Lupus Erythematosus

		All ED visits (those that resulted in admission to the hospital and those that did not)	Only hospital visits that originated in the ED	Only ED visits that ended in discharge (no hospital admission)	Standard errors		
					All ED Visits	Admitted to the hospital from the ED	Discharged from the ED
All discharges		20,331 (100.00%)	10,104 (100.00%)	10,227 (100.00%)	900	587	508
Age (mean)		36.56	36.54	36.59	0.37	0.37	0.37
Age group	<1	*	*	*	*	*	*
	1–17	1,192 (5.87%)	732 (61.35%)	461 (38.65%)	167	120 (3.93%)	73 (3.93%)
	18–44	13,552 (66.65%)	6,509 (48.03%)	7,043 (51.97%)	667	421 (1.76%)	398 (1.76%)
	45–64	4,762 (23.42%)	2,323 (48.79%)	2,439 (51.21%)	249	161 (2.19%)	164 (2.19%)
	65–84	796 (3.91%)	515 (64.73%)	281 (35.27%)	86	57 (4.49%)	53 (4.49%)
	85+	*	*	*	*	*	*
Sex	Male	1,990 (9.79%)	1,219 (61.24%)	771 (38.76%)	134	103 (3.05%)	80 (3.05%)
	Female	18,341 (90.21%)	8,886 (48.45%)	9,456 (51.55%)	828	530 (1.61%)	484 (1.61%)
Region	Northeast	3,908 (19.22%)	2,438 (62.40%)	1,469 (37.60%)	412	347 (3.85%)	166 (3.85%)
	Midwest	2,869 (14.11%)	1,333 (46.48%)	1,535 (53.52%)	281	179 (3.20%)	154 (3.20%)
	South	9,249 (45.49%)	4,129 (44.64%)	5,120 (55.36%)	640	366 (2.32%)	404 (2.32%)
	West	4,306 (21.18%)	2,203 (51.17%)	2,102 (48.83%)	391	242 (2.61%)	208 (2.61%)

* Denotes missing values

Lupus follows the same patterns as other estrogen-induced conditions. It is more prevalent in the South and the West and manifests most in females at 90.2% with males having a rate of 9.8%. It is found most in menstruating women at 66.7% in ages 18–44.

TABLE 64
2008 National statistics—first-listed diagnosis only

Patient and hospital characteristics for
ICD-9-CM first-listed diagnosis code
340 Multiple Sclerosis

		All ED visits (those that resulted in admission to the hospital and those that did not)	Only hospital visits that originated in the ED	Only ED visits that ended in discharge (no hospital admission)	Standard errors		
					All ED Visits	Admitted to the hospital from the ED	Discharged from the ED
All discharges		29,125 (100.00%)	16,039 (100.00%)	13,086 (100.00%)	1,105	789	553
Age (mean)		43.44	44.45	42.20	0.27	0.27	0.27
Age group	1–17	402 (1.38%)	205 (50.86%)	198 (49.14%)	76	52 (8.85%)	52 (8.85%)
	18–44	15,213 (52.23%)	7,755 (50.97%)	7,458 (49.03%)	674	466 (1.68%)	378 (1.68%)
	45–64	11,783 (40.46%)	7,065 (59.96%)	4,718 (40.04%)	502	362 (1.53%)	259 (1.53%)
	65–84	1,689 (5.80%)	986 (58.36%)	703 (41.64%)	136	86 (3.92%)	100 (3.92%)
	85+	*	*	*	*	*	*
	Missing	*	*	*	*	*	*
Sex	Male	7,513 (25.80%)	4,347 (57.85%)	3,167 (42.15%)	346	246 (1.89%)	204 (1.89%)
	Female	21,611 (74.20%)	11,692 (54.10%)	9,919 (45.90%)	871	612 (1.46%)	461 (1.46%)
Region	Northeast	7,151 (24.55%)	4,482 (62.67%)	2,669 (37.33%)	622	482 (3.21%)	301 (3.21%)
	Midwest	6,596 (22.65%)	3,442 (52.17%)	3,155 (47.83%)	482	316 (2.49%)	267 (2.49%)
	South	10,765 (36.96%)	5,901 (54.82%)	4,863 (45.18%)	704	503 (2.04%)	322 (2.04%)
	West	4,613 (15.84%)	2,214 (48.00%)	2,399 (52.00%)	324	195 (2.48%)	201 (2.48%)

* Denotes missing values

Many scientists believe that Multiple Sclerosis (MS) may be due to estrogen dominance. In 2008, discharges for MS were more prevalent in the South, followed by the Northeast, the Midwest, and the West. Women had the highest rate, 74.2%, and males 25.8%. The discharge rate was highest in the prime-age group, 52.2%, and older adults, 40.5%. The 65–84 age group had a rate of 5.8% and the very young, ages 1–17, were at 1.4%.

TABLE 65
2008 National statistics—first-listed diagnosis only

Patient and hospital characteristics for
ICD-9-CM first-listed diagnosis code
704.00 Alopecia Nos

| | | All ED visits (those that resulted in admission to the hospital and those that did not) | Only hospital visits that originated in the ED | Only ED visits that ended in discharge (no hospital admission) | Standard errors | | |
					All ED Visits	Admitted to the hospital from the ED	Discharged from the ED
All discharges		2,145 (100.00%)	—	2,145 (100.00%)	144	—	144
Age (mean)		22.63	—	22.63	1.02	1.02	1.02
Age group	<1	*		*	*		*
	1–17	806 (37.59%)		806 (100.00%)	77		77 (0.00%)
	18–44	1,074 (50.05%)		1,074 (100.00%)	97		97 (0.00%)
	45–64	202 (9.40%)		202 (100.00%)	35		35 (0.00%)
	65–84	*		*	*		*
Sex	Male	825 (38.44%)		825 (100.00%)	73		73 (0.00%)
	Female	1,320 (61.56%)		1,320 (100.00%)	104		104 (0.00%)
Region	Northeast	561 (26.14%)		561 (100.00%)	84		84 (0.00%)
	Midwest	486 (22.64%)		486 (100.00%)	56		56 (0.00%)
	South	725 (33.79%)		725 (100.00%)	69		69 (0.00%)
	West	374 (17.43%)		374 (100.00%)	76		76 (0.00%)

* Denotes missing values

TABLE 66

Patient and hospital characteristics for ICD-9-CM first-listed diagnosis code 704.8 Hair Diseases Nec

		All ED visits (those that resulted in admission to the hospital and those that did not)	Only hospital visits that originated in the ED	Only ED visits that ended in discharge (no hospital admission)	Standard errors		
					All ED Visits	Admitted to the hospital from the ED	Discharged from the ED
All discharges		79,815 (100.00%)	397 (100.00%)	79,418 (100.00%)	2,850	44	2,845
Age (mean)		28.02	41.81	27.95	0.25	0.25	0.25
Age group	<1	904 (1.13%)	*	898 (99.40%)	86	*	86 (0.60%)
	1–17	15,718 (19.69%)	*	15,700 (99.89%)	759	*	759 (0.06%)
	18–44	51,127 (64.06%)	217 (0.42%)	50,911 (99.58%)	1,954	32 (0.06%)	1,949 (0.06%)
	45–64	10,359 (12.98%)	123 (1.19%)	10,235 (98.81%)	480	24 (0.23%)	477 (0.23%)
	65–84	1,566 (1.96%)	*	1,545 (98.66%)	101	*	100 (0.60%)
	85+	142 (0.18%)	*	129 (90.59%)	28	*	27 (5.24%)
Sex	Male	40,626 (50.90%)	217 (0.53%)	40,409 (99.47%)	1,510	30 (0.08%)	1,508 (0.08%)
	Female	39,185 (49.10%)	180 (0.46%)	39,005 (99.54%)	1,438	33 (0.08%)	1,433 (0.08%)
	Missing	*	*	*	*	*	*
Region	Northeast	15,211 (19.06%)	125 (0.82%)	15,086 (99.18%)	1,222	25 (0.17%)	1,217 (0.17%)
	Midwest	21,145 (26.49%)	76 (0.36%)	21,069 (99.64%)	1,440	19 (0.09%)	1,439 (0.09%)
	South	30,953 (38.78%)	138 (0.44%)	30,816 (99.56%)	1,892	24 (0.08%)	1,891 (0.08%)
	West	12,506 (15.67%)	*	12,448 (99.54%)	989	*	982 (0.15%)

* Denotes missing values

TABLE 67

Patient and hospital characteristics for ICD-9-CM first-listed diagnosis code 698.1 Pruritus Of Genitalia

		All ED visits (those that resulted in admission to the hospital and those that did not)	Only hospital visits that originated in the ED	Only ED visits that ended in discharge (no hospital admission)	Standard errors		
					All ED Visits	Admitted to the hospital from the ED	Discharged from the ED
All discharges		5,030 (100.00%)	—	5,030 (100.00%)	339	—	339
Age (mean)		29.51	—	29.51	0.57	0.57	0.57
Age group	<1	*		*	*		*
	1–17	879 (17.48%)		879 (100.00%)	88		88 (0.00%)
	18–44	3,249 (64.59%)		3,249 (100.00%)	240		240 (0.00%)
	45–64	731 (14.53%)		731 (100.00%)	78		78 (0.00%)
	65–84	148 (2.95%)		148 (100.00%)	30		30 (0.00%)
	85+	*		*	*		*
Sex	Male	924 (18.36%)		924 (100.00%)	93		93 (0.00%)
	Female	4,107 (81.64%)		4,107 (100.00%)	286		286 (0.00%)
Region	Northeast	951 (18.91%)		951 (100.00%)	170		170 (0.00%)
	Midwest	1,272 (25.29%)		1,272 (100.00%)	151		151 (0.00%)
	South	2,149 (42.73%)		2,149 (100.00%)	209		209 (0.00%)
	West	657 (13.07%)		657 (100.00%)	139		139 (0.00%)

* Denotes missing values

Hormone Imbalance Syndrome

TABLE 68

Patient and hospital characteristics for ICD-9-CM first-listed diagnosis code 698.8 Pruritic Conditions Nec

		All ED visits (those that resulted in admission to the hospital and those that did not)	Only hospital visits that originated in the ED	Only ED visits that ended in discharge (no hospital admission)	Standard errors		
					All ED Visits	Admitted to the hospital from the ED	Discharged from the ED
All discharges		6,493 (100.00%)	239 (100.00%)	6,254 (100.00%)	358	37	356
Age (mean)		39.01	53.44	38.46	0.58	0.58	0.58
Age group	<1	*	*	*	*	*	*
	1–17	975 (15.01%)	*	951 (97.54%)	87	*	87 (1.09%)
	18–44	2,958 (45.55%)	58 (1.96%)	2,900 (98.04%)	190	16 (0.55%)	190 (0.55%)
	45–64	1,650 (25.41%)	72 (4.34%)	1,578 (95.66%)	117	19 (1.13%)	114 (1.13%)
	65–84	748 (11.51%)	*	686 (91.70%)	66	*	62 (2.55%)
	85+	135 (2.08%)	*	112 (83.03%)	27	*	24 (7.87%)
Sex	Male	2,208 (34.00%)	89 (4.05%)	2,119 (95.95%)	151	21 (0.92%)	148 (0.92%)
	Female	4,282 (65.95%)	149 (3.48%)	4,133 (96.52%)	251	30 (0.70%)	250 (0.70%)
	Missing	*	*	*	*	*	*
Region	Northeast	1,203 (18.52%)	86 (7.19%)	1,116 (92.81%)	151	22 (2.04%)	152 (2.04%)
	Midwest	1,510 (23.25%)	*	1,475 (97.71%)	173	*	170 (1.08%)
	South	2,695 (41.50%)	86 (3.19%)	2,609 (96.81%)	242	19 (0.71%)	239 (0.71%)
	West	1,086 (16.73%)	*	1,054 (97.08%)	132	*	133 (1.43%)

* Denotes missing values

TABLE 69

Patient and hospital characteristics for ICD-9-CM first-listed diagnosis code 698.9 Pruritic Disorder Nos

		All ED visits (those that resulted in admission to the hospital and those that did not)	Only hospital visits that originated in the ED	Only ED visits that ended in discharge (no hospital admission)	Standard errors		
					All ED Visits	Admitted to the hospital from the ED	Discharged from the ED
All discharges		46,892 (100.00%)	160 (100.00%)	46,732 (100.00%)	2,021	27	2,017
Age (mean)		39.70	50.68	39.66	0.40	0.40	0.40
Age group	<1	136 (0.29%)	*	136 (100.00%)	25	*	25 (0.00%)
	1–17	6,311 (13.46%)	*	6,298 (99.80%)	463	*	461 (0.11%)
	18–44	21,274 (45.37%)	56 (0.26%)	21,218 (99.74%)	989	16 (0.08%)	986 (0.08%)
	45–64	13,191 (28.13%)	41 (0.31%)	13,149 (99.69%)	637	12 (0.09%)	637 (0.09%)
	65–84	5,167 (11.02%)	*	5,128 (99.25%)	243	*	242 (0.25%)
	85+	814 (1.74%)	*	803 (98.61%)	72	*	72 (0.83%)
Sex	Male	15,781 (33.65%)	*	15,732 (99.69%)	743	*	742 (0.09%)
	Female	31,106 (66.34%)	111 (0.36%)	30,995 (99.64%)	1,363	22 (0.07%)	1,360 (0.07%)
	Missing	*	*	*	*	*	*
Region	Northeast	9,659 (20.60%)	*	9,629 (99.69%)	1,450	*	1,450 (0.13%)
	Midwest	11,106 (23.68%)	*	11,078 (99.74%)	743	*	741 (0.10%)
	South	18,359 (39.15%)	70 (0.38%)	18,289 (99.62%)	1,063	17 (0.09%)	1,057 (0.09%)
	West	7,769 (16.57%)	*	7,736 (99.58%)	549	*	548 (0.17%)

* Denotes missing values

TABLE 70

2006 National statistics—principal diagnosis only

Outcomes by patient and hospital characteristics for
ICD-9-CM principal diagnosis code
218.0 Submucous Leiomyoma

		Total number of discharges	LOS (length of stay), days (median)	Charges, $ (median)	Costs, $ (median)	Aggregate costs
All discharges		29,330 (100.00%)	2.0	15,200	5,510	180,513,446
Age group	18–44	14,263 (48.63%)	2.0	15,066	5,435	86,555,700
	45–64	14,561 (49.65%)	2.0	15,241	5,570	90,359,177
	65–84	468 (1.60%)	3.0	16,457	6,454	3,327,788
	85+	*	*	*	*	*
	Missing	*	*	*	*	*
Sex	Female	29,236 (99.68%)	2.0	15,192	5,509	179,891,572
	Missing	93 (0.32%)	3.0	24,957	7,161	621,874
Median income for zip code	Low	7,883 (26.88%)	2.0	14,962	5,504	48,683,898
	Not low	20,654 (70.42%)	2.0	15,313	5,498	126,420,961
	Missing	793 (2.70%)	3.0	12,850	6,184	5,408,587
Region	Northeast	7,649 (26.08%)	2.0	14,699	5,603	47,259,724
	Midwest	4,651 (15.86%)	2.0	14,710	5,777	30,156,862
	South	11,400 (38.87%)	2.0	13,644	5,160	65,048,583
	West	5,630 (19.20%)	2.0	20,988	6,173	38,048,277

* Denotes missing values

Submucous fibroid tumor follows the same patterns as other estrogen-induced conditions noted above. It is more prevalent in the South and the Northeast, the West, and the Midwest and manifests most in older women, ages 45–64, who made up 49.7% of the discharges in 2008. This may suggest that women do not lose their estrogen in their 50s and 60s. Therefore, beware of estrogen supplementation in older women. Even after TAH/BSO, these women may still be producing estrogen if they have intact adrenal glands, skin cells, and are obese.

TABLE 71

Outcomes by patient and hospital characteristics for ICD-9-CM principal diagnosis code 218.1 Intramural Leiomyoma

		Total number of discharges	LOS (length of stay), days (median)	Charges, $ (median)	Costs, $ (median)	Aggregate costs
All discharges		65,370 (100.00%)	2.0	15,133	5,492	399,431,992
Age group	18–44	31,979 (48.92%)	2.0	14,909	5,407	191,536,699
	45–64	32,424 (49.60%)	2.0	15,324	5,553	200,897,932
	65–84	890 (1.36%)	2.0	16,730	6,251	6,462,091
	85+	*	*	*	*	*
	Missing	*	2.0	20,643	5,424	315,535
Sex	Female	65,185 (99.72%)	2.0	15,120	5,492	398,296,802
	Missing	185 (0.28%)	2.0	22,483	5,424	1,135,190
Median income for zip code	Low	15,114 (23.12%)	2.0	14,965	5,469	94,156,667
	Not low	48,646 (74.42%)	2.0	15,241	5,488	294,174,855
	Missing	1,610 (2.46%)	2.0	12,672	5,814	11,100,470
Region	Northeast	13,973 (21.37%)	2.0	13,419	5,466	85,026,247
	Midwest	13,427 (20.54%)	2.0	14,943	5,692	84,170,322
	South	24,555 (37.56%)	2.0	13,938	5,115	140,312,562
	West	13,415 (20.52%)	2.0	20,617	6,016	89,922,861

* Denotes missing values

Intramural fibroid tumors follow the same patterns as other estrogen-induced conditions noted above. It is more prevalent in the South and the Northeast, the West, and the Midwest and manifests most in older women, ages 45–64, who made up 49.6% of the discharges in 2008. This again suggests that women do not lose their estrogen in their 50s and 60s. Therefore beware of estrogen supplementation in older women.

TABLE 72

Outcomes by patient and hospital characteristics for ICD-9-CM principal diagnosis code 218.2 Subserous Leiomyoma

		Total number of discharges	LOS (length of stay), days (median)	Charges, $ (median)	Costs, $ (median)	Aggregate costs
All discharges		21,209 (100.00%)	2.0	15,597	5,596	131,754,085
Age group	18–44	11,179 (52.71%)	2.0	15,445	5,506	68,476,149
	45–64	9,600 (45.26%)	2.0	15,624	5,647	60,092,017
	65–84	380 (1.79%)	2.0	17,929	6,086	2,626,132
	85+	*	*	*	*	*
	Missing	*	*	*	*	*
Sex	Female	21,035 (99.18%)	2.0	15,530	5,586	130,479,345
	Missing	175 (0.82%)	2.0	26,112	7,197	1,274,740
Median income for zip code	Low	4,701 (22.17%)	2.0	15,492	5,597	29,049,562
	Not low	16,103 (75.93%)	2.0	15,616	5,577	99,784,357
	Missing	404 (1.91%)	2.0	15,124	6,519	2,920,166
Region	Northeast	4,707 (22.19%)	2.0	14,813	5,656	30,208,760
	Midwest	3,924 (18.50%)	2.0	15,207	5,812	25,173,677
	South	7,572 (35.70%)	2.0	13,968	5,144	43,156,248
	West	5,007 (23.61%)	2.0	19,500	6,111	33,215,400

* Denotes missing values

Subserous fibroid tumor has the same pattern as others in regional prevalence and is seen more in prime-age females, ages 18–44, at 52.7% followed by older women with 45.3%.

TABLE 73

Outcomes by patient and hospital characteristics for
ICD-9-CM principal diagnosis code
218.9 Uterine Leiomyoma Nos

		Total number of discharges	LOS (length of stay), days (median)	Charges, $ (median)	Costs, $ (median)	Aggregate costs
All discharges		88,080 (100.00%)	2.0	15,651	5,547	550,778,268
Age group	1–17	*	*	*	*	*
	18–44	45,866 (52.07%)	2.0	15,374	5,422	279,288,396
	45–64	40,919 (46.46%)	2.0	15,892	5,665	261,039,229
	65–84	1,105 (1.26%)	3.0	17,244	6,204	9,083,044
	85+	*	*	*	*	*
	Missing	141 (0.16%)	2.0	24,613	6,831	951,332
Sex	Female	87,524 (99.37%)	2.0	15,620	5,546	547,356,531
	Missing	557 (0.63%)	2.0	21,187	6,261	3,421,737
Median income for zip code	Low	21,894 (24.86%)	2.0	15,244	5,432	135,664,401
	Not low	64,511 (73.24%)	2.0	15,812	5,574	403,395,476
	Missing	1,675 (1.90%)	2.0	14,153	5,878	11,718,390
Region	Northeast	14,420 (16.37%)	2.0	15,792	5,594	94,334,753
	Midwest	18,665 (21.19%)	2.0	14,319	5,779	116,929,171
	South	37,360 (42.42%)	2.0	15,045	5,246	221,617,010
	West	17,636 (20.02%)	2.0	18,934	6,043	117,897,333

* Denotes missing values

Uterine fibroid tumors nos follow the same patterns as other estrogen-induced conditions noted above. They were more prevalent in the South and Midwest followed by the West and the Northeast and manifest most in prime-age females, ages 18–44, making up 52.0% of the discharges in 2006; they comprise 46.5% of the discharges in older females, ages 45–64. The very old, 65–84, had 1.3% of the discharges.

TABLE 74

Outcomes by patient and hospital characteristics for ICD-9-CM principal diagnosis code 218.9 Uterine Leiomyoma Nos

		Total number of discharges	LOS (length of stay), days (median)	Charges, $ (median)	Costs, $ (median)	Aggregate costs
All discharges		100,390 (100.00%)	2.0	19,170	6,203	701,589,380
Age group	1–17	*	*	*	*	*
	18–44	49,362 (49.17%)	2.0	18,816	6,082	337,151,963
	45–64	49,023 (48.83%)	2.0	19,513	6,321	349,542,545
	65–84	1,585 (1.58%)	2.0	18,742	6,183	11,503,812
	85+	71 (0.07%)	4.0	35,745	8,850	941,992
	Missing	*	2.0	24,040	6,571	2,382,620
Sex	Female	99,569 (99.18%)	2.0	19,110	6,200	695,952,870
	Missing	820 (0.82%)	2.0	30,639	6,452	5,636,510
Median income for zip code	Low	24,137 (24.04%)	2.0	17,631	5,990	163,819,487
	Not low	74,208 (73.92%)	2.0	19,808	6,264	523,048,882
	Missing	2,044 (2.04%)	2.0	20,132	6,372	14,721,011
Region	Northeast	15,223 (15.16%)	2.0	17,046	5,568	95,132,791
	Midwest	20,527 (20.45%)	2.0	17,878	6,667	152,371,243
	South	41,134 (40.97%)	2.0	18,339	5,940	273,119,973
	West	23,506 (23.41%)	2.0	26,768	6,911	180,965,374

* Denotes missing values

The bulk of fibroid tumor discharges in 2008 occurred in the South, the West, the Midwest and the Northeast. Prime-age females ages 18–44 had the highest rate at 49.2%, followed by older adult females ages 45–64 with 48.8%. Even females ages 65–84 were diagnosed with some fibroid tumors, the rate standing at 1.58%. This indicates that menopause does not end estrogen dominance.

TABLE 75

2008 National statistics—principal diagnosis only

Outcomes by patient and hospital characteristics for
ICD-9-CM principal diagnosis code
174.9 Malign Neopl Breast Nos

		Total number of discharges	LOS (length of stay), days (median)	Charges, $ (median)	Costs, $ (median)	Aggregate costs
All discharges		32,563 (100.00%)	2.0	21,772	7,101	300,541,676
Age group	18–44	4,719 (14.49%)	2.0	27,929	9,503	53,087,118
	45–64	14,839 (45.57%)	2.0	24,409	8,038	150,392,502
	65–84	11,213 (34.43%)	2.0	18,218	6,060	85,131,132
	85+	1,708 (5.24%)	2.0	15,235	5,137	10,971,318
	Missing	*	2.0	31,746	9,126	959,606
Sex	Female	32,384 (99.45%)	2.0	21,740	7,105	299,199,225
	Missing	179 (0.55%)	1.0	27,428	5,771	1,342,451
Median income for zip code	Low	7,895 (24.24%)	2.0	18,365	6,315	64,400,942
	Not low	24,014 (73.75%)	2.0	22,914	7,452	229,670,976
	Missing	654 (2.01%)	2.0	21,859	7,347	6,469,759
Region	Northeast	4,149 (12.74%)	2.0	22,637	6,747	36,177,837
	Midwest	8,161 (25.06%)	2.0	20,169	7,611	79,603,243
	South	13,472 (41.37%)	2.0	20,469	6,673	119,913,401
	West	6,782 (20.83%)	2.0	27,077	7,601	64,847,195

* Denotes missing values

Breast cancer discharges in 2008, were more prevalent in the South, 41.4%, and the Midwest at 25.1%, followed by the West at 20.8% and the Northeast at 12.7%. These findings are in line with the high estrogen-producing chemicals used in farmlands in the South and the Midwest. There were 32,563 total discharges in 2008 that cost 300 million dollars in 2008.

TABLE 76

2006 National statistics—related diagnoses or procedures

Principal diagnosis = 174.9 Malign Neopl Breast Nos

ICD-9-CM secondary diagnosis code and name		Total number of discharges	Aggregate charges, $ (the "national bill")	Standard errors	
				Total number of discharges	Aggregate charges, $ (the "national bill")
Principal diagnosis = 174.9 Malign Neopl Breast Nos		23,788	524,253,104	1,142	30,382,359
401.9	Hypertension Nos	8,656	174,394,994	453	10,351,976
196.3	Mal Neo Lymph-Axilla/Arm	4,855	103,709,987	330	7,515,488
250.00	Dmii Wo Cmp Nt St Uncntr (after Oct 1, 1997)	2,894	57,361,552	185	4,262,404
530.81	Esophageal Reflux	2,153	45,968,136	158	3,758,561
198.5	Secondary Malig Neo Bone	2,109	58,143,553	146	5,606,795
244.9	Hypothyroidism Nos	1,957	41,963,889	143	3,353,272
305.1	Tobacco Use Disorder	1,682	35,130,885	131	3,263,269
272.4	Hyperlipidemia Nec/Nos	1,458	30,880,780	131	3,057,380
197.7	Second Malig Neo Liver	1,333	37,891,056	105	4,292,576
V15.82	History Of Tobacco Use	1,263	26,375,850	104	2,466,281
311	Depressive Disorder Nec	1,220	28,028,881	105	2,916,543
272.0	Pure Hypercholesterolemia	1,210	23,345,781	106	2,287,699
496	Chr Airway Obstruct Nec	1,123	22,903,482	87	2,158,205
197.0	Secondary Malig Neo Lung	1,095	35,563,773	95	4,897,391
493.90	Asth W/O Stat Asthm Nos (after Oct 1, 2001)	1,088	24,551,219	81	2,174,189
285.9	Anemia Nos	1,069	30,214,974	87	3,395,969
V16.3	Family Hx-Breast Malig	981	27,096,933	94	3,366,653
233.0	Ca In Situ Breast	934	21,855,052	117	3,096,630
715.90	Osteoarthros Nos-Unspec	926	16,820,595	87	1,854,814
428.0	Chf Nos (after Oct 1, 2002)	919	25,996,982	79	5,280,479

In this table, malignant neoplasm of breast Nos (not otherwise specified) ICD-9 code 174.9 is the primary diagnosis. The associated secondary diagnoses are reported by order of importance. This table gives you an idea of the group of diseases that go together.

TABLE 77

2006 National statistics—principal diagnosis only

Outcomes by patient and hospital characteristics for
ICD-9-CM principal diagnosis code
185 Malign Neopl Prostate

		Total number of discharges	LOS (length of stay), days (median)	Charges, $ (median)	Costs, $ (median)	Aggregate costs	Aggregate charges, $ (the "national bill")
All discharges		88,908 (100.00%)	2.0	22,342	7,959	790,861,938	2,290,596,019
Age group	<1	*	*	*	*	*	*
	1–17	*	*	*	*	*	*
	18–44	925 (1.04%)	2.0	23,843	8,084	7,778,131	21,906,547
	45–64	47,464 (53.39%)	2.0	23,055	8,206	428,202,772	1,237,799,316
	65–84	36,819 (41.41%)	2.0	21,609	7,681	325,141,122	943,136,338
	85+	3,549 (3.99%)	3.0	14,986	5,750	28,128,456	82,001,573
	Missing	*	2.0	30,950	8,487	1,106,675	4,048,579
Sex	Male	88,489 (99.53%)	2.0	22,302	7,963	787,403,141	2,278,016,039
	Missing	*	2.0	29,826	7,557	3,458,797	12,579,981
Median income for zip code	Low	17,460 (19.64%)	2.0	21,355	7,586	152,793,998	448,486,454
	Not low	69,135 (77.76%)	2.0	22,572	8,037	616,678,116	1,784,069,334
	Missing	2,313 (2.60%)	2.0	21,239	8,266	21,389,824	58,040,232
Region	Northeast	15,616 (17.56%)	2.0	21,351	7,512	144,310,648	416,260,350
	Midwest	20,088 (22.59%)	2.0	22,297	8,374	180,209,144	480,622,087
	South	33,246 (37.39%)	2.0	20,659	7,513	272,247,042	808,727,093
	West	19,958 (22.45%)	2.0	26,812	8,882	194,095,104	584,986,489

* Denotes missing values

TABLE 78

2008 National statistics—principal diagnosis only

Outcomes by patient and hospital characteristics for
ICD-9-CM principal diagnosis code
185 Malign Neopl Prostate

		Total number of discharges	LOS (length of stay), days (median)	Charges, $ (median)	Costs, $ (median)	Aggregate costs
All discharges		107,906 (100.00%)	2.0	28,337	9,393	1,119,047,290
Age group	1–17	*	*	*	*	*
	18–44	1,140 (1.06%)	2.0	29,690	9,705	11,955,112
	45–64	61,266 (56.78%)	2.0	29,058	9,620	643,966,925
	65–84	42,109 (39.02%)	2.0	27,559	9,180	434,528,160
	85+	3,107 (2.88%)	3.0	16,639	5,556	25,051,947
	Missing	268 (0.25%)	2.0	41,497	11,306	3,147,028
Sex	Male	107,100 (99.25%)	2.0	28,243	9,385	1,109,969,209
	Missing	806 (0.75%)	2.0	43,897	10,979	9,078,081
Median income for zip code	Low	20,496 (18.99%)	2.0	26,142	8,948	203,578,956
	Not low	84,620 (78.42%)	2.0	28,758	9,494	884,800,615
	Missing	2,789 (2.59%)	2.0	29,992	9,524	30,667,720
Region	Northeast	19,209 (17.80%)	2.0	27,385	7,802	183,103,515
	Midwest	26,651 (24.70%)	2.0	26,679	10,451	296,871,211
	South	38,806 (35.96%)	2.0	27,312	8,956	376,891,047
	West	23,241 (21.54%)	2.0	34,084	10,488	262,181,518

* Denotes missing values

Prostate cancer was prevalent in the South and Midwest at rates comparable to those of breast cancer in 2006 and 2008. In the case of prostate cancer, it is the older adults, ages 45–64, who had the highest rate in 2006 and 2008 at 53.4% and 56.8%, followed by the 65–84 age group, at 41.4% and 39.0%, and those over 85 at 4% and 2.9%. The testosterone loss and estrogen dominance in men is highest among older adults ages 45+. Note that there were 107,906 total discharges that cost 1.1 billion dollars in 2008.

TABLE 79

2008 National statistics—related diagnoses or procedures

Principal diagnosis = 185 Malign Neopl Prostate

CCS secondary diagnosis category and name		Total number of discharges	LOS (length of stay), days (median)	Charges, $ (median)	Aggregate charges, $ (the "national bill")
Principal diagnosis = 185 Malign Neopl Prostate		107,906	2.0	28,337	3,514,086,954
98	Essential hypertension	49,352	2.0	28,119	1,607,289,466
53	Hyperlipidemia	30,724	2.0	27,880	993,666,848
663	Screening and history of mental health and substance abuse codes	22,184	2.0	28,617	723,901,206
259	Residual codes, unclassified	16,302	2.0	29,240	554,194,554
138	Esophageal disorders	15,329	2.0	28,090	498,188,000
49	Diabetes mellitus without complication	13,796	2.0	28,187	458,337,491
101	Coronary atherosclerosis	12,087	2.0	27,273	388,804,835
163	Genitourinary symptoms and ill-defined conditions	10,359	2.0	21,951	312,798,568
257	Other aftercare	9,003	2.0	24,757	260,507,138
58	Other nutritional, endocrine, and metabolic disorders	8,677	2.0	28,802	308,867,997
42	Secondary malignancies	7,217	4.0	23,898	237,658,699
155	Other gastrointestinal disorders	7,028	2.0	30,329	265,261,815
59	Anemia	6,884	4.0	29,666	263,062,491
106	Cardiac dysrhythmias	6,478	2.0	29,044	234,349,778
238	Complications of surgical procedures or medical care	6,434	4.0	39,582	316,657,273
164	Hyperplasia of prostate	6,195	2.0	24,184	179,508,600
162	Other disease of bladder and urethra	5,285	2.0	22,982	152,956,830
143	Abdominal hernia	5,201	2.0	31,065	188,584,030
55	Fluid and electrolyte disorders	5,018	4.0	32,515	220,251,343
203	Osteoarthritis	4,975	2.0	27,465	160,229,268

TABLE 80

2006 National statistics—related diagnoses or procedures

Principal diagnosis = 185 Malign Neopl Prostate

ICD-9-CM secondary diagnosis code and name		Total number of discharges	Aggregate charges, $ (the "national bill")	Standard errors	
				Total number of discharges	Aggregate charges, $ (the "national bill")
Principal diagnosis = 185 Malign Neopl Prostate		88,908	2,290,596,019	4,926	146,641,425
401.9	Hypertension Nos	39,690	1,010,464,627	2,186	64,083,725
272.4	Hyperlipidemia Nec/Nos	10,924	279,594,745	978	26,941,834
530.81	Esophageal Reflux	10,698	257,892,922	785	21,160,573
250.00	Dmii Wo Cmp Nt St Uncntr (after Oct 1, 1997)	10,125	256,970,074	549	15,861,025
272.0	Pure Hypercholesterolemia	9,626	244,419,317	700	20,671,423
V15.82	History Of Tobacco Use	9,466	241,880,399	824	25,244,824
305.1	Tobacco Use Disorder	7,751	199,466,501	497	14,504,377
414.01	Crnry Athrscl Native Vessel	6,206	167,156,561	371	12,114,879
198.5	Secondary Malig Neo Bone	4,059	127,721,985	202	11,181,423
599.7	Hematuria	3,974	109,640,623	197	7,337,208
285.1	Ac Posthemorrhag Anemia	3,881	118,488,266	309	9,165,495
496	Chr Airway Obstruct Nec	3,766	103,252,499	215	7,319,936
285.9	Anemia Nos	3,740	116,833,265	221	8,108,917
788.20	Retention Urine Nos	3,576	77,984,942	189	5,406,558
414.00	Cor Ath Unsp Vsl Ntv/Gft	3,470	82,399,772	233	6,160,217
V45.81	Aortocoronary Bypass	3,460	85,450,095	244	7,126,408
427.31	Atrial Fibrillation	3,385	105,663,070	198	8,611,586
412	Old Myocardial Infarct	3,062	76,774,299	214	6,399,115
560.1	Paralytic Ileus	2,954	109,915,199	247	10,053,569
278.00	Obesity Nos	2,928	74,797,061	342	8,203,963

Tables 79 and 80 show some of the comorbidities associated with prostate cancer in 2006 and 2008. Most of these comorbidities are also associated with breast cancer and obesity. Hence prostate cancer and breast cancer are highly associated with obesity, which in turn is associated with hormone disruption.

TABLE 81

2006 National statistics—related diagnoses or procedures

Principal diagnosis = 179 Malig Neopl Uterus Nos

ICD-9-CM secondary diagnosis code and name	Total number of discharges	Aggregate charges, $ (the "national bill")	Standard errors	
			Total number of discharges	Aggregate charges, $ (the "national bill")
Principal diagnosis = 179 Malig Neopl Uterus Nos	**1,816**	**52,017,959**	**138**	**7,669,658**
401.9 Hypertension Nos	650	17,158,087	73	2,357,182
250.00 Dmii Wo Cmp Nt St Uncntr (after Oct 1, 1997)	317	8,633,414	49	1,690,180
285.9 Anemia Nos	188	5,252,686	32	1,093,300
276.51 Dehydration	187	6,114,365	32	1,544,211
599.0 Urin Tract Infection Nos	176	8,345,565	31	1,766,731
244.9 Hypothyroidism Nos	162	4,558,929	28	1,140,490
197.6 Sec Mal Neo Peritoneum	149	*	28	*
530.81 Esophageal Reflux	148	4,706,386	28	1,190,794
197.0 Secondary Malig Neo Lung	130	3,325,829	25	973,871
272.4 Hyperlipidemia Nec/Nos	120	2,723,663	24	642,365
278.00 Obesity Nos	111	2,679,974	26	774,811
272.0 Pure Hypercholesterolemia	108	2,217,390	22	531,760
560.1 Paralytic Ileus	107	5,156,147	22	1,273,929
285.1 Ac Posthemorrhag Anemia	97	*	21	*
591 Hydronephrosis	96	3,458,037	21	994,154
218.9 Uterine Leiomyoma Nos	95	2,437,257	22	662,958
627.1 Postmenopausal Bleeding (after Oct 1, 2000)	94	2,020,910	21	527,599
V66.7 Encountr Palliative Care	93	*	22	*
V10.3 Hx Of Breast Malignancy	88	2,224,411	25	709,041

* Denotes missing values

The uterine cancer comorbidities are highly correlated with obesity comorbidities.

TABLE 82

2006 National statistics—principal diagnosis only

Outcomes by patient and hospital characteristics for
ICD-9-CM principal diagnosis code
179 Malig Neopl Uterus Nos

		Total number of discharges	LOS (length of stay), days (median)	Charges, $ (median)	Costs, $ (median)	Aggregate costs	Aggregate charges, $ (the "national bill")
All discharges		1,816 (100.00%)	3.0	19,627	6,738	17,215,181	52,017,959
Age group	18–44	172 (9.46%)	3.0	22,232	6,496	1,554,270	4,367,896
	45–64	689 (37.95%)	3.0	21,116	6,862	6,271,612	17,920,799
	65–84	745 (41.03%)	4.0	19,627	6,768	7,214,304	22,781,955
	85+	210 (11.56%)	4.0	*	*	*	*
Sex	Female	1,816 (100.00%)	3.0	19,627	6,738	17,215,181	52,017,959
Median income for zip code	Low	546 (30.05%)	4.0	19,229	6,517	5,521,225	17,578,450
	Not low	1,222 (67.26%)	3.0	20,525	6,853	11,138,840	33,338,913
	Missing	*	*	*	*	*	*
Region	Northeast	279 (15.34%)	4.0	*	7,976	4,284,633	*
	Midwest	447 (24.62%)	3.0	15,794	6,585	3,308,415	8,397,530
	South	831 (45.77%)	4.0	19,219	6,513	6,996,848	21,233,076
	West	259 (14.27%)	3.0	22,763	7,208	2,625,285	8,163,373

* Denotes missing values

Uterine cancer has patterns similar to prostate cancer and is more prevalent in the South and the Midwest. This cancer is also more prevalent in women 45+.

TABLE 83

2006 National statistics—principal diagnosis only

Outcomes by patient and hospital characteristics for
ICD-9-CM principal diagnosis code
600.01 Bph W Urinary Obstructn

		Total number of discharges	LOS (length of stay), days (median)	Charges, $ (median)	Costs, $ (median)	Aggregate costs	Aggregate charges, $ (the "national bill")
All discharges		40,093 (100.00%)	2.0	11,600	4,345	219,090,669	625,529,168
Age group	18–44	124 (0.31%)	2.0	10,256	3,690	562,666	1,747,327
	45–64	7,965 (19.87%)	2.0	11,001	4,137	39,210,362	111,638,218
	65–84	27,765 (69.25%)	2.0	11,711	4,367	153,552,856	442,146,220
	85+	4,197 (10.47%)	2.0	12,012	4,759	25,526,095	69,157,245
	Missing	*	*	*	*	*	*
Sex	Male	39,944 (99.63%)	2.0	11,579	4,341	218,253,568	622,306,712
	Missing	148 (0.37%)	*	21,162	5,624	837,101	3,222,456
Median income for zip code	Low	9,059 (22.60%)	2.0	11,750	4,287	49,530,133	143,831,161
	Not low	29,996 (74.82%)	2.0	11,572	4,348	162,177,937	463,570,830
	Missing	1,038 (2.59%)	2.0	11,294	4,559	7,382,599	18,127,177
Region	Northeast	8,066 (20.12%)	2.0	11,056	4,596	52,251,554	140,718,783
	Midwest	9,858 (24.59%)	2.0	10,371	4,339	51,766,054	124,731,945
	South	13,809 (34.44%)	2.0	11,878	4,108	69,688,148	211,343,888
	West	8,359 (20.85%)	2.0	14,092	4,489	45,384,913	148,734,552

* Denotes missing values

Benign prostatic hypertrophy (BPH) has patterns similar to prostate cancer and is more prevalent in the South and the Midwest. BPH is also more prevalent in men aged 45 and over and the highest rate is found in the 65–84 age group.

TABLE 84

2006 National statistics—related diagnoses or procedures

Principal diagnosis = 600.01 Bph W Urinary Obstructn

ICD-9-CM secondary diagnosis code and name		Total number of discharges	Aggregate charges, $ (the "national bill")	Standard errors	
				Total number of discharges	Aggregate charges, $ (the "national bill")
Principal diagnosis = 600.01 Bph W Urinary Obstructn		40,093	625,529,168	1,656	28,206,543
401.9	Hypertension Nos	19,290	293,042,152	870	14,956,280
250.00	Dmii Wo Cmp Nt St Uncntr (after Oct 1, 1997)	7,027	111,634,949	337	5,916,580
414.01	Crnry Athrscl Native Vssl	5,067	83,198,581	277	5,443,099
599.7	Hematuria	5,039	104,590,019	248	6,352,671
272.4	Hyperlipidemia Nec/Nos	4,563	70,965,835	308	5,273,978
530.81	Esophageal Reflux	4,405	59,426,035	276	4,234,458
496	Chr Airway Obstruct Nec	3,676	59,420,291	195	3,536,205
427.31	Atrial Fibrillation	3,591	69,541,427	212	5,423,942
272.0	Pure Hypercholesterolemia	3,533	53,019,529	222	3,825,626
V15.82	History Of Tobacco Use	3,436	50,966,912	242	4,008,208
414.00	Cor Ath Unsp Vsl Ntv/Gft	3,191	51,807,226	205	3,808,927
V45.81	Aortocoronary Bypass	3,142	48,314,839	206	3,360,273
599.0	Urin Tract Infection Nos	3,008	73,117,167	160	5,296,281
601.1	Chronic Prostatitis	2,480	38,984,188	199	3,994,361
305.1	Tobacco Use Disorder	2,412	33,977,139	156	2,449,120
428.0	Chf Nos (after Oct 1, 2002)	2,404	48,706,631	143	3,524,926
412	Old Myocardial Infarct	2,301	32,935,841	173	2,551,216
596.8	Bladder Disorder Nec	2,153	32,074,547	211	3,072,331
285.9	Anemia Nos	1,989	43,017,364	129	3,671,294
594.1	Bladder Calculus Nec	1,898	34,575,936	120	2,900,080

The BPH comorbidities tightly correlate with obesity comorbidities.

TABLE 85

2006 National statistics—related diagnoses or procedures

Principal diagnosis = 278.01 Morbid Obesity

ICD-9-CM secondary diagnosis code and name		Total number of discharges	Aggregate charges, $ (the "national bill")	Standard errors	
				Total number of discharges	Aggregate charges, $ (the "national bill")
Principal diagnosis = 278.01 Morbid Obesity		96,371	3,520,016,040	7,811	307,693,342
V85.4	Bmi 40 And Over, adult	48,669	1,689,064,505	5,031	178,458,143
401.9	Hypertension Nos	48,465	1,750,750,672	4,016	159,505,577
530.81	Esophageal Reflux	33,247	1,160,643,983	2,995	110,920,479
250.00	Dmii Wo Cmp Nt St Uncntr (after Oct 1, 1997)	26,354	972,219,156	2,237	90,083,078
780.57	Oth Unspcf Sleep Apnea	18,828	668,125,208	1,843	69,534,105
327.23	Obstructive Sleep Apnea	17,136	643,271,473	1,927	73,577,311
311	Depressive Disorder Nec	16,603	557,141,160	1,563	52,861,082
493.90	Asth W/O Stat Asthm Nos (after Oct 1, 2001)	15,231	531,733,326	1,364	51,518,804
272.0	Pure Hypercholesterolemia	15,175	545,980,325	1,714	64,772,531
272.4	Hyperlipidemia Nec/Nos	13,522	457,744,495	1,409	48,589,442
715.90	Osteoarthros Nos-Unspec	11,902	407,362,437	1,697	51,788,563
244.9	Hypothyroidism Nos	9,148	326,374,614	847	33,270,629
625.6	Fem Stress Incontinence	9,110	306,929,922	1,292	42,351,026
571.8	Chronic Liver Dis Nec	8,404	258,973,892	1,908	55,533,039
V15.82	History Of Tobacco Use	7,908	264,499,810	987	31,604,376
568.0	Peritoneal Adhesions	7,422	314,944,619	891	39,650,817
553.3	Diaphragmatic Hernia	4,703	171,204,380	546	22,939,407
716.90	Arthropathy Nos-Unspec	4,323	154,353,965	676	27,508,341
724.2	Lumbago	4,238	152,047,145	701	26,592,247
724.5	Backache Nos	3,990	126,545,818	673	20,014,185

The 2006 morbid obesity comorbidities.

TABLE 86

2006 National statistics—related diagnoses or procedures

Principal diagnosis = 493.90 Asth W/O Stat Asthm Nos
(after Oct 1, 2001)

ICD-9-CM secondary diagnosis code and name		Total number of discharges	Aggregate charges, $ (the "national bill")	Standard errors	
				Total number of discharges	Aggregate charges, $ (the "national bill")
Principal diagnosis = 493.90 Asth W/O Stat Asthm Nos (after Oct 1, 2001)		28,302	289,139,919	1,177	15,253,077
401.9	Hypertension Nos	6,612	90,774,605	324	5,814,266
530.81	Esophageal Reflux	2,820	35,313,136	170	2,774,643
250.00	Dmii Wo Cmp Nt St Uncntr (after Oct 1, 1997)	2,633	34,597,558	150	2,528,448
272.4	Hyperlipidemia Nec/Nos	2,227	32,553,772	148	2,786,346
799.02	Hypoxemia	2,071	18,274,644	180	1,658,716
486	Pneumonia, Organism Nos	1,823	18,856,291	144	2,138,284
305.1	Tobacco Use Disorder	1,767	18,941,594	129	1,619,386
382.9	Otitis Media Nos	1,760	12,427,310	263	2,484,348
465.9	Acute Uri Nos	1,703	12,618,504	126	1,124,795
276.51	Dehydration	1,598	15,683,545	123	1,505,422
428.0	Chf Nos (after Oct 1, 2002)	1,569	24,724,654	109	2,780,807
244.9	Hypothyroidism Nos	1,491	21,572,713	111	2,091,574
278.00	Obesity Nos	1,377	19,633,029	104	1,827,458
414.01	Crnry Athrscl Native Vssl	1,238	18,059,465	97	1,752,499
311	Depressive Disorder Nec	1,162	15,393,059	87	1,520,321
427.31	Atrial Fibrillation	1,127	17,533,934	98	1,955,271
276.8	Hypopotassemia	1,054	15,943,615	87	1,984,559
300.00	Anxiety State Nos	1,047	13,414,807	90	1,404,255
272.0	Pure Hypercholesterolemia	927	12,435,941	86	1,393,170
079.99	Viral Infection Nos	923	7,198,409	138	1,233,067

Comorbidities of asthma diagnosis (493.90) correlate with obesity comorbidities and are therefore closely associated with obesity induced asthma through adipocyte production of TNF-α and IL-6.

TABLE 87

2006 National statistics—related diagnoses or procedures

Principal diagnosis = 276.8 Hypopotassemia

ICD-9-CM secondary diagnosis code and name		Total number of discharges	Aggregate charges, $ (the "national bill")	Standard errors	
				Total number of discharges	Aggregate charges, $ (the "national bill")
Principal diagnosis = 276.8 Hypopotassemia		29,290	423,836,126	866	17,601,671
401.9	Hypertension Nos	12,284	167,226,503	454	8,275,726
276.51	Dehydration	4,981	73,353,975	201	4,536,591
250.00	Dmii Wo Cmp Nt St Uncntr (after Oct 1, 1997)	4,626	66,589,349	211	3,919,102
428.0	Chf Nos (after Oct 1, 2002)	4,528	76,015,234	203	4,786,163
305.1	Tobacco Use Disorder	3,500	44,326,286	188	3,128,895
275.2	Dis Magnesium Metabolism	3,440	55,753,596	206	4,507,689
530.81	Esophageal Reflux	3,404	44,025,221	177	3,097,671
496	Chr Airway Obstruct Nec	3,280	53,542,830	161	3,976,770
272.4	Hyperlipidemia Nec/Nos	3,134	44,168,502	186	3,395,741
599.0	Urin Tract Infection Nos	3,116	60,511,764	153	4,562,984
244.9	Hypothyroidism Nos	3,031	43,290,234	150	2,944,453
276.1	Hyposmolality	2,987	47,613,092	147	3,523,730
427.31	Atrial Fibrillation	2,912	50,578,453	153	3,877,476
285.9	Anemia Nos	2,760	48,419,088	142	3,901,027
311	Depressive Disorder Nec	2,756	35,958,309	144	2,629,785
414.01	Crnry Athrscl Natve Vssl	2,681	40,561,853	162	3,416,859
787.91	Diarrhea	2,270	37,101,997	126	2,957,394
780.79	Malaise And Fatigue Nec	1,702	20,868,669	107	1,987,066
780.39	Convulsions Nec	1,526	28,916,693	108	3,059,848
414.00	Cor Ath Unsp Vsl Ntv/Gft	1,423	19,821,559	97	1,880,480

Low potassium comorbidities also correlate well with obesity comorbidities. Note that hypothyroidism, hypertension, type 2 diabetes, hyperlipidemia, GERD, and depressive disorders are related to low potassium and obesity.

TABLE 88

2006 National statistics—principal diagnosis only

Outcomes by patient and hospital characteristics for
ICD-9-CM principal diagnosis code
276.8 Hypopotassemia

		Total number of discharges	LOS (length of stay), days (median)	Charges, $ (median)	Costs, $ (median)	Aggregate costs	Aggregate charges, $ (the "national bill")
All discharges		29,290 (100.00%)	3.0	9,247	3,685	152,684,436	423,836,126
Age group	<1	*	*	*	*	*	*
	1–17	494 (1.69%)	2.0	7,683	3,380	3,173,865	8,040,172
	18–44	5,659 (19.32%)	2.0	7,919	3,054	24,318,017	66,729,696
	45–64	10,049 (34.31%)	3.0	9,571	3,815	55,194,780	152,543,533
	65–84	10,062 (34.35%)	3.0	9,958	3,932	54,123,438	152,287,106
	85+	2,976 (10.16%)	3.0	9,483	3,929	15,567,236	43,516,437
	Missing	*	*	*	*	*	*
Sex	Male	8,699 (29.70%)	3.0	9,760	3,842	48,126,722	134,791,859
	Female	20,574 (70.24%)	3.0	9,079	3,594	104,509,170	288,890,493
	Missing	*	*	*	*	*	*
Median income for zip code	Low	9,813 (33.50%)	3.0	8,235	3,320	45,318,079	123,283,685
	Not low	18,755 (64.03%)	3.0	9,890	3,840	103,001,286	291,172,476
	Missing	722 (2.46%)	3.0	8,661	3,928	4,365,071	9,379,965
Region	Northeast	5,297 (18.08%)	3.0	11,370	4,525	36,632,471	103,957,007
	Midwest	7,071 (24.14%)	3.0	8,004	3,625	33,536,041	77,806,831
	South	12,025 (41.06%)	3.0	8,677	3,200	53,790,626	151,397,500
	West	4,898 (16.72%)	2.0	12,633	4,158	28,725,298	90,674,788

* Denotes missing values

Low potassium was more prevalent in females, 70.2%, and seem to increase with age starting at 19.3% in the 18–44 age group followed by 34.3% in the 45–64 age group and 34.4% in the 65–84 age group. Low potassium was also more prevalent in the South and the Midwest followed by the Northeast and the West. Potassium is important in the conversion of T4 to T3 and its lack will therefore lead to hypothyroidism and obesity.

TABLE 89

Outcomes by patient and hospital characteristics for ICD-9-CM principal diagnosis code 251.2 Hypoglycemia Nos

		Total number of discharges	LOS (length of stay), days (median)	Charges, $ (median)	Costs, $ (median)	Aggregate costs	Aggregate charges, $ (the "national bill")
All discharges		5,984 (100.00%)	2.0	8,844	3,395	30,651,515	86,585,012
Age group	<1	118 (1.97%)	3.0	*	*	*	*
	1–17	766 (12.79%)	2.0	5,855	2,348	2,540,742	6,406,958
	18–44	1,063 (17.77%)	2.0	8,332	3,150	4,808,410	14,172,288
	45–64	1,405 (23.48%)	2.0	10,580	3,825	7,610,950	21,338,944
	65–84	1,865 (31.17%)	2.0	9,381	3,679	10,634,884	29,299,951
	85+	763 (12.74%)	3.0	11,218	4,127	4,075,685	11,485,796
	Missing	*	*	*	*	*	*
Sex	Male	2,377 (39.72%)	2.0	8,405	3,356	11,518,090	32,028,107
	Female	3,584 (59.90%)	2.0	9,166	3,401	19,049,577	54,233,119
	Missing	*	*	*	*	*	*
Median income for zip code	Low	1,995 (33.35%)	3.0	8,752	3,458	10,083,133	29,446,590
	Not low	3,846 (64.28%)	2.0	8,959	3,371	19,845,925	55,776,946
	Missing	142 (2.37%)	2.0	7,550	3,440	722,457	1,361,477
Region	Northeast	1,271 (21.23%)	2.0	10,587	3,867	8,840,418	26,499,391
	Midwest	1,478 (24.71%)	2.0	7,322	3,260	6,335,438	15,473,712
	South	2,340 (39.11%)	2.0	8,272	3,127	10,848,582	29,989,997
	West	895 (14.95%)	2.0	12,185	3,749	4,627,077	14,621,912

* Denotes missing values

TABLE 90

2006 National statistics—related diagnoses or procedures

Principal diagnosis = 251.2 Hypoglycemia Nos

ICD-9-CM secondary diagnosis code and name	Total number of discharges	LOS (length of stay), days (median)	Charges, $ (median)	Aggregate charges, $ (the "national bill")
Principal diagnosis = 251.2 Hypoglycemia Nos	5,984	2.0	8,844	86,585,012
401.9 Hypertension Nos	1,757	3.0	10,001	23,237,646
276.51 Dehydration	665	3.0	9,042	11,223,447
244.9 Hypothyroidism Nos	616	3.0	12,961	9,919,415
428.0 Chf Nos (after Oct 1, 2002)	609	3.0	13,394	12,899,700
780.39 Convulsions Nec	591	2.0	10,366	9,599,073
530.81 Esophageal Reflux	574	3.0	10,485	9,135,049
780.2 Syncope And Collapse	541	2.0	9,812	7,224,084
599.0 Urin Tract Infection Nos	520	3.0	10,799	8,614,242
496 Chr Airway Obstruct Nec	519	3.0	10,874	9,883,056
272.4 Hyperlipidemia Nec/Nos	513	2.0	10,515	7,090,878
427.31 Atrial Fibrillation	471	3.0	14,344	9,885,085
305.1 Tobacco Use Disorder	458	2.0	8,405	5,566,115
414.01 Crnry Athrscl Natve Vssl	457	3.0	13,282	7,532,463
276.8 Hypopotassemia	436	2.0	10,299	8,887,663
311 Depressive Disorder Nec	421	2.0	10,181	5,941,262
285.9 Anemia Nos	400	3.0	13,745	7,033,249
403.91 Hyp Renal Nos W Ren Fail (after Oct 1, 2005)	364	3.0	13,779	8,828,233
294.8 Organic Brain Synd Nec (after Oct 1, 2004)	354	3.0	9,887	4,442,892
493.90 Asth W/O Stat Asthm Nos (after Oct 1, 2001)	332	2.0	6,813	4,106,280
414.00 Cor Ath Unsp Vsl Ntv/Gft	327	2.0	8,634	3,538,633

Hypoglycemia and comorbidities.

TABLE 91

Outcomes by patient and hospital characteristics for ICD-9-CM principal diagnosis code 250.02 Dmii Wo Cmp Uncntrld (after Oct 1, 1997)

		Total number of discharges	LOS (length of stay), days (median)	Charges, $ (median)	Costs, $ (median)	Aggregate costs	Aggregate charges, $ (the "national bill")
All discharges		45,493 (100.00%)	3.0	8,699	3,329	210,320,767	590,883,626
Age group	1–17	442 (0.97%)	2.0	6,275	2,290	1,365,478	3,608,815
	18–44	10,554 (23.20%)	2.0	7,305	2,749	40,627,984	116,050,707
	45–64	19,755 (43.42%)	3.0	8,960	3,364	90,613,050	253,222,325
	65–84	12,610 (27.72%)	3.0	9,589	3,778	65,393,286	182,898,909
	85+	2,124 (4.67%)	4.0	9,517	3,965	12,298,929	35,025,639
	Missing	*	*	*	*	*	*
Sex	Male	22,319 (49.06%)	3.0	8,362	3,181	100,224,237	278,004,951
	Female	23,132 (50.85%)	3.0	9,015	3,462	109,990,638	312,525,474
	Missing	*	*	*	*	*	*
Median income for zip code	Low	19,643 (43.18%)	3.0	8,355	3,180	86,511,174	244,149,890
	Not low	23,946 (52.64%)	3.0	9,062	3,384	110,832,972	324,481,632
	Missing	1,904 (4.19%)	3.0	8,189	4,408	12,976,621	22,252,103
Region	Northeast	11,977 (26.33%)	3.0	11,133	4,577	76,128,865	206,859,644
	Midwest	9,147 (20.11%)	3.0	7,065	3,106	35,614,631	85,183,706
	South	19,346 (42.52%)	3.0	7,816	2,863	71,550,556	208,253,088
	West	5,023 (11.04%)	2.0	11,718	3,682	27,026,715	90,587,187

* Denotes missing values

Hormone Imbalance Syndrome

TABLE 92

Outcomes by patient and hospital characteristics for
ICD-9-CM principal diagnosis code
250.11 Dmi Keto Nt St Uncntrld

		Total number of discharges	LOS (length of stay), days (median)	Charges, $ (median)	Costs, $ (median)	Aggregate costs	Aggregate charges, $ (the "national bill")
All discharges		47,598 (100.00%)	2.0	10,265	3,972	251,165,745	691,647,916
Age group	<1	*	3.0	16,915	6,442	567,222	1,522,835
	1–17	12,258 (25.75%)	2.0	8,192	3,263	49,644,417	129,018,706
	18–44	27,650 (58.09%)	2.0	10,381	4,012	141,705,056	390,536,696
	45–64	6,573 (13.81%)	3.0	13,207	5,135	50,747,247	146,398,232
	65–84	903 (1.90%)	4.0	14,900	6,136	7,537,746	21,335,604
	85+	69 (0.15%)	4.0	17,609	7,811	615,347	1,738,646
	Missing	68 (0.14%)	2.0	11,037	4,812	348,710	1,097,198
Sex	Male	23,230 (48.80%)	2.0	9,927	3,830	117,925,397	320,792,290
	Female	24,134 (50.70%)	2.0	10,667	4,122	131,868,561	366,282,551
	Missing	235 (0.49%)	2.0	17,735	5,075	1,371,787	4,573,075
Median income for zip code	Low	15,361 (32.27%)	2.0	10,222	3,832	76,292,501	214,413,671
	Not low	31,079 (65.29%)	2.0	10,278	4,041	168,378,298	460,423,439
	Missing	1,158 (2.43%)	2.0	10,543	4,294	6,494,946	16,810,806
Region	Northeast	8,370 (17.58%)	2.0	10,624	4,223	50,028,847	140,183,937
	Midwest	11,262 (23.66%)	2.0	9,608	3,892	56,315,499	138,992,581
	South	19,265 (40.47%)	2.0	9,566	3,648	90,225,919	245,309,050
	West	8,701 (18.28%)	2.0	13,519	4,718	54,595,480	167,162,348

TABLE 93

Outcomes by patient and hospital characteristics for ICD-9-CM principal diagnosis code 250.13 Dmi Ketoacd Uncontrold

		Total number of discharges	LOS (length of stay), days (median)	Charges, $ (median)	Costs, $ (median)	Aggregate costs	Aggregate charges, $ (the "national bill")
All discharges		44,211 (100.00%)	3.0	11,205	4,242	267,316,676	762,942,609
Age group	<1	*	*	*	*	*	*
	1–17	7,095 (16.05%)	2.0	8,717	3,325	30,797,541	80,858,455
	18–44	28,346 (64.11%)	2.0	11,057	4,134	159,936,301	458,416,676
	45–64	7,414 (16.77%)	3.0	14,864	5,548	63,494,712	185,942,542
	65–84	1,164 (2.63%)	4.0	17,296	6,943	11,334,455	32,116,702
	85+	113 (0.26%)	5.0	*	*	*	*
	Missing	*	2.0	11,309	5,037	280,625	805,338
Sex	Male	21,437 (48.49%)	2.0	10,521	3,997	122,331,297	341,952,572
	Female	22,630 (51.19%)	3.0	11,911	4,472	144,168,041	418,631,149
	Missing	144 (0.33%)	2.0	17,002	5,870	817,338	2,358,889
Median income for zip code	Low	15,686 (35.48%)	3.0	11,062	4,147	88,471,668	257,253,036
	Not low	27,363 (61.89%)	3.0	11,291	4,272	169,855,722	487,130,364
	Missing	1,163 (2.63%)	3.0	10,481	4,958	8,989,286	18,559,209
Region	Northeast	7,209 (16.30%)	3.0	13,368	5,021	59,142,252	167,779,833
	Midwest	9,612 (21.74%)	2.0	9,435	3,974	51,201,098	125,528,502
	South	19,593 (44.32%)	3.0	10,446	3,916	103,267,883	292,037,064
	West	7,798 (17.64%)	2.0	15,674	5,096	53,705,444	177,597,209

* Denotes missing values

TABLE 94

Outcomes by patient and hospital characteristics for
ICD-9-CM principal diagnosis code
250.60 Dmii Neuro Nt St Uncntrl (after Oct 1, 1997)

		Total number of discharges	LOS (length of stay), days (median)	Charges, $ (median)	Costs, $ (median)	Aggregate costs	Aggregate charges, $ (the "national bill")
All discharges		38,546 (100.00%)	4.0	15,370	5,571	315,952,530	912,188,875
Age group	18–44	6,694 (17.37%)	3.0	12,763	4,695	43,508,431	127,001,775
	45–64	18,443 (47.85%)	4.0	15,746	5,744	157,317,773	450,471,656
	65–84	12,056 (31.28%)	4.0	16,462	5,952	104,029,316	302,766,870
	85+	1,354 (3.51%)	5.0	14,544	5,419	11,097,009	31,948,574
Sex	Male	17,497 (45.39%)	4.0	15,614	5,665	149,182,505	426,193,723
	Female	21,040 (54.58%)	4.0	15,257	5,505	166,698,845	485,734,625
	Missing	*	*	*	*	*	*
Median income for zip code	Low	12,265 (31.82%)	4.0	14,392	5,181	95,617,863	282,425,185
	Not low	25,309 (65.66%)	4.0	15,897	5,764	212,220,745	610,289,507
	Missing	972 (2.52%)	4.0	13,618	5,604	8,113,921	19,474,182
Region	Northeast	7,569 (19.64%)	4.0	17,380	6,574	74,054,804	206,762,406
	Midwest	8,175 (21.21%)	4.0	13,907	5,458	62,160,343	166,872,138
	South	16,323 (42.35%)	4.0	14,095	5,121	122,713,414	352,691,941
	West	6,479 (16.81%)	4.0	19,088	6,049	57,023,969	185,862,389

* Denotes missing values

TABLE 95

2006 National statistics—principal diagnosis only

Outcomes by patient and hospital characteristics for ICD-9-CM principal diagnosis code 401.0 Malignant Hypertension

		Total number of discharges	LOS (length of stay), days (median)	Charges, $ (median)	Costs, $ (median)	Aggregate costs	Aggregate charges, $ (the "national bill")
All discharges		25,450 (100.00%)	2.0	10,937	4,057	138,040,640	402,750,445
Age group	<1	*	*	*	*	*	*
	1–17	105 (0.41%)	4.0	*	*	*	*
	18–44	4,643 (18.25%)	2.0	10,647	3,807	23,648,886	68,972,311
	45–64	10,280 (40.39%)	2.0	11,415	4,220	55,808,983	164,650,517
	65–84	8,302 (32.62%)	2.0	10,790	4,029	46,317,610	134,180,375
	85+	2,104 (8.27%)	3.0	9,747	3,871	10,633,325	30,078,540
	Missing	*	*	*	*	*	*
Sex	Male	9,244 (36.32%)	2.0	11,049	4,022	50,619,822	145,469,442
	Female	16,189 (63.61%)	2.0	10,907	4,066	87,366,055	257,056,026
	Missing	*	*	*	*	*	*
Median income for zip code	Low	9,381 (36.86%)	2.0	9,988	3,718	44,434,179	130,303,874
	Not low	15,374 (60.41%)	2.0	11,778	4,296	89,171,209	262,567,442
	Missing	695 (2.73%)	3.0	10,649	4,273	4,435,252	9,879,129
Region	Northeast	4,864 (19.11%)	2.0	13,875	5,174	34,620,477	103,653,489
	Midwest	5,017 (19.71%)	2.0	9,569	4,022	26,782,849	68,093,852
	South	12,995 (51.06%)	2.0	10,188	3,705	61,999,349	180,666,552
	West	2,573 (10.11%)	2.0	14,731	4,682	14,637,965	50,336,552

* Denotes missing values

TABLE 96

Outcomes by patient and hospital characteristics for ICD-9-CM principal diagnosis code 401.9 Hypertension Nos

		Total number of discharges	LOS (length of stay), days (median)	Charges, $ (median)	Costs, $ (median)	Aggregate costs	Aggregate charges, $ (the "national bill")
All discharges		81,210 (100.00%)	2.0	9,909	3,676	387,531,437	1,099,464,030
Age group	<1	*	*	*	*	*	*
	1–17	556 (0.68%)	2.0	9,743	3,635	3,031,978	8,799,441
	18–44	13,460 (16.57%)	2.0	9,753	3,580	60,550,134	173,871,574
	45–64	32,718 (40.29%)	2.0	10,096	3,704	156,501,517	443,798,709
	65–84	26,803 (33.00%)	2.0	9,904	3,698	130,657,644	371,971,478
	85+	7,622 (9.39%)	3.0	9,365	3,586	36,216,770	99,550,894
	Missing	*	*	*	*	*	*
Sex	Male	30,045 (37.00%)	2.0	9,940	3,694	150,153,027	426,109,908
	Female	51,109 (62.93%)	2.0	9,874	3,664	237,188,247	672,759,248
	Missing	*	1.0	6,471	2,055	190,164	594,873
Median income for zip code	Low	30,675 (37.77%)	2.0	9,416	3,484	138,191,832	400,171,762
	Not low	47,468 (58.45%)	2.0	10,316	3,753	230,164,340	666,170,954
	Missing	3,067 (3.78%)	2.0	7,883	4,548	19,175,266	33,121,314
Region	Northeast	17,881 (22.02%)	2.0	10,517	4,271	103,526,417	284,132,365
	Midwest	16,100 (19.83%)	2.0	8,879	3,666	72,322,270	184,899,359
	South	37,846 (46.60%)	2.0	9,482	3,391	161,706,958	469,468,067
	West	9,383 (11.55%)	2.0	13,013	4,086	49,975,793	160,964,240

* Denotes missing values

TABLE 97

2006 National statistics—first-listed diagnosis only

Patient and hospital characteristics for ICD-9-CM first-listed diagnosis code 401.0 Malignant Hypertension

		All ED visits (those that resulted in admission to the hospital and those that did not)	Only hospital visits that originated in the ED	Only ED visits that ended in discharge (no hospital admission)	Standard errors		
					All ED Visits	Admitted to the hospital from the ED	Discharged from the ED
All discharges		37,639 (100.00%)	21,763 (100.00%)	15,876 (100.00%)	1,799	1,015	1,187
Age (mean)		59.65	60.58	58.36	0.35	0.35	0.35
Age group	<1	*	*	*	*	*	*
	1–17	*	*	*	*	*	*
	18–44	7,531 (20.01%)	3,926 (52.13%)	3,605 (47.87%)	430	226 (2.09%)	299 (2.09%)
	45–64	15,131 (40.20%)	8,888 (58.74%)	6,243 (41.26%)	773	470 (1.94%)	488 (1.94%)
	65–84	11,781 (31.30%)	6,848 (58.13%)	4,933 (41.87%)	640	351 (2.07%)	431 (2.07%)
	85+	3,096 (8.23%)	2,033 (65.68%)	1,063 (34.32%)	212	156 (3.20%)	133 (3.20%)
Median income for zip code	Low	14,533 (38.61%)	7,678 (52.83%)	6,855 (47.17%)	1,092	599 (2.96%)	770 (2.96%)
	Not low	22,307 (59.27%)	13,626 (61.08%)	8,681 (38.92%)	1,157	689 (1.75%)	683 (1.75%)
	Missing	799 (2.12%)	458 (57.41%)	340 (42.59%)	96	57 (4.89%)	65 (4.89%)
Region	Northeast	6,895 (18.32%)	4,856 (70.43%)	2,039 (29.57%)	828	511 (3.77%)	435 (3.77%)
	Midwest	7,004 (18.61%)	4,150 (59.25%)	2,854 (40.75%)	702	448 (2.84%)	360 (2.84%)
	South	18,705 (49.70%)	10,292 (55.02%)	8,413 (44.98%)	1,247	711 (2.68%)	862 (2.68%)
	West	5,034 (13.38%)	2,465 (48.95%)	2,570 (51.05%)	709	249 (5.50%)	590 (5.50%)

* Denotes missing values

TABLE 98

Patient and hospital characteristics for ICD-9-CM first-listed diagnosis code 401.9 Hypertension Nos

		All ED visits (those that resulted in admission to the hospital and those that did not)	Only hospital visits that originated in the ED	Only ED visits that ended in discharge (no hospital admission)	Standard errors		
					All ED Visits	Admitted to the hospital from the ED	Discharged from the ED
All discharges		559,934 (100.00%)	59,057 (100.00%)	500,877 (100.00%)	14,329	2,258	13,235
Age (mean)		57.23	60.89	56.80	0.21	0.21	0.21
Age group	<1	95 (0.02%)	*	66 (68.98%)	24	*	19 (11.25%)
	1–17	2,531 (0.45%)	320 (12.66%)	2,211 (87.34%)	204	62 (1.82%)	163 (1.82%)
	18–44	137,287 (24.52%)	10,598 (7.72%)	126,688 (92.28%)	4,528	541 (0.32%)	4,231 (0.32%)
	45–64	225,626 (40.30%)	23,303 (10.33%)	202,323 (89.67%)	6,603	998 (0.38%)	6,120 (0.38%)
	65–84	161,741 (28.89%)	19,138 (11.83%)	142,603 (88.17%)	4,144	794 (0.41%)	3,756 (0.41%)
	85+	32,640 (5.83%)	5,668 (17.36%)	26,972 (82.64%)	922	272 (0.70%)	805 (0.70%)
	Missing	*		*	*		*
Median income for zip code	Low	200,083 (35.73%)	20,690 (10.34%)	179,394 (89.66%)	7,926	1,188 (0.44%)	7,174 (0.44%)
	Not low	346,266 (61.84%)	37,102 (10.71%)	309,164 (89.29%)	10,931	1,632 (0.39%)	10,059 (0.39%)
	Missing	13,584 (2.43%)	1,265 (9.31%)	12,320 (90.69%)	605	103 (0.68%)	565 (0.68%)
Region	Northeast	79,372 (14.18%)	10,171 (12.81%)	69,200 (87.19%)	6,161	924 (0.88%)	5,573 (0.88%)
	Midwest	112,712 (20.13%)	13,273 (11.78%)	99,440 (88.22%)	6,335	1,031 (0.75%)	5,796 (0.75%)
	South	273,532 (48.85%)	27,738 (10.14%)	245,794 (89.86%)	9,811	1,602 (0.51%)	9,127 (0.51%)
	West	94,318 (16.84%)	7,875 (8.35%)	86,443 (91.65%)	5,565	783 (0.72%)	5,216 (0.72%)

* Denotes missing values

The bulk of hypertension in 2006 was also found in females in the South and the Midwest, followed by the West and the Northeast. The rate was higher for older people, ages 45–64 who saw a rate of 40.3% followed by the 65–84 age group at 28.9%, and finally the prime-age group, 18–44, with 24.5%. The very old had 5.8%.

Summary

Tables 31–98 have provided evidence on conditions that have been reported to be due to estrogen excess in the body. Many of these conditions have high prevalence in women due to the increased endogenous estrogen production that couples with xenoestrogens (pesticides and herbicides, and the myriad of estrogenic products in cosmetics-see books such as: *Toxic Beauty: How Cosmetics and Personal Care Products Endanger Your Health... And What You Can Do About It,* Samuel S. Epstein & Randall Fitzgerald, Ben Bella Books, 2009 and *A Consumer's Dictionary of Cosmetic Ingredients,* 7th edition, Ruth Winter 2009) adds to plant based estrogens to create havoc in women. This super-estrogen dominance in women manifests as the multiple symptoms reported on pages 96–98. The next section will shed some light on endogenous estrogen production process in women and men.

Sources of Endogenous Estrogens

Most endogenous estrogens in women are produced during the menstrual cycle but can also be produced by the adrenal glands and by conversion of testosterone to estrogens. Aromatase is the enzyme that facilitates the conversion of testosterone to estrogen. Obesity increases the activity of aromatase and hence obese men and women tend to have more estrogens than lean individuals. Men produce estrogen by converting testosterone to the estrogens via aromatase. Estrogen is responsible for the gynecomastia that men develop with increasing age, obesity, and alcohol abuse.

Estrogens in women and men are not benign and the consequences will be covered in the following chapter. Chapter 5 will cover the production of endogenous hormones and consequences.

PROGESTERONE DEFICIENCY, ESTROGEN DOMINANCE, LEPTIN RESISTANCE, INSULIN RESISTANCE AND OBESITY

Our good hormones come from what is known as bad (LDL) cholesterol which generates Pregnenolone. Pregnenolone divides into two other hormones, progesterone and DHEA (DeHydroEpiAndrosterone); these two in turn produce estradiol, estrone and testosterone. When we get older, we lose some of these hormones and others increase. The changes in hormones cause a hormonal disequilibrium which is the source of many diseases and symptoms treated by all physicians. The diagram on the next page is a rough illustration of endogenous hormone production cascade.

ORIGIN OF HORMONES, THEIR INTERACTIONS AND CONSEQUENCES

Cholesterol (LDL)

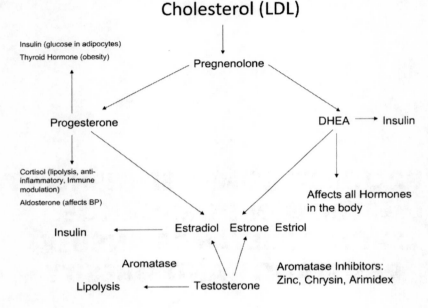

WHAT CAUSES ESTROGEN DOMINANCE?
* Endogenous estrogens
* Exogenous estrogens
    - Xenoestrogens: Herbicide, Pesticides (as listed on pages 81–87) and other household chemicals including cosmetics and cosmeceuticals (see the books referenced at page 185)

Phytoestrogens: Plant estrogens (five old bay seasoning ingredients: bay leaf, celery, nutmeg, cloves, cinnamon), Alfalfa Sprouts, Cottonseed Oil, Cumin, Tea, Tea Tree Oil, Oregano, Melaleuca products, Dates, Thyme, Peppermint, Tumeric, Fenugreek, Feverfew, Pomegranate, Flax oil, Wheat (weak Phytoestrogen), Garlic, Hemp Oil, Red Clover, Hops (beer), Rosemary, Caffeine, Coffee, Coffee Decaf, Safflower, Safflower Oil, Canola Oil,

Chamomile, Chamomile tea, Licorice, Soy, Chocolate and its main product cocoa, Clover, Mint, Sunflower Oil, Sunflower Seeds, only to name a few... (see additional xenoestrogens and phytoestrogens list by Peter Eckhart, MD, *www. Woomhoo.com*)

Progesterone Deficiency and Consequences

Both men and women produce progesterone. While progesterone is produced by the adrenal glands and testis in men, the progesterone in women is produced during the menstrual cycle by the ovaries and a small amount by the adrenal glands. The progesterone gene can be inherited from the mother and low progesterone in the mother can lead to low progesterone in the daughter or son. When girls inherit the low progesterone gene, they developed progesterone deficiency symptoms early in life. Right after menarche, the young girl starts experiencing menorrhagia (heavy menstrual periods) and/or dysmenorrhea (painful menstrual cramps) often accompanied by nausea, vomiting and diarrhea. This is quite debilitating for many young girls of the world. These women also often have difficulty conceiving and if they conceive, they have difficulty carrying the pregnancy to term. They tend to have multiple miscarriages and if an astute OB/GYN physician realizes the low progesterone problem and injects even synthetic progesterone, the pregnancy can go to term. If the low progesterone woman becomes pregnant, the first trimester could represent a real challenge. She will have nausea and vomiting throughout the pregnancy, but these symptoms are worse in the first trimester when the progesterone production is still average. During the second trimester, the progesterone is produced by the placenta, about 400 mg/day, and that helps to alleviate the nausea and vomiting problem. After delivery, when the placenta is gone, the progesterone production ceases and the woman becomes depressed. This may explain much of the post-partum depression experienced by women. The low progesterone also causes many symptoms and some of these symptoms are the same as the estrogen dominance symptoms:

- Dysmenorrhea
- Menorrhagia
- Infertility
- Anovulatory menstrual cycles
- Irregular periods
- Endometriosis
- Early miscarriage
- Carbohydrate cravings
- Breast tenderness
- Ovarian cysts
- Puffiness/bloating
- Water retention
- Lower body temperature.
- Internally anxious, outwardly calm
- Premenstrual backache
- Frequent complaining
- Endless crying
- Breast and/or ovarian cysts
- Defective luteal phase
- Fibroid tumors
- Excessive facial and body hair on women
- Infanticide fears
- Feelings of loneliness
- Maltreatment of newborn baby, harmful, violent thoughts
- Absence of maternal instinct and behavior
- Nausea during pregnancy
- Night sweats
- PCOS (polycystic ovarian Syndrome)
- Pre-eclampsia
- Rejection of baby

- Feelings of resentment
- Early aging of skin
- Feelings of uselessness
- Vaginal thinning, dryness, and itching
- Miscarriage
- Temporary psychosis
- Breast tenderness and/or mastitis
- Premenstrual breast tenderness
- Follicular keratoses ("goose bumps") on backs of arms and legs
- Hot flashes/flushes
- Erratic menstrual cycle
- Excessive menstrual flow
- Lack of menstrual periods
- Depression after childbirth
- Depression during peri-menopause/menopause
- Irregular menstrual flow
- Period pains and/or ovulation cramps
- Easily upset, quick to cry
- Depression
- Panic attacks or panicky feelings
- Sense of confusion
- Feelings of unreality
- Exhaustion
- Feelings of guilt
- Tricotilomania (Hair pulling)
- Hallucinations
- Histrionic behavior
- Infertility
- Feelings of insecurity
- Internally upset by criticism
- Suicidal thoughts or attempts
- Binges

- Thinning of Hair /hair loss (women)
- Lack of self confidence and esteem
- SAD (seasonal affective disorder)
- Sleep disturbances
- Emotional balance upset by stress
- Irrational fears
- Flaking, brittle, and weak nails
- Water retention
- Feelings of anger
- Mood swings
- Anxiety
- Abdominal bloating
- Agitation
- Agoraphobia
- Blood clots
- Brown patches on cheeks
- Bruising and capillary breakage
- Chronic fatigue
- Claustrophobia
- Lethargy
- Rage
- Self mutilation
- Verbal and physical violence
- Dark rings under the eyes
- Eating or drinking to alleviate depression
- Difficulty in getting up after enough sleep
- Dizziness
- Tired all the time
- Frequent or regular migraines
- Feelings of tension
- Cravings for sweet foods
- Procrastination
- Asthma

- Loss of libido
- Short term memory loss
- Clumsiness
- Acne
- Insomnia
- Nervousness
- Palpitations
- Inability to concentrate
- Hypoglycemia
- Manic behavior
- Obsessions without compulsions
- Cracked heels
- Endometriosis
- Low libido
- Osteoporosis
- Paranoia
- Prostate problems
- Spaced out
- Weight gain at puberty/childbirth/menopause
- Feelings of aggression
- Quick reaction or over-reaction to alcohol
- Forgeting what you're about to say
- Fuzzy brain
- Alcohol abuse
- Cold hands and feet
- Quick tempered
- Frequent or regular headaches
- Irritability
- Dry skin
- Incontinence
- Personality changes
- Regular epileptic fits
- Psoriasis

- Shaking or trembling
- Itching skin
- Varicose veins
- Low blood pressure
- Constipation
- Allergies or sensitivities to foods or chemicals
- Brown spots on back of hands
- Fainting spells
- Burning eyes
- Misty vision
- Painful eyes

Common Effects of Progesterone Deficiency

- Cortisol decreases
- Thyroid function decreases
- TSH measure is not enough
- T4 does not always convert to T3
- Measure these three in thyroid function test
- Insulin increases
- Initially hypoglycemia occurs
- Adrenaline is produced to increase glucose
- Glucagon is produced to increase glucose
- Carbohydrate consumption increases
- Excess carbohydrates is pushed into adipocytes
- Filled adipocytes produce leptin, adiponectin, visfatin, and apelin
- Lepin effect on the hypothylamus
- Leptin resistance and depression/anxiety

- Insulin resistance
- Leptin/Insulin resistance and type 2 diabetes
- Leptin resistance and ghrelin/NPY
- Leptin resistance and Bios Life Slim
- Leptin resistance and MaxWLx
- Adipocytes make inflammatory cytokines
- Adipocytes help skin cells and adrenal glands to produce estradiol and estrone
- Estrogens increase both insulin and thyroid binding globulin
- Estrogen affects mast cells and basophils to release allergy causing mediators
- Too much thyroid-binding globulin causes a decrease in thyroid function

Effect of Insulin on Cholesterol

- Fatty acids and glucose are used to make cholesterol
- Fatty acids and glucose convert to acetyl-CoA via beta-oxidation and glycolysis
- Rate-limiting enzyme is HMG-CoA Reductase
- Insulin potentiates HMG-CoA reductase
- Statin drugs are HMG-CoA reductase inhibitors
- Type 2 diabetics with high glucose, increased fat, and insulin resistance will make more cholesterol.

The diagram on the following page shows the cholesterol making process.

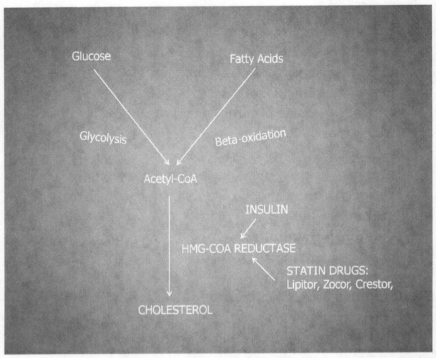

In this diagram, HMG-COA reductase is the rate-limiting enzyme in the making of cholesterol and insulin is a catalyst for HMG-COA reductase. Statin drugs are HMG-COA reductase inhibitors.

INSULIN AND HYPERTENSION
- Insulin causes salt retention
- Salt retention increases blood pressure
- Half of all patients with hypertension have insulin resistance

Insulin Resistance
- Insulin is the number one fat maker
- Insulin directs excess glucose into adipocytes
- Insulin resistance occurs when adipocytes cannot accommodate glucose

- Two measures of insulin resistance worth knowing:
  - *The Homeostatic Model Assessment of Insulin Resistance* (HOMA)
  - *The Quantitative Insulin Sensitivity Check Index* (QUICKI)

HOMA and Quick Calculations

HOMA or HOMA-IR= insulin (µU/m) x [glucose (mmol/L)/22.5)]

Patients with a HOMA score of 2.6 or above are considered to have insulin resistance

QUICKI =1/log(insulin)(µU/m) + log[fasting glucose (mg/dl)]

Patients with a QUICKI score of 0.33 or above are considered to have insulin resistanc

Laboratory Work

When you suspect hormone deficiency, you should order progesterone, DHEA, DHEA-S, androstenedione, estradiol, estrone, cortisol, aldosterone (if patient has hypertension or hypotension), fasting insulin, leptin level if patient is obese, lipid panel, comprehensive metabolic panel, total and free testosterone, dihydrotestosterone (DHT), sex hormone binding globulin (SHBG), FSH and LH, homocysteine, high sensitivity CRP, TSH, free T4 and free T3, Somatomedin–C (IGF-1), and IGFBP3, for both men and women and add PSA for males. The test for lipids that will be appropriate in the future will be oxidized LDL cholesterol. Some laboratories are now performing this test. It is important to look at the proportion of LDL that is oxidized because that portion is what is dangerous and LDL does not have to be elevated to oxidize. Remember that LDL is needed for production of steroid hormones. Hence lowering total LDL may be detrimental to the body. Preventing oxidation of LDL using antioxidants makes more sense.

Hormone Interrelationship

- Decrease in progesterone, DHEA and increase in estradiol and estrone tend to increase insulin.

- Progesterone modulates thyroid hormone activity by keeping potassium and zinc in cells. Potassium and zinc are known to help convert T4 into T3 for increased metabolism.

- Decrease in progesterone leads to estrogen dominance and estrogen dominance leads to an increase in insulin and further decrease in thyroid hormone activity. (Never rely on TSH alone. It is not uncommon to find elevated or decreased TSH level in the face of normal T4 and T3 and it is more common to find low free T3 in the face of Normal free T4 and TSH.) It is also frequent to see women on Synthroid with more weight problems, which suggests a suboptimal treatment of hypothyroidism.

Why Many Women and Men Gain Weight in Their Late Thirties and Beyond

PROGESTERONE DEFICIENCY AND OBESITY

Decrease in progesterone leads to:
- increased insulin
- decreased thyroid hormone activity
- the interaction of these two events leads to obesity.

Estradiol increases insulin and decreases thyroid function with same result.

Symptoms of Progesterone Deficiency and Estrogen Dominance

- Premenstrual breast tenderness
- Premenstrual mood swings
- Premenstrual fluid retention and weight gain
- Premenstrual headaches
- Migraine headaches
- Severe menstrual cramps
- Heavy periods with clotting
- Irregular menstrual cycles
- Uterine fibroid tumors
- Ovarian cysts
- Fibrocystic breast disease
- Endometriosis
- Infertility problems
- More than one miscarriage
- Joint pain
- Muscle pain
- Decreased libido
- Anxiety and panic attacks, or depression
- Hot flashes
- Difficulty sleeping

Estrogen Excess or Dominance and Obesity

- Increased estrogen leads to an increase in insulin and increase in thyroid binding globulin (TBG), which results in low metabolism and increased fat making.
- Oral but not transdermal estradiol increases TBG, whereas testosterone lowers TBG.
- Testosterone increases T3/T4 ratios. Estradiol does not affect T3/T4 ratios, irrespective of the route of administration.
- Therefore, the T4 substitution dose in women with primary hypothyroidism, characterized by impaired endogenous

T4 production, must be increased when oral estrogens are administered.

Effect of DHEA Deficiency on Insulin
- Decrease in DHEA leads to increased insulin and thus potentiates lipogenesis.
- Insulin increase not only leads to diabetes, but also leads to increased blood pressure secondary to salt retention by renal tubules.
- DHEA decreases with age and stress.
- DHEA and progesterone together increase testosterone and estradiol and estrone. Decrease in DHEA most often leads to decrease in testosterone. Estrogens may be normal because they are also produced by sources other than DHEA (adipocytes, skin cells, and adrenal glands).

Progesterone Deficiency and Inflammatory Diseases
- Premenstrual asthma (PMA)
- Premenstrual migraines
- Premenstrual dermatitis
- Non-allergic rhinitis and enhanced seasonal/perennial allergic rhinitis
- Fibromyalgia
- Interstitial cystitis (know that IC is a mast cell disease and is more prevalent in women than men; see the IC statistics from HCUP database. I suspect that estrogen dominance in women causes IC. When estrogen binds to its receptor-α on the mast cell, it causes mast cell degranulation in the detrusor muscle of the bladder that leads to the IC symptoms. Hence balancing estrogen by giving adequate amounts of progesterone and DIM and I-3-C may help IC patients)
- Arthritis
- Loin pain Hematuria(possibly)

- Endometriosis
- Multiple sclerosis (possibly)
- Non-allergic Rhinitis, and Seasonal/Perennial Allergic Rhinitis
- Obesity and asthma
- What obesity and asthma have in common?
- Premenstrual asthma
- Asthma discharge observations

Estrogens and Benign Tumors and Many Other Conditions in Women

- Fibroid tumors
- Fibrocystic breast disease
- Ovarian cysts
- Cervical dysplasia (non-HPV related)
- Endometriosis

Estrogens and Cancer

- Studies of estrogen metabolism have led to the hypothesis that reaction of certain estrogen metabolites, predominantly catechol estrogen-3,4-quinones with DNA, can generate the critical mutations initiating breast, prostate, and other cancers
- The endogenous estrogens estrone (E1) and estradiol (E2) are oxidized to catechol estrogens (CE), 2-and-4-hydroxylated estrogens, which can be further oxidized to CE quinones that are involved in breast and prostate cancer.

Estrogen is associated with the following cancers and perhaps many more:

- Breast cancer
- Uterine cancer
- Ovarian cancer

- Cervical cancer
- Vaginal cancer
- Colon cancer
- Prostate cancer

Estrogen and Progesterone Receptors in Breast Cancer

- ER positive/PR positive (estrogen-receptor-positive breast cancer is more prevalent than other types of breast cancer).
- ER positive/PR negative
- ER negative/PR positive
- ER negative/PR negative

Hormone Imbalance Types

- Based on my clinical evaluation of patients who present with hormone imbalance, the laboratory results show twelve different hormonal patterns. The first group has no deficiency and there are very few of these individuals. The second group only lacks progesterone; the third group lacks both progesterone and estradiol; the fourth group

PROGESTERONE	ESTRADIOL	DHEA	TESTOSTERONE
+	+	+	+
−	+	+	+
−	−	+	+
−	−	−	+
−	−	−	−
+	+	+	−
+	+	−	−
+	−	−	−
+	−	+	−
+	−	−	+
−	+	−	+
−	+	+	−

lacks progesterone, estradiol and DHEA. The fifth group lacks progesterone, estradiol, DHEA, and testosterone. Those individuals also often lack Pregnenolone. You can follow through the table and see all the possible hormone deficiency combinations.

If a woman does not have a low progesterone to begin with, as she gets older, she tends to lose her progesterone because of anovulatory menstrual cycles. Women also lose their progesterone because of progesterone-containing birth control pills (progestins) that suppress the natural production of progesterone. Women produce progesterone during their menstrual cycle as follows:

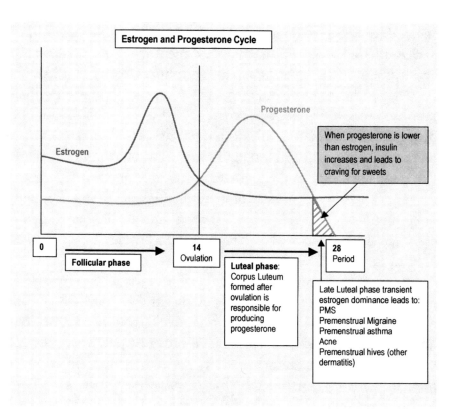

Estrogen and Progesterone Cycle

Progesterone

Estrogen

When progesterone is lower than estrogen, insulin increases and leads to craving for sweets

0

Follicular phase

14
Ovulation

Luteal phase:
Corpus Luteum
formed after
ovulation is
responsible for
producing
progesterone

28
Period

Late Luteal phase transient
estrogen dominance leads to:
PMS
Premenstrual Migraine
Premenstrual asthma
Acne
Premenstrual hives (other
dermatitis)

Progesterone is produced after ovulation. In women who have a normal cycle of twenty eight days, the fourteenth day is known as ovulation or when the egg (ovum) is released from the ovary. When the egg is released, the pocket where the egg came from does not disappear. It becomes yellow and is known as the "yellow body" or Corpus Luteum in Latin. The female menstrual cycle is therefore divided into three phases: Pre-ovulatory phase or follicular phase, ovulatory phase and post-ovulatory phase also known as the luteal phase because of the activity of the Corpus Luteum. Before ovulation, the estrogens estradiol, estrone, and estriol increase, reach their peak around the ovulation time and decline thereafter. The progesterone is flat prior to ovulation but right after ovulation it starts to increase and peaks about seven days before the period. Three to five days (but sometimes a week) before the period, many women develop premenstrual syndrome (PMS) or premenstrual dysphoric disorder (PMDD).

The syndrome or disorder consists of uneasy feeling, emotional lability, bloating, acne, premenstrual asthma exacerbations for post pubertal women with asthma, premenstrual migraines, pre-menstrual dermatitis (hives), and most women around the world crave sugary foods, and chocolate is only one of them. The sugar craving is due to the activity of insulin which is the sugar craving hormone. Insulin increases when progesterone decreases below estrogen in the last week of the menstrual cycle. This transient insulin increase is responsible for the sugar craving.

Women tend to have anovulatory menstrual cycles in their late twenties, early thirties, mid thirties and beyond. This leads to progressive dwindling of the protective hormone progesterone and the ensuing unopposed estrogen leads to a persistent, instead of transient, insulin increase. This permanent insulin increase in turn leads to constant craving for sweets. Eating sweets or high sugar content foods lead to increase in the blood glucose.

The insulin has to quickly dispose of the glucose so as to prevent it from spilling in the blood. The quicker way of getting rid of the glucose in the blood is to put it into the fat cells. Fat cells convert the glucose into fatty acids for storage and the end result is obesity. Hence, it is not surprising to see women gain weight after age thirty five or even sooner if their progesterone deficiency starts earlier.

When progesterone decreases, thyroid function also decreases which compounds the weight gain problem.

How does thyroid function connect to progesterone?

Progesterone aids in the retention of zinc, potassium and selenium in our cells.

Zinc, potassium and selenium allow the thyroid hormone T4 to enter the cell and then to be converted to the active form T3 that is used for metabolism. Low progesterone decreases this mineral retention in cells. As a result, T4 does not convert to T3. Patients with hypothyroidism are given a T4 equivalent Levothyroxine (Synthroid). If the patient has low progesterone as occurs in menopausal women, then this treatment remains ineffective. These patients do not readily lose the weight and if T3 is measured, it is found to be low. T3 may be within the standardized specified range carved in stone, per orthodox medicine standards that "no one" should deviate from. The TSH in this case is often greater than 2. If 0.49–4.47 is the normal range, and 0.49 is considered perfectly optimal thyroid function, then anything above 0.49 is not perfect. Anything above this perfect number is signaling that the body needs a little more thyroid to optimally achieve metabolism. Unfortunately, our rigid standard of care once again does not even consider the patients' symptoms of continued fatigue and difficulty of losing weight despite the thyroid supplementation. We continue to treat the patients with the same medications even though the results are not there. This leads to frustration and patients seek alternative therapies on their own.

Increased estrogen leads to increased thyroid binding globulin that binds both T4 and T3 tightly and does not relinquish them for metabolism. Some scientists have therefore suggested that women be supplemented with thyroid medication when they are on birth control pills. These pills tend to prevent ovulation and therefore decrease the progesterone level in the users. Hence, many of these women on these pills tend to gain weight.

Since progesterone is known to be an antagonist to estrogen, when progesterone decreases and estrogen level remains the same or increases, then estrogen dominance arises that leads to the increase in the thyroid binding globulin, which in turns leads to suppression of the thyroid function.

Estrogen is also associated with copper. Copper is required for the synthesis and release of estrogen and also forms enzymes in the liver which help to break down leftover estrogen into harmless substances. Estrogen can cause copper retention if zinc or progesterone levels are too low or calcium level is high. Since copper contributes to the increase in estrogen, an increase in copper level in the body may therefore decrease thyroid function.

If calcium and copper increase together, they can have a detrimental effect on thyroid function. Progesterone, by antagonizing estrogen and allowing potassium, selenium and zinc to remain in cells, reverses all these negative mineral effects on the thyroid function. Unfortunately, TSH, measured by most physicians to test for the thyroid function, often does not capture this imbalance.

Remember that the decrease in progesterone also leads to estrogen dominance that in turn leads to an increase in insulin. Insulin causes craving for carbohydrates and is also responsible for putting glucose into adipocytes. Initially, when insulin increases, the blood glucose decreases which prompts craving for carbohydrates (sugar-containing foods). In order to replenish the decreased glucose, adrenaline is also produced and most people become "hyper." When glucose is plentiful, the insulin puts it into fat cells and people start gaining weight. When the fat cells are filled, they signal to the brain that they have enough of the glucose by producing hormones such as leptin which, in effect, tells the hypothalamus to put a break on the appetite and sugar cravings (Bios Life Slim®—listed in the *Physicians' Desk Reference* (PDR)—boosts leptin so as to help adipocytes communicate better with the hypothalamus). After a while, the message is lost and most people continue to gain the weight. When the fat cells are filled and do not want the glucose, this glucose spills into the blood, and high levels of glucose in the blood is what is known as diabetes (insulin resistance).

Fat cells also produce adipokines such as TNF-α, Interleukin-6, and many others that lead to inflammatory processes such as asthma, allergic rhinitis, and aches and pains. That is why most obese individuals experience these symptoms. One adipokine, adiponectin, is known to be inversely related to asthma symptoms. The fat cells also produce estrogens (estradiol and estrone) which in turn increase the insulin level and decrease the thyroid function (by increasing the thyroid binding globulin) and therefore lead to more weight gain. Too much estrogen is not good for the body. For women, the decrease in progesterone and increase in estrogens lead to several benign tumors such as fibroid tumors, fibrocystic breast disease, ovarian cysts, polycystic ovarian syndrome, LAM (lymphagiomyomatosis), and the malignant tumors such as breast, vaginal, cervical, uterine, ovarian, and colon cancers, among others. Benign but devastating tumors such as fibroid tumors are a source of heavy and often prolonged bleeding (dysfunctional uterine bleeding) and anemia, which lead to hysterectomies (surgical removal of the uterus). Both men and women lose their testosterone with age, and this leads in turn to low libido, decreased muscle mass, increased insulin, and abdominal weight gain.

When men lose their progesterone to estrogens via the enzyme aromatase in their mid fifties and beyond, or if they abuse alcohol, or if they are obese, many tend to grow what is colloquially known as "man boobs" or gynecomastia. Men in their fifties with high estrogen levels and without their protective testosterone are at risk for prostate cancer and colon cancer and perhaps many other cancers. Xenoestrogens and phytoestrogens, coupled with endogenous estrogens, have similar effects in both men and women. Younger men do not develop prostate cancer because of the protective effect of testosterone.

Estrogens also cause benign tumors in women as mentioned in previous pages. In men prostate enlargement, called benign prostatic hypertrophy, may be due to too much estrogen. This condition is usually linked to dihydrotestosterone, a more potent form of testosterone blamed for causing male pattern baldness and prostate enlargement. The HCUP data used in this study showed higher BPH discharges in the South and the Midwest where use of estrogen-causing chemicals are higher than in the Northeast and the West. Hence, endogenous estrogens, xenoestrogens, and phytoestrogens have an impact on the prostate in terms of hypertrophy or cancer.

DHEA

DHEA is the mother of all hormones and affects all other hormones in the body. It is also known as the longevity hormone. Studies have shown that people who have more of it tend to live longer on average compared to people who have less of it. A decrease in DHEA, which occurs with age and stress, has direct effects on the overall well-being of humans. A decrease in DHEA leads to a decrease in testosterone and an increase in insulin. An increase in insulin tends to cause not only diabetes but also salt retention in kidney tubules, and salt retention leads to hypertension.

Reason for High Cholesterol

When the steroid hormones are low, the body wants to produce them. So it naturally raises the ingredient that is needed to make those hormones, and that is why cholesterol increases. An increase in cholesterol, especially LDL cholesterol, should therefore be a signal to test for the hormones.

Cholesterol Production and Consequences

Cholesterol is made in the liver out of fat and glucose, and insulin serves as the fuel to the rate limiting enzyme HMG-CoA reductase. This is why many diabetics have cholesterol problems and why obese men and women (who invariably have hormone imbalance) also have fatty liver. In the making of cholesterol, occasionally cholesterol stones are formed and lodge in the gallbladder and gallbladder neck, preventing the flow of bile. This leads to cholecystitis (inflammation of the gallbladder) which is one of the main reasons for a cholecystectomy (surgical removal of the gallbladder). In medical school, we learned that cholecystitis is often found in "Females, Fat, Fertile, and Forty." The only thing peculiar about age forty in women is anovulatory menstrual cycles that lead to progesterone deficiency. As you know, progesterone deficiency leads to estrogen dominance, and this eventually leads to obesity. Hence the four "Fs" perfectly fit the hormone imbalance state in women. Most women with hormone imbalance have already had a cholecystectomy when they present to clinic. From the HCUP database, it appears that women have slightly more cholesterol than men (see Table 99 on page 211). However, coronary artery disease and myocardial infarction are much higher in men than women, as depicted in Tables 100–114.

SUMMARY OF ENDOGENOUS HORMONE IMBALANCE PROCESSES AND CONSEQUENCES

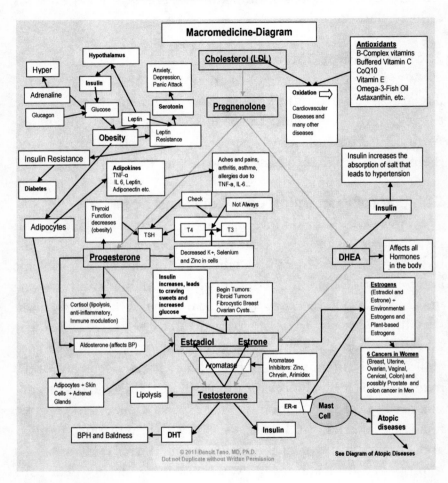

Macromedicine-Diagram

Hypothalamus

Hyper

Insulin

Adrenaline

Glucagon

Glucose

Leptin

Obesity

Leptin Resistance

Anxiety, Depression, Panic Attack

Serotonin

Cholesterol (LDL)

Pregnenolone

Antioxidants
B-Complex vitamins
Buffered Vitamin C
CoQ10
Vitamin E
Omega-3-Fish Oil
Astaxanthin, etc.

Oxidation

Cardiovascular Diseases and many other diseases

Insulin Resistance

Diabetes

Adipocytes

Adipokines
TNF-α
IL 6, Leptin,
Adiponectin etc.

Aches and pains, arthritis, asthma, allergies due to TNF-a, IL-6…

Thyroid Function decreases (obesity)

Check

Not Always

TSH

T4

T3

Insulin increases the absorption of salt that leads to hypertension

Insulin

Progesterone

Decreased K+, Selenium and Zinc in cells

DHEA

Affects all Hormones in the body

Insulin increases, leads to craving sweets and increased glucose

Begin Tumors:
Fibroid Tumors
Fibrocystic Breast
Ovarian Cysts…

Cortisol (lipolysis, anti-inflammatory, Immune modulation)

Aldosterone (affects BP)

Estrogens
(Estradiol and Estrone) +
Environmental Estrogens and Plant-based Estrogens

Adipocytes + Skin Cells + Adrenal Glands

Lipolysis

Estradiol   **Estrone**

Aromatase

Aromatase Inhibitors: Zinc, Chrysin, Arimidex

6 Cancers in Women
(Breast, Uterine, Ovarian, Vaginal, Cervical, Colon) and possibly Prostate and colon cancer in Men

Testosterone

ER-α

Mast Cell

Atopic diseases

BPH and Baldness

DHT

Insulin

See Diagram of Atopic Diseases

© 2011 Benoit Tano, MD, Ph.D.
Dot not Duplicate without Written Permission

TABLE 99

Patient and hospital characteristics for ICD-9-CM first-listed diagnosis code 272.4 Hyperlipidemia Nec/Nos

		All ED visits (those that resulted in admission to the hospital and those that did not)	Only hospital visits that originated in the ED	Only ED visits that ended in discharge (no hospital admission)	Standard errors		
					All ED Visits	Admitted to the hospital from the ED	Discharged from the ED
All discharges		1,861 (100.00%)	197 (100.00%)	1,664 (100.00%)	272	32	269
Age (mean)		56.70	60.18	56.28	0.97	0.97	0.97
Age group	<1	*	*	*	*	*	*
	1–17	*	*	*	*	*	*
	18–44	378 (20.32%)	*	360 (95.16%)	73	*	73 (2.31%)
	45–64	732 (39.35%)	94 (12.83%)	638 (87.17%)	111	21 (3.11%)	109 (3.11%)
	65–84	654 (35.14%)	84 (12.89%)	570 (87.11%)	99	20 (3.31%)	97 (3.31%)
	85+	*	*	*	*	*	*
Sex	Male	889 (47.78%)	74 (8.38%)	815 (91.62%)	148	17 (2.25%)	147 (2.25%)
	Female	972 (52.22%)	122 (12.57%)	850 (87.43%)	137	26 (2.86%)	134 (2.86%)
Median income for zip code	Low	593 (31.87%)	49 (8.26%)	544 (91.74%)	150	14 (3.00%)	149 (3.00%)
	Not low	1,207 (64.88%)	142 (11.78%)	1,065 (88.22%)	137	27 (2.40%)	135 (2.40%)
	Missing	*	*	*	*	*	*
Region	Northeast	*	*	*	*	*	*
	Midwest	394 (21.16%)	*	375 (95.25%)	66	*	64 (2.24%)
	South	648 (34.82%)	103 (15.86%)	545 (84.14%)	74	21 (3.12%)	70 (3.12%)
	West	350 (18.80%)	*	314 (89.92%)	70	*	67 (4.53%)

* Denotes missing values

This shows that hyperlipidemia is more prevalent in women, and the reported data show that the South and the Midwest have the highest rates.

TABLE 100

2008 National statistics—first-listed diagnosis only

Patient and hospital characteristics for ICD-9-CM first-listed diagnosis code 414.00 Cor Ath Unsp Vsl Ntv/Gft

		All ED visits (those that resulted in admission to the hospital and those that did not)	Only hospital visits that originated in the ED	Only ED visits that ended in discharge (no hospital admission)	Standard errors		
					All ED Visits	Admitted to the hospital from the ED	Discharged from the ED
All discharges		59,149 (100.00%)	42,291 (100.00%)	16,858 (100.00%)	2,522	2,245	835
Age (mean)		67.24	67.88	65.63	0.23	0.23	0.23
Age group	1–17	*	*	*	*	*	*
	18–44	2,439 (4.12%)	1,592 (65.26%)	847 (34.74%)	191	160 (3.06%)	88 (3.06%)
	45–64	22,387 (37.85%)	15,327 (68.47%)	7,059 (31.53%)	1,107	990 (1.77%)	405 (1.77%)
	65–84	28,406 (48.02%)	20,895 (73.56%)	7,511 (26.44%)	1,211	1,070 (1.28%)	395 (1.28%)
	85+	5,908 (9.99%)	4,477 (75.78%)	1,431 (24.22%)	305	263 (1.83%)	126 (1.83%)
Sex	Male	35,741 (60.43%)	25,462 (71.24%)	10,279 (28.76%)	1,448	1,263 (1.31%)	515 (1.31%)
	Female	23,395 (39.55%)	16,829 (71.93%)	6,566 (28.07%)	1,170	1,053 (1.60%)	382 (1.60%)
	Missing	*	*	*	*	*	*
Median income for zip code	Low	19,468 (32.91%)	13,707 (70.41%)	5,762 (29.59%)	1,456	1,311 (2.11%)	380 (2.11%)
	Not low	37,711 (63.76%)	26,984 (71.56%)	10,727 (28.44%)	1,523	1,267 (1.36%)	625 (1.36%)
	Missing	1,969 (3.33%)	1,600 (81.22%)	370 (18.78%)	431	426 (4.63%)	57 (4.63%)
Region	Northeast	12,369 (20.91%)	10,875 (87.93%)	1,493 (12.07%)	1,634	1,586 (1.78%)	180 (1.78%)
	Midwest	12,375 (20.92%)	7,737 (62.52%)	4,638 (37.48%)	928	734 (2.73%)	427 (2.73%)
	South	26,506 (44.81%)	17,766 (67.03%)	8,740 (32.97%)	1,545	1,292 (2.07%)	645 (2.07%)
	West	7,900 (13.36%)	5,912 (74.84%)	1,987 (25.16%)	662	563 (2.72%)	257 (2.72%)

* Denotes missing values

Coronary artery disease is, however, more prevalent in men (particularly older men) and increases with age; ages 45–64: 37.9% and ages 65–84: 48%. The South has more prevalence followed by the Midwest and Northeast.

TABLE 101

Patient and hospital characteristics for ICD-9-CM first-listed diagnosis code 414.01 Crnry Athrscl Natve Vssl

		All ED visits (those that resulted in admission to the hospital and those that did not)	Only hospital visits that originated in the ED	Only ED visits that ended in discharge (no hospital admission)	Standard errors		
					All ED Visits	Admitted to the hospital from the ED	Discharged from the ED
All discharges		323,705 (100.00%)	278,682 (100.00%)	45,022 (100.00%)	14,559	12,668	3,082
Age (mean)		64.43	64.72	62.59	0.17	0.17	0.17
Age group	1–17	*	*	*	*	*	*
	18–44	18,337 (5.66%)	14,982 (81.70%)	3,355 (18.30%)	896	732 (1.12%)	280 (1.12%)
	45–64	146,105 (45.14%)	123,978 (84.86%)	22,127 (15.14%)	6,864	5,837 (0.79%)	1,617 (0.79%)
	65–84	139,189 (43.00%)	121,953 (87.62%)	17,236 (12.38%)	6,520	5,811 (0.68%)	1,226 (0.68%)
	85+	20,029 (6.19%)	17,769 (88.72%)	2,259 (11.28%)	1,038	942 (0.83%)	199 (0.83%)
	Missing	*	*	*	*	*	*
Sex	Male	190,455 (58.84%)	163,809 (86.01%)	26,646 (13.99%)	8,696	7,541 (0.69%)	1,835 (0.69%)
	Female	133,140 (41.13%)	114,874 (86.28%)	18,267 (13.72%)	6,029	5,280 (0.75%)	1,311 (0.75%)
	Missing	*	*	*	*	*	*
Median income for zip code	Low	91,452 (28.25%)	77,640 (84.90%)	13,813 (15.10%)	6,075	5,148 (0.96%)	1,331 (0.96%)
	Not low	222,437 (68.72%)	192,132 (86.38%)	30,305 (13.62%)	10,565	9,298 (0.72%)	2,140 (0.72%)
	Missing	9,815 (3.03%)	8,911 (90.79%)	904 (9.21%)	1,449	1,429 (1.54%)	107 (1.54%)
Region	Northeast	54,377 (16.80%)	50,800 (93.42%)	3,577 (6.58%)	5,794	5,514 (1.19%)	718 (1.19%)
	Midwest	70,932 (21.91%)	57,522 (81.10%)	13,409 (18.90%)	5,940	4,663 (1.74%)	1,865 (1.74%)
	South	151,035 (46.66%)	126,436 (83.71%)	24,599 (16.29%)	11,125	9,512 (0.98%)	2,274 (0.98%)
	West	47,361 (14.63%)	43,924 (92.74%)	3,437 (7.26%)	4,398	4,225 (1.16%)	578 (1.16%)

* Denotes missing values

TABLE 102

Patient and hospital characteristics for ICD-9-CM first-listed diagnosis code 414.02 Crn Ath Atlg Vn Bps Grft

		All ED visits (those that resulted in admission to the hospital and those that did not)	Only hospital visits that originated in the ED	Only ED visits that ended in discharge (no hospital admission)	Standard errors		
					All ED Visits	Admitted to the hospital from the ED	Discharged from the ED
All discharges		11,476 (100.00%)	10,645 (100.00%)	831 (100.00%)	758	716	106
Age (mean)		67.45	67.68	64.43	0.27	0.27	0.27
Age group	18–44	253 (2.20%)	206 (81.54%)	*	37	33 (6.09%)	*
	45–64	4,249 (37.03%)	3,935 (92.62%)	314 (7.38%)	307	288 (1.31%)	61 (1.31%)
	65–84	6,398 (55.75%)	5,955 (93.07%)	443 (6.93%)	441	417 (0.88%)	63 (0.88%)
	85+	572 (4.99%)	545 (95.30%)	*	70	68 (2.19%)	*
	Missing	*	*	*	*	*	*
Sex	Male	8,254 (71.92%)	7,602 (92.11%)	652 (7.89%)	548	517 (0.99%)	90 (0.99%)
	Female	3,218 (28.04%)	3,043 (94.56%)	175 (5.44%)	245	236 (0.95%)	32 (0.95%)
	Missing	*	*	*	*	*	*
Median income for zip code	Low	3,170 (27.62%)	2,900 (91.47%)	270 (8.53%)	304	276 (1.47%)	56 (1.47%)
	Not low	8,093 (70.52%)	7,533 (93.08%)	560 (6.92%)	546	523 (0.88%)	76 (0.88%)
	Missing	213 (1.85%)	213 (100.00%)	*	36	36 (0.00%)	*
Region	Northeast	1,072 (9.34%)	1,023 (95.46%)	*	229	222 (2.45%)	*
	Midwest	3,116 (27.15%)	2,879 (92.40%)	237 (7.60%)	408	387 (1.65%)	56 (1.65%)
	South	5,606 (48.85%)	5,117 (91.28%)	489 (8.72%)	535	496 (1.18%)	79 (1.18%)
	West	1,683 (14.66%)	1,627 (96.67%)	*	263	261 (1.91%)	*

* Denotes missing values

TABLE 103

Patient and hospital characteristics for ICD-9-CM first-listed diagnosis code 410.01 Ami Anterolateral, Init

		All ED visits (those that resulted in admission to the hospital and those that did not)	Only hospital visits that originated in the ED	Only ED visits that ended in discharge (no hospital admission)	Standard errors		
					All ED Visits	Admitted to the hospital from the ED	Discharged from the ED
All discharges		13,337 (100.00%)	10,596 (100.00%)	2,741 (100.00%)	596	584	164
Age (mean)		63.36	64.13	60.41	0.33	0.33	0.33
Age group	18–44	1,412 (10.59%)	1,077 (76.25%)	335 (23.75%)	102	92 (2.66%)	41 (2.66%)
	45–64	5,945 (44.57%)	4,555 (76.62%)	1,390 (23.38%)	308	298 (1.83%)	103 (1.83%)
	65–84	4,690 (35.17%)	3,810 (81.23%)	881 (18.77%)	243	235 (1.61%)	72 (1.61%)
	85+	1,290 (9.67%)	1,154 (89.51%)	135 (10.49%)	90	85 (1.85%)	25 (1.85%)
Sex	Male	8,795 (65.94%)	6,745 (76.70%)	2,050 (23.30%)	414	403 (1.66%)	136 (1.66%)
	Female	4,542 (34.06%)	3,851 (84.78%)	691 (15.22%)	238	228 (1.38%)	62 (1.38%)
Median income for zip code	Low	3,387 (25.40%)	2,587 (76.37%)	800 (23.63%)	216	194 (2.33%)	87 (2.33%)
	Not low	9,558 (71.67%)	7,744 (81.02%)	1,814 (18.98%)	467	454 (1.45%)	130 (1.45%)
	Missing	392 (2.94%)	265 (67.64%)	127 (32.36%)	53	45 (5.81%)	26 (5.81%)
Region	Northeast	2,395 (17.96%)	1,836 (76.66%)	559 (23.34%)	259	242 (3.48%)	82 (3.48%)
	Midwest	3,400 (25.49%)	2,624 (77.17%)	776 (22.83%)	323	309 (2.76%)	83 (2.76%)
	South	5,355 (40.15%)	4,324 (80.74%)	1,031 (19.26%)	378	383 (2.13%)	94 (2.13%)
	West	2,187 (16.40%)	1,812 (82.87%)	375 (17.13%)	201	200 (3.20%)	67 (3.20%)

TABLE 104

Patient and hospital characteristics for ICD-9-CM first-listed diagnosis code 410.10 Ami Anterior Wall, Unspec

		All ED visits (those that resulted in admission to the hospital and those that did not)	Only hospital visits that originated in the ED	Only ED visits that ended in discharge (no hospital admission)	Standard errors		
					All ED Visits	Admitted to the hospital from the ED	Discharged from the ED
All discharges		1,209 (100.00%)	276 (100.00%)	933 (100.00%)	126	51	115
Age (mean)		62.82	67.41	61.47	0.85	0.85	0.85
Age group	18–44	75 (6.21%)	*	67 (89.90%)	18	*	17 (6.84%)
	45–64	621 (51.40%)	117 (18.80%)	504 (81.20%)	79	24 (3.86%)	75 (3.86%)
	65–84	447 (37.00%)	118 (26.28%)	330 (73.72%)	63	33 (6.30%)	54 (6.30%)
	85+	65 (5.39%)	*	*	18	*	*
Sex	Male	878 (72.68%)	175 (19.93%)	703 (80.07%)	103	38 (4.09%)	95 (4.09%)
	Female	330 (27.32%)	101 (30.44%)	230 (69.56%)	48	28 (6.80%)	38 (6.80%)
Median income for zipcode	Low	280 (23.14%)	*	204 (73.10%)	43	*	35 (7.59%)
	Not low	901 (74.57%)	196 (21.71%)	706 (78.29%)	110	40 (4.38%)	105 (4.38%)
	Missing	*	*	*	*	*	*
Region	Northeast	245 (20.29%)	*	211 (86.18%)	57	*	55 (5.33%)
	Midwest	281 (23.23%)	49 (17.48%)	*	79	15 (5.85%)	*
	South	446 (36.88%)	134 (29.97%)	312 (70.03%)	64	39 (7.21%)	53 (7.21%)
	West	237 (19.59%)	*	178 (75.11%)	49	*	42 (10.08%)

* Denotes missing values

TABLE 105

Patient and hospital characteristics for ICD-9-CM first-listed diagnosis code 410.11 Ami Anterior Wall, Init

		All ED visits (those that resulted in admission to the hospital and those that did not)	Only hospital visits that originated in the ED	Only ED visits that ended in discharge (no hospital admission)	Standard errors		
					All ED Visits	Admitted to the hospital from the ED	Discharged from the ED
All discharges		43,112 (100.00%)	37,562 (100.00%)	5,550 (100.00%)	1,731	1,743	287
Age (mean)		64.24	64.52	62.34	0.22	0.22	0.22
Age group	1–17	*	*	*	*	*	*
	18–44	3,769 (8.74%)	3,288 (87.25%)	481 (12.75%)	213	208 (1.45%)	54 (1.45%)
	45–64	19,213 (44.57%)	16,444 (85.59%)	2,769 (14.41%)	825	827 (1.02%)	166 (1.02%)
	65–84	15,352 (35.61%)	13,456 (87.65%)	1,896 (12.35%)	680	678 (1.00%)	139 (1.00%)
	85+	4,769 (11.06%)	4,364 (91.50%)	405 (8.50%)	232	226 (0.97%)	46 (0.97%)
Sex	Male	28,259 (65.55%)	24,313 (86.04%)	3,946 (13.96%)	1,185	1,192 (0.96%)	225 (0.96%)
	Female	14,853 (34.45%)	13,248 (89.20%)	1,604 (10.80%)	617	613 (0.83%)	112 (0.83%)
Median income for zip code	Low	10,595 (24.58%)	9,078 (85.69%)	1,516 (14.31%)	624	612 (1.42%)	140 (1.42%)
	Not low	31,442 (72.93%)	27,547 (87.61%)	3,895 (12.39%)	1,358	1,351 (0.84%)	222 (0.84%)
	Missing	1,075 (2.49%)	937 (87.11%)	139 (12.89%)	127	122 (2.89%)	31 (2.89%)
Region	Northeast	7,226 (16.76%)	6,242 (86.38%)	984 (13.62%)	720	710 (1.94%)	117 (1.94%)
	Midwest	10,569 (24.51%)	8,917 (84.37%)	1,651 (15.63%)	723	722 (1.71%)	155 (1.71%)
	South	17,260 (40.04%)	15,246 (88.33%)	2,014 (11.67%)	1,235	1,240 (1.27%)	171 (1.27%)
	West	8,057 (18.69%)	7,157 (88.82%)	900 (11.18%)	656	689 (1.91%)	123 (1.91%)

* Denotes missing values

TABLE 106

Patient and hospital characteristics for ICD-9-CM first-listed diagnosis code 410.21 Ami Inferolateral, Init

		All ED visits (those that resulted in admission to the hospital and those that did not)	Only hospital visits that originated in the ED	Only ED visits that ended in discharge (no hospital admission)	Standard errors		
					All ED Visits	Admitted to the hospital from the ED	Discharged from the ED
All discharges		10,789 (100.00%)	8,608 (100.00%)	2,181 (100.00%)	478	461	164
Age (mean)		63.03	63.21	62.33	0.35	0.35	0.35
Age group	1–17	*	*	*	*	*	*
	18–44	988 (9.16%)	811 (82.04%)	178 (17.96%)	77	73 (2.95%)	31 (2.95%)
	45–64	5,017 (46.50%)	3,906 (77.85%)	1,111 (22.15%)	258	236 (2.02%)	110 (2.02%)
	65–84	3,830 (35.50%)	3,093 (80.75%)	737 (19.25%)	199	192 (1.77%)	67 (1.77%)
	85+	949 (8.80%)	798 (84.05%)	151 (15.95%)	80	75 (2.85%)	29 (2.85%)
Sex	Male	7,090 (65.72%)	5,602 (79.00%)	1,489 (21.00%)	333	317 (1.67%)	119 (1.67%)
	Female	3,699 (34.28%)	3,006 (81.27%)	693 (18.73%)	192	183 (1.87%)	71 (1.87%)
Median income for zip code	Low	2,543 (23.57%)	2,004 (78.81%)	539 (21.19%)	192	160 (3.44%)	103 (3.44%)
	Not low	7,980 (73.96%)	6,397 (80.17%)	1,582 (19.83%)	380	368 (1.55%)	119 (1.55%)
	Missing	267 (2.47%)	207 (77.44%)	*	42	37 (6.30%)	*
Region	Northeast	1,801 (16.69%)	1,510 (83.88%)	290 (16.12%)	194	191 (3.07%)	52 (3.07%)
	Midwest	2,679 (24.83%)	1,962 (73.24%)	717 (26.76%)	248	236 (3.48%)	89 (3.48%)
	South	4,538 (42.06%)	3,619 (79.75%)	919 (20.25%)	315	300 (2.57%)	119 (2.57%)
	West	1,771 (16.42%)	1,516 (85.60%)	255 (14.40%)	175	173 (2.70%)	45 (2.70%)

* Denotes missing values

TABLE 107

Patient and hospital characteristics for
ICD-9-CM first-listed diagnosis code
410.31 Ami Inferopost, Initial

		All ED visits (those that resulted in admission to the hospital and those that did not)	Only hospital visits that originated in the ED	Only ED visits that ended in discharge (no hospital admission)	Standard errors		
					All ED Visits	Admitted to the hospital from the ED	Discharged from the ED
All discharges		6,994 (100.00%)	6,126 (100.00%)	868 (100.00%)	371	361	88
Age (mean)		63.30	63.38	62.76	0.36	0.36	0.36
Age group	18–44	491 (7.02%)	439 (89.44%)	*	56	53 (3.04%)	*
	45–64	3,402 (48.65%)	2,971 (87.32%)	431 (12.68%)	207	200 (1.52%)	52 (1.52%)
	65–84	2,612 (37.35%)	2,271 (86.92%)	342 (13.08%)	160	155 (1.71%)	45 (1.71%)
	85+	488 (6.98%)	446 (91.23%)	*	55	52 (3.15%)	*
Sex	Male	4,883 (69.83%)	4,241 (86.85%)	642 (13.15%)	269	261 (1.40%)	67 (1.40%)
	Female	2,110 (30.17%)	1,885 (89.31%)	226 (10.69%)	135	130 (1.73%)	38 (1.73%)
Median income for zip code	Low	1,577 (22.55%)	1,371 (86.95%)	206 (13.05%)	159	150 (2.17%)	35 (2.17%)
	Not low	5,288 (75.61%)	4,638 (87.71%)	650 (12.29%)	290	282 (1.47%)	78 (1.47%)
	Missing	129 (1.84%)	117 (90.68%)	*	30	29 (5.34%)	*
Region	Northeast	1,476 (21.11%)	1,281 (86.80%)	195 (13.20%)	188	185 (2.94%)	41 (2.94%)
	Midwest	2,008 (28.72%)	1,775 (88.36%)	234 (11.64%)	169	166 (2.14%)	43 (2.14%)
	South	2,461 (35.19%)	2,107 (85.59%)	355 (14.41%)	242	234 (2.51%)	60 (2.51%)
	West	1,048 (14.98%)	963 (91.94%)	84 (8.06%)	122	118 (2.23%)	24 (2.23%)

* Denotes missing values

TABLE 108

Patient and hospital characteristics for
ICD-9-CM first-listed diagnosis code
410.41 Ami Inferior Wall, Init

		All ED visits (those that resulted in admission to the hospital and those that did not)	Only hospital visits that originated in the ED	Only ED visits that ended in discharge (no hospital admission)	Standard errors		
					All ED Visits	Admitted to the hospital from the ED	Discharged from the ED
All discharges		62,514 (100.00%)	51,145 (100.00%)	11,369 (100.00%)	2,297	2,325	511
Age (mean)		62.62	62.76	61.99	0.18	0.18	0.18
Age group	1–17	*	*	*	*	*	*
	18–44	5,234 (8.37%)	4,228 (80.78%)	1,006 (19.22%)	265	252 (1.59%)	84 (1.59%)
	45–64	31,187 (49.89%)	25,403 (81.45%)	5,784 (18.55%)	1,223	1,227 (1.15%)	302 (1.15%)
	65–84	21,416 (34.26%)	17,522 (81.82%)	3,893 (18.18%)	841	843 (1.14%)	208 (1.14%)
	85+	4,668 (7.47%)	3,988 (85.42%)	681 (14.58%)	229	210 (1.38%)	70 (1.38%)
Sex	Male	42,935 (68.68%)	35,043 (81.62%)	7,892 (18.38%)	1,637	1,649 (1.07%)	374 (1.07%)
	Female	19,575 (31.31%)	16,097 (82.24%)	3,477 (17.76%)	747	747 (1.12%)	192 (1.12%)
	Missing	*	*	*	*	*	*
Median income for zip code	Low	15,445 (24.71%)	12,370 (80.09%)	3,075 (19.91%)	856	823 (1.54%)	220 (1.54%)
	Not low	45,543 (72.85%)	37,577 (82.51%)	7,967 (17.49%)	1,812	1,815 (1.10%)	426 (1.10%)
	Missing	1,526 (2.44%)	1,198 (78.53%)	328 (21.47%)	151	144 (3.25%)	49 (3.25%)
Region	Northeast	9,851 (15.76%)	7,860 (79.80%)	1,990 (20.20%)	903	886 (2.44%)	196 (2.44%)
	Midwest	16,035 (25.65%)	12,522 (78.09%)	3,513 (21.91%)	1,038	1,032 (2.07%)	279 (2.07%)
	South	25,438 (40.69%)	21,258 (83.57%)	4,180 (16.43%)	1,624	1,649 (1.55%)	289 (1.55%)
	West	11,191 (17.90%)	9,505 (84.93%)	1,686 (15.07%)	865	915 (2.57%)	248 (2.57%)

* Denotes missing values

TABLE 109

Patient and hospital characteristics for ICD-9-CM first-listed diagnosis code 410.51 Ami Lateral Nec, Initial

		All ED visits (those that resulted in admission to the hospital and those that did not)	Only hospital visits that originated in the ED	Only ED visits that ended in discharge (no hospital admission)	Standard errors		
					All ED Visits	Admitted to the hospital from the ED	Discharged from the ED
All discharges		6,033 (100.00%)	5,077 (100.00%)	956 (100.00%)	299	291	96
Age (mean)		64.57	64.75	63.62	0.47	0.47	0.47
Age group	1–17	*	*	*	*	*	*
	18–44	491 (8.14%)	390 (79.45%)	101 (20.55%)	58	52 (4.14%)	22 (4.14%)
	45–64	2,620 (43.42%)	2,228 (85.04%)	392 (14.96%)	158	152 (2.02%)	54 (2.02%)
	65–84	2,268 (37.60%)	1,918 (84.53%)	351 (15.47%)	134	127 (1.92%)	45 (1.92%)
	85+	642 (10.65%)	538 (83.70%)	105 (16.30%)	58	53 (3.60%)	25 (3.60%)
Sex	Male	3,868 (64.12%)	3,254 (84.11%)	615 (15.89%)	221	213 (1.95%)	77 (1.95%)
	Female	2,165 (35.88%)	1,824 (84.24%)	341 (15.76%)	119	112 (1.97%)	45 (1.97%)
Median income for zip code	Low	1,430 (23.69%)	1,161 (81.19%)	269 (18.81%)	127	115 (3.35%)	53 (3.35%)
	Not low	4,483 (74.30%)	3,818 (85.17%)	665 (14.83%)	239	231 (1.55%)	69 (1.55%)
	Missing	121 (2.00%)	99 (81.65%)	*	24	22 (7.56%)	*
Region	Northeast	888 (14.72%)	757 (85.24%)	131 (14.76%)	123	115 (3.77%)	36 (3.77%)
	Midwest	1,497 (24.82%)	1,236 (82.55%)	261 (17.45%)	129	123 (3.05%)	47 (3.05%)
	South	2,522 (41.80%)	2,094 (83.03%)	428 (16.97%)	213	210 (2.37%)	54 (2.37%)
	West	1,126 (18.66%)	990 (87.96%)	*	111	109 (4.48%)	*

* Denotes missing values

TABLE 110
Patient and hospital characteristics for ICD-9-CM first-listed diagnosis code 410.71 Subendo Infarct, Initial

		All ED visits (those that resulted in admission to the hospital and those that did not)	Only hospital visits that originated in the ED	Only ED visits that ended in discharge (no hospital admission)	Standard errors		
					All ED Visits	Admitted to the hospital from the ED	Discharged from the ED
All discharges		310,656 (100.00%)	296,570 (100.00%)	14,085 (100.00%)	10,329	10,236	744
Age (mean)		70.31	70.60	64.25	0.17	0.17	0.17
Age group	1–17	*	*	*	*	*	*
	18–44	13,437 (4.33%)	12,264 (91.27%)	1,173 (8.73%)	531	515 (0.64%)	85 (0.64%)
	45–64	95,144 (30.63%)	89,085 (93.63%)	6,059 (6.37%)	3,357	3,300 (0.39%)	355 (0.39%)
	65–84	144,054 (46.37%)	138,449 (96.11%)	5,605 (3.89%)	4,991	4,966 (0.26%)	348 (0.26%)
	85+	58,010 (18.67%)	56,768 (97.86%)	1,242 (2.14%)	2,189	2,169 (0.17%)	99 (0.17%)
Sex	Male	172,280 (55.46%)	163,653 (94.99%)	8,627 (5.01%)	5,935	5,878 (0.29%)	460 (0.29%)
	Female	138,372 (44.54%)	132,917 (96.06%)	5,454 (3.94%)	4,524	4,487 (0.25%)	328 (0.25%)
	Missing	*	*	*	*	*	*
Median income for zip code	Low	83,259 (26.80%)	78,802 (94.65%)	4,457 (5.35%)	4,443	4,353 (0.46%)	377 (0.46%)
	Not low	219,329 (70.60%)	210,023 (95.76%)	9,306 (4.24%)	7,968	7,878 (0.27%)	554 (0.27%)
	Missing	8,068 (2.60%)	7,746 (96.00%)	323 (4.00%)	814	812 (0.67%)	46 (0.67%)
Region	Northeast	65,256 (21.01%)	63,454 (97.24%)	1,802 (2.76%)	4,739	4,692 (0.34%)	215 (0.34%)
	Midwest	66,742 (21.48%)	62,790 (94.08%)	3,952 (5.92%)	4,397	4,293 (0.62%)	405 (0.62%)
	South	125,412 (40.37%)	119,384 (95.19%)	6,028 (4.81%)	7,164	7,131 (0.42%)	432 (0.42%)
	West	53,246 (17.14%)	50,943 (95.67%)	2,304 (4.33%)	3,685	3,672 (0.78%)	396 (0.78%)

* Denotes missing values

TABLE 111

Patient and hospital characteristics for ICD-9-CM first-listed diagnosis code 410.72 Subendo Infarct, Subseq

		All ED visits (those that resulted in admission to the hospital and those that did not)	Only hospital visits that originated in the ED	Only ED visits that ended in discharge (no hospital admission)	Standard errors		
					All ED Visits	Admitted to the hospital from the ED	Discharged from the ED
All discharges		1,242 (100.00%)	1,076 (100.00%)	166 (100.00%)	91	83	37
Age (mean)		70.84	70.69	71.84	0.96	0.96	0.96
Age group	18–44	70 (5.62%)	61 (87.60%)	*	18	17 (8.26%)	*
	45–64	350 (28.22%)	318 (90.82%)	*	43	40 (3.28%)	*
	65–84	537 (43.24%)	460 (85.68%)	*	55	51 (4.09%)	*
	85+	284 (22.91%)	236 (82.98%)	*	39	35 (5.70%)	*
Sex	Male	689 (55.51%)	596 (86.49%)	93 (13.51%)	63	58 (3.43%)	26 (3.43%)
	Female	553 (44.49%)	479 (86.78%)	73 (13.22%)	56	52 (3.61%)	21 (3.61%)
Median income for zip code	Low	271 (21.84%)	252 (92.88%)	*	36	35 (3.52%)	*
	Not low	897 (72.22%)	754 (84.07%)	143 (15.93%)	77	69 (3.52%)	35 (3.52%)
	Missing	*	*	*	*	*	*
Region	Northeast	261 (21.00%)	236 (90.31%)	*	40	39 (4.20%)	*
	Midwest	186 (14.97%)	145 (77.79%)	*	33	27 (7.77%)	*
	South	459 (36.95%)	409 (89.16%)	*	52	49 (3.22%)	*
	West	336 (27.08%)	286 (85.18%)	*	55	47 (6.97%)	*

* Denotes missing values

TABLE 112
Patient and hospital characteristics for ICD-9-CM first-listed diagnosis code 410.81 Ami Nec, Initial

		All ED visits (those that resulted in admission to the hospital and those that did not)	Only hospital visits that originated in the ED	Only ED visits that ended in discharge (no hospital admission)	Standard errors		
					All ED Visits	Admitted to the hospital from the ED	Discharged from the ED
All discharges		6,556 (100.00%)	4,750 (100.00%)	1,806 (100.00%)	525	489	191
Age (mean)		68.04	69.69	63.72	0.60	0.60	0.60
Age group	18–44	400 (6.09%)	234 (58.59%)	165 (41.41%)	50	38 (6.57%)	34 (6.57%)
	45–64	2,355 (35.92%)	1,589 (67.47%)	766 (32.53%)	236	215 (3.91%)	92 (3.91%)
	65–84	2,644 (40.33%)	1,928 (72.90%)	716 (27.10%)	230	211 (3.29%)	90 (3.29%)
	85+	1,158 (17.66%)	999 (86.32%)	158 (13.68%)	115	110 (3.09%)	37 (3.09%)
Sex	Male	3,835 (58.50%)	2,665 (69.49%)	1,170 (30.51%)	335	311 (3.35%)	125 (3.35%)
	Female	2,721 (41.50%)	2,085 (76.62%)	636 (23.38%)	218	202 (2.94%)	84 (2.94%)
Median income for zip code	Low	1,851 (28.24%)	1,237 (66.80%)	615 (33.20%)	308	289 (6.20%)	99 (6.20%)
	Not low	4,448 (67.84%)	3,315 (74.53%)	1,133 (25.47%)	366	339 (2.96%)	135 (2.96%)
	Missing	257 (3.92%)	*	59 (22.83%)	69	*	17 (7.71%)
Region	Northeast	1,840 (28.06%)	1,408 (76.53%)	*	311	275 (7.10%)	*
	Midwest	1,136 (17.33%)	663 (58.39%)	473 (41.61%)	111	88 (4.92%)	70 (4.92%)
	South	2,551 (38.90%)	1,898 (74.40%)	653 (25.60%)	386	376 (4.45%)	82 (4.45%)
	West	1,030 (15.70%)	781 (75.84%)	249 (24.16%)	132	120 (4.82%)	53 (4.82%)

* Denotes missing values

Myocardial infarction (MI) is also more prevalent in men than women and it is more prevalent in the South and the Midwest followed by the Northeast and the West. This trend is the same for all types of MI.

TABLE 113
Patient and hospital characteristics for ICD-9-CM first-listed diagnosis code 410.90 Ami Nos, Unspecified

		All ED visits (those that resulted in admission to the hospital and those that did not)	Only hospital visits that originated in the ED	Only ED visits that ended in discharge (no hospital admission)	Standard errors		
					All ED Visits	Admitted to the hospital from the ED	Discharged from the ED
All discharges		10,231 (100.00%)	622 (100.00%)	9,609 (100.00%)	848	91	835
Age (mean)		64.53	71.34	64.09	0.50	0.50	0.50
Age group	1–17	*	*	*	*	*	*
	18–44	908 (8.88%)	*	875 (96.37%)	109	*	108 (1.31%)
	45–64	4,408 (43.08%)	178 (4.03%)	4,230 (95.97%)	416	44 (1.00%)	410 (1.00%)
	65–84	3,677 (35.94%)	248 (6.75%)	3,429 (93.25%)	336	51 (1.39%)	329 (1.39%)
	85+	1,233 (12.05%)	163 (13.21%)	1,070 (86.79%)	106	30 (2.32%)	100 (2.32%)
Sex	Male	6,603 (64.53%)	327 (4.95%)	6,276 (95.05%)	575	60 (0.92%)	566 (0.92%)
	Female	3,624 (35.42%)	295 (8.14%)	3,329 (91.86%)	306	47 (1.33%)	299 (1.33%)
	Missing	*	*	*	*	*	*
Median income for zip code	Low	2,932 (28.66%)	223 (7.61%)	2,709 (92.39%)	306	57 (1.77%)	288 (1.77%)
	Not low	7,091 (69.31%)	390 (5.50%)	6,701 (94.50%)	714	63 (0.99%)	709 (0.99%)
	Missing	208 (2.03%)	*	199 (95.78%)	43	*	43 (2.99%)
Region	Northeast	1,620 (15.83%)	*	1,556 (96.09%)	265	*	261 (1.38%)
	Midwest	3,231 (31.58%)	207 (6.41%)	3,023 (93.59%)	652	52 (1.85%)	645 (1.85%)
	South	3,585 (35.04%)	226 (6.30%)	3,359 (93.70%)	329	47 (1.32%)	322 (1.32%)
	West	1,796 (17.55%)	*	1,671 (93.01%)	340	*	332 (2.96%)

* Denotes missing values

TABLE 114

Patient and hospital characteristics for ICD-9-CM first-listed diagnosis code 410.91 Ami Nos, Initial

		All ED visits (those that resulted in admission to the hospital and those that did not)	Only hospital visits that originated in the ED	Only ED visits that ended in discharge (no hospital admission)	Standard errors		
					All ED Visits	Admitted to the hospital from the ED	Discharged from the ED
All discharges		58,739 (100.00%)	26,769 (100.00%)	31,970 (100.00%)	1,698	1,068	1,217
Age (mean)		67.70	72.01	64.09	0.23	0.23	0.23
Age group	1–17	*	*	*	*	*	*
	18–44	4,122 (7.02%)	1,282 (31.10%)	2,840 (68.90%)	190	88 (1.91%)	166 (1.91%)
	45–64	21,048 (35.83%)	7,261 (34.50%)	13,787 (65.50%)	659	375 (1.57%)	578 (1.57%)
	65–84	23,673 (40.30%)	11,381 (48.08%)	12,292 (51.92%)	778	473 (1.40%)	547 (1.40%)
	85+	9,871 (16.81%)	6,840 (69.29%)	3,032 (30.71%)	397	324 (1.44%)	177 (1.44%)
Sex	Male	35,868 (61.06%)	14,748 (41.12%)	21,120 (58.88%)	1,051	638 (1.40%)	823 (1.40%)
	Female	22,862 (38.92%)	12,017 (52.56%)	10,846 (47.44%)	742	495 (1.34%)	467 (1.34%)
	Missing	*	*	*	*	*	*
Median income for zipcode	Low	18,813 (32.03%)	8,370 (44.49%)	10,443 (55.51%)	1,007	564 (1.82%)	656 (1.82%)
	Not low	38,434 (65.43%)	17,789 (46.28%)	20,646 (53.72%)	1,246	768 (1.48%)	919 (1.48%)
	Missing	1,492 (2.54%)	610 (40.91%)	881 (59.09%)	114	66 (3.35%)	87 (3.35%)
Region	Northeast	8,041 (13.69%)	3,409 (42.40%)	4,632 (57.60%)	623	358 (3.15%)	448 (3.15%)
	Midwest	15,307 (26.06%)	5,810 (37.96%)	9,497 (62.04%)	793	374 (1.86%)	613 (1.86%)
	South	24,040 (40.93%)	11,246 (46.78%)	12,794 (53.22%)	1,114	738 (2.28%)	828 (2.28%)
	West	11,351 (19.32%)	6,304 (55.53%)	5,048 (44.47%)	790	572 (2.96%)	468 (2.96%)

* Denotes missing values

Summary of Cholesterol Production and Consequences

Coronary artery disease and myocardial infarction (MI) are also more prevalent in the South and the Midwest followed by the Northeast and the West. This trend is the same for all types of MI. MI occurs as men get older. The groups that get prostate cancer because of high estrogen levels are the same groups prone to MI. These groups tend to have low testosterone. This makes sense because low testosterone leads to high insulin that leads to ventral obesity in men and, hence, high risk of MI. Testosterone is often lost to estrogens in older men and that is the time when they develop the gynecomastia ("man boobs"). When estrogen increases, insulin increases. Men at that time crave for sweets, just like women do in their late luteal phase, and therefore become obese. The high endogenous estrogens in aging men coupled with the environmental estrogens lead to obesity, prostate cancer, and benign prostatic hypertrophy. Men with low testosterone and high estrogen problems also have many of the symptoms listed for women with estrogen dominance. Most common symptoms are fatigue, irritability, apathy, lack of ambition, decreased libido (no testosterone, no libido for both men and women), anxiety, nervousness, depression, weight gain (pot bellies—and beer can make it worse due to hops which is a phytoestrogen), high blood pressure, diabetes, and hypercholesterolemia. These conditions represent the bulk of what primary care physicians treat. They are mostly hormone related, and the hormones are not checked by most of these physicians. I have seen some physicians starting patients on testosterone gels and injections when patients complain of low libido, without even measuring the testosterone level. Some healthcare providers measure the testosterone level and start their patients on testosterone replacement therapy but they never check the estradiol, estrone or DHT levels. Most of these patients end up converting their testosterone gel or injections into estrone and some estradiol; others convert the testosterone to DHT. These by-products of testosterone can cause more harm by causing prostate enlargement or even prostate cancer if the estrogens become too high and remain imbalanced over a long period of time. It is important to measure the hormones (see lab work list on page 195) prior to starting anyone on hormones. Once a patient is on bio-identical hormones, then follow-up should

SUMMARY OF ENDOGENOUS HORMONE IMBALANCE PROCESSES AND CONSEQUENCES

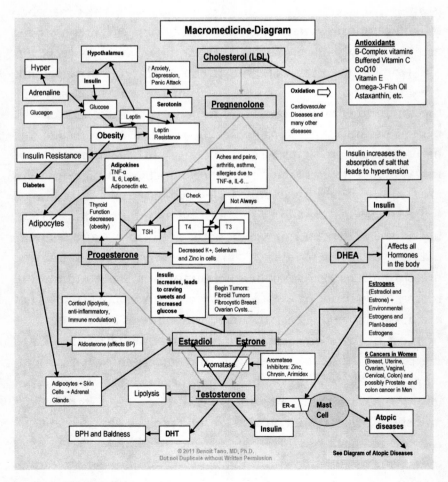

© 2010 Benoit Tano, MD, PhD

be every three months and the patient should have full access to the physician for adjustment of the hormones. Remember to re-measure some of the hormones by six months or sooner if the patient still complains of symptoms.

The End Results of Endogenous Hormone Production Imbalance Are the Following:

- Progesterone deficiency
- Estrogen dominance
- Thyroid deficiency
- Leptin resistance
- Insulin resistance
- Hyperlipidemia
- DHEA deficiency
- Testosterone deficiency

While obesity and its comorbidities are increasing rapidly worldwide, allergic diseases also seem to follow the same pattern. In the case of growing atopic diseases, environmental pollution and the estrogen epidemic seem to greatly contribute to this growing phenomenon. The next chapter will shed some light on this growing problem.

CHAPTER 6

THE ESTROGEN EPIDEMIC AND ATOPIC DISEASES

- Allergy in childhood
- Estrogen dominance and adult onset allergies
    - Allergic Rhinitis
    - Chronic Sinusitis
    - Food Allergy
    - Medication Allergy
    - Urticaria and Angioedema

The 2010 Allergy and Asthma Statistics as reported by the American Academy of Allergy Asthma & Immunology-AAAAI (obtained from the CDC annual reports):

General
- A nationwide survey found that more than half (54.6%) of all US citizens test positive to one or more allergens.[6]
- In a recent survey, over fifty percent of homes had at least six detectable allergens present.[23]

- Allergic diseases affect as many as 40 to 50 million Americans.[24]

Allergic Rhinitis

- In 2006, eight percent of adults and over nine percent of children had been diagnosed with hay fever in the past twelve months.[1, 2]
- There were more than 12 million physician office visits because of allergic rhinitis in 2006.[3]
- Allergic rhinitis affects between ten percent and thirty percent of all adults and as many as forty percent of children.[4]
- The prevalence of rhinitis is around thirty five percent in Europe and Australasia, according to the European Community Respiratory Health Survey (ECRHS).[5]
- From 2000 to 2005, the cost of treating allergic rhinitis almost doubled from $6.1 billion (in 2005 dollars) to $11.2 billion. More than half of that was spent on prescription medications.[10]
- Immunotherapy helps reduce hay fever symptoms in about eighty five percent of people with allergic rhinitis.[24]
- Allergic Rhinitis is estimated to affect approximately 60 million people in the United States, and its prevalence is increasing.[27]

Sinusitis

- Sinusitis accounts for approximately twenty percent of office visits to specialists in allergy and immunology.[21]
- Approximately twelve percent of Americans under the age of forty five have symptoms of chronic sinusitis.[21]
- In one study, fifty five percent of patients with sinusitis also had a history of allergic rhinitis.[21]
- Sinusitis is one of the leading forms of chronic disease, with an estimated 18 million cases and at least 30 million courses of antibiotics per year.[22]

* About 40,000 people have sinus surgery every year.[22]

Drug Allergy
* Anaphylactic reactions to penicillin cause 400 deaths each year.[7]
* Between six percent and ten percent of adverse drug reactions are allergic or immunologic in nature.[15]
* Between twenty nine percent and sixty five percent of patients with HIV/AIDS are allergic to sulfonamide drugs, compared to two percent to four percent of other individuals.[16]
* Penicillin is the most common cause of drug-induced anaphylaxis.[20]

Skin Allergies
* About twenty seven percent of children who have a food allergy also have eczema or a skin allergy.[8]
* Contact dermatitis leads to approximately 5.7 million doctor visits each year.[18]
* More than 3,700 substances have been identified as contact allergens.[18]
* Atopic dermatitis affects between ten percent and twenty percent of children and one percent to three percent of adults.[19]
* As many as fifteen percent to twenty four percent of people in the United States will experience acute urticaria (hives) and/or angioedema at some point in their lives.[25]

Food Allergy
* In 2007, approximately 3 million children under the age of eighteen were reported to have a food or digestive allergy in the previous twelve months.[8]
* The prevalence of food allergy among children under the age of eighteen increased eighteen percent from 1997 to 2007.[8]

- Kids with a food allergy are two to four times more likely to have conditions such as asthma and other allergies.[8]

- Food allergies affect about six percent of children under the age of three.[11]

- Six and a half million Americans (or 2.3 percent of the general population) are allergic to seafood.[12]

- More than 3 million people in the United States report being allergic to peanuts, tree nuts or both.[13]

- More than three percent of adults have one or more food allergies.[14]

- Food allergies account for thirty five to fifty percent of all cases of anaphylaxis.[20]

- Food allergies affect approximately six percent of young children and three to four percent of adults in the US population.[27]

- Milk allergy is the most common childhood food allergy, affecting 2.5 percent of children less than age three. Eighty percent of milk allergy is outgrown by age sixteen.[30]

- Egg allergy is the second most common food allergy in children, affecting 1.5–3.2 percent of children. Sixty eight of egg allergy is outgrown by age sixteen.[31]

- Peanut allergy affects 1.2 percent of children. Approximately twenty percent of children outgrow it by age six.[32]

- Tree nut allergy (almonds, walnuts, etc.) affects 1.2 percent of the population. Approximately nine percent of children outgrow tree nut allergy by age six.[33]

- Peanut allergy doubled in children from 1997–2002.[34]

- Most peanut allergic patients can safely eat other legumes such as soy or beans (ninety five percent), but they can have concurrent allergy to tree nuts such as walnuts or pecans (twenty five to fifty percent).[32]

- Skin contact and inhalation exposure to peanut butter are unlikely to cause systemic reactions or anaphylaxis.[35]

- Anaphylaxis occurs in twenty percent of allergic reactions to peanuts and tree nuts.[36]

- It is estimated that the number of cases of anaphylaxis from foods in the US increased from 21,000 per year in 1999 to 51,000 per year in 2008, based on long term population studies of anaphylaxis from the Mayo Clinic in Minnesota.[29, 37]

- From 2003 to 2006, food allergies resulted in approximately 317,000 visits to hospital emergency departments, outpatient clinics and physicians' offices, according to Branum and colleagues, using data from multiple US national surveys collected by the National Center for Health Statistics.[38]

- Food allergy related hospital admissions increased from 2,600 per year (1998–2000) to 9,500 per year (2004–2006), according to a study from Branum and colleagues.[38]

- It is estimated that food allergies cause approximately 150 to 200 fatalities per year, based on data from a five year study of anaphylaxis in Minnesota from the Mayo Clinic.[39]

- Fatal food anaphylaxis is most often caused by peanuts (fifty to sixty two percent) and tree nuts (fifteen to thirty percent).[40]

- Risk factors for fatal anaphylaxis include failure or delay in administration of epinephrine, history of asthma and teenagers.[41, 42]

Insect Sting Allergy

- At least forty people in the United States die each year as the result of insect stings.[17]

- Life-threatening reactions to insect stings occur in 0.4 percent to 0.8 percent of children and three percent of adults.[17]

- The estimated annual economic impact of imported fire ants is $1.2 billion in Texas alone.[26]

Latex Allergy

- Latex allergy affects between five percent and fifteen percent of healthcare workers, but less than one percent of the general population.[9]
- Between twenty four percent and sixty percent of people with spina bifida have latex allergy.[9]

Sources:

1. Pleis JR, Lethbridge-Çejku M. Summary health statistics for US Adults: National Health Interview Survey, 2006. National Center for Health Statistics. Vital Health Stat 10(235), 2007.

2. Bloom B, Cohen RA. Summary Health Statistics for US Children: National Health Interview Survey, 2006. National Center for Health Statistics. Vital Health Stat 10(234), 2007.

3. Cherry DK, Hing E, Woodwell DA, Rechtsteiner EA. National Ambulatory Medical Care Survey: 2006 Summary. National Health Statistics Reports; No 3. Hyattsville, MD: National Center for Health Statistics, 2008.

4. The Diagnosis and Management of Rhinitis: An Updated Practice Parameter. Joint Task Force on Practice Parameters. *J Allergy Clin Immunol.* 2008; 122: S1–S84.

5. Janson C et al. The European Community Respiratory Health Survey: what are the main results so far? *European Respiratory Journal.* 2001; 18:598–611.

6. Arbes SJ et al. Prevalences of positive skin test responses to 10 common allergens in the US population: Results from the Third National Health and Nutrition Examination Survey. *J Allergy Clin Immunol,* 2005; 116:377–383.

7. Neugut AL, Ghatak AT and Miller RL. Anaphylaxis in the United States: An investigation into its epidemiology. *Archives of Internal Medicine* 61 (1): 15–21, 2001.

8. Branum AM, Lukacs SL. Food Allergy among U.S. children: Trends in prevalence and hospitalizations. NCHS data brief, no 10. Hyattsville, MD: National Center for Health Statistics, 2008.

9. Poley GE and Slater JE. Latex allergy. *J Allergy Clin Immunol,* 2000; 105:1054–1062.

10. Soni A. Allergic rhinitis: Trends in use and expenditures, 2000 to 2005. Statistical Brief #204, Agency for Healthcare Research and Quality, 2008.

11. Sampson HA. Food allergy. *J Allergy Clin Immunol,* 2003; 111:S540–S547.

12. Munoz-Furlong A, Sampson HA, Sicherer SH. Prevalence of self-reported seafood allergy in the US [abstract] *J Allergy Clin Immunol,* 2004;113(suppl):S100.

13. Sicherer SH, Munoz-Furlong A, Sampson HA. Prevalence of peanut and tree nut allergy in the United States determined by means of a random digit dial telephone survey: A 5-year follow-up study. *J Allergy Clin Immunol,* 2003;112:1203–1207.

14. Sampson HA. Update on food allergy. *J Allergy Clin Immunol,* 2004; 113:805–819.

15. Gruchalla R. Understanding drug allegies. *J Allergy Clin Immunol,* 2000;105:S637–44.

16. Greenberger PA. Drug allergy. *J Allergy Clin Immunol,* 2006; 117:S464–S470

17. Stinging insect hypersensitivity: A practice parameter update. *J Allergy Clin Immunol,* 2004; 114:869–886.

18. Contact dermatitis: A practice parameter. Ann *Allergy Asthma Immunol,* 2006; 97:S1–S38.

19. Disease management of atopic dermatitis: An updated practice parameter. Ann *Allergy Asthma Immunol*, 2004; 93:S1–S21.

20. The diagnosis and management of anaphylaxis: An updated practice parameter. *J Allergy Clin Immunol*, 2005; 115:S483–523.

21. Hamilos DL. Chronic sinusitis. *J Allergy Clin Immunol*, 2000;106:213–27.

22. Platts-Mills TAE, Rosenwasser LJ. Chronic sinusitis consensus and the way forward. *J Allergy Clin Immunol*, 2004; 114: 1359–1361.

23. Salo PM et al. Exposure to multiple indoor allergens in US homes and its relationship to asthma. *J Allergy Clin Immunol*, 2008; 121: 678–684.e2.

24. Airborne allergens: Something in the air. National Institute of Allergy and Infectious Diseases. NIH Publication No. 03-7045, 2003.

25. Urticaria: Part 1. *Annals of Allergy, Asthma and Immunology*, 2000; 85:525–531.

26. Texas Imported Fire Ant Research and Management Project Web site. *http://fireant.tamu.edu*. Accessed June 12, 2009.

27. Nathan RA. The burden of allergic rhinitis. *Allergy Asthma Proc*, 2007;28:3–9.

28. Sicherer SH, Sampson HA. Food allergy. *J Allergy Clin Immunol*, 2006;117:S470–5.

29. Yocum MW, et al. Epidemiology of anaphylaxis in Olmsted County: a population-based study. *J Allergy Clin Immunol*, 1999;104;451–6.

30. Sicherer SH, Sampson HA. Food allergy. *J Allergy Clin Immunol*, 2006;117:S470–5.

31. Savage JH, et al. The natural history of egg allergy. *J Allergy Clin Immunol*, 2007;120:1413–7.

32. Sicherer SH, Sampson HA. Peanut allergy: emerging concepts and approaches for an apparent epidemic. *J Allergy Clin Immunol*, 2007;120:491–503.

33. Fleischer DM, et al. The natural history of tree nut allergy. *J Allergy Clin Immunol*, 2005;116:1087–93.

34. Sicherer SH, et al. Prevalence of peanut and tree nut allergy in the United States determined by means of a random digit dial telephone survey: a 5-year follow-up study. *J Allergy Clin Immunol*, 2003;112:1203–7.

35. Simonte SJ, et al. Relevance of casual contact with peanut butter in children with peanut allergy. *J Allergy Clin Immunol*, 2003;112:180–2.

36. Sicherer SH, et al. Clinical features of acute allergic reactions to peanut and tree nuts in children. *Pediatrics 1998*;102(1) e6.

37. Decker, W, et al. The etiology and incidence of anaphylaxis in Rochester, Minnesota: A report from the Rochester Epidemiology Project. *J Allergy Clin Immunol*, 2008;122:1161–5.

38. Branum AM, et al. Food allergy among children in the United States. *Pediatrics 2009*;124:1549–1555.

39. Sampson HA. Anaphylaxis and emergency treatment. *Pediatrics 2003*;111:1601–08.

40. Keet CA, Wood RA. Food allergy and anaphylaxis. *Immunol Allergy Clin N Am*, 2007;27:193–212.

41. Bock SA, et al. Fatalities due to anaphylactic reactions to food. *J Allergy Clin Immunol*, 2001;107:191–3.

42. Sampson HA, et al. Fatal and near-fatal anaphylactic reactions to food in children and adolescents. *New Engl J Med, 1992*;327: 380–4.

Asthma Statistics

- Approximately 34.1 million Americans have been diagnosed with asthma by a health professional during their lifetime.[1]

- An estimated 300 million people worldwide suffer from asthma, with 250,000 annual deaths attributed to the disease.[2]

- Workplace conditions, such as exposure to fumes, gases or dust, are responsible for eleven percent of asthma cases worldwide.[2]

- About seventy percent of asthmatics also have allergies.[2]

- The prevalence of asthma increased seventy five percent from 1980–1994.[3]

- Asthma rates in children under the age of five have increased more than 160 percent from 1980–1994.[3]

- It is estimated that the number of people with asthma will grow by more than 100 million by 2025.[2]

- Asthma accounts for approximately 500,000 hospitalizations each year.[5]

- Thirteen million school days are missed each year due to asthma.[5]

- Asthma accounts for about 10.1 million missed work days for adults annually.[5]

- Asthma was responsible for 3,384 deaths in the United States in 2005.[6]

- The annual economic cost of asthma is $19.7 billion. Direct costs make up $14.7 billion of that total, and indirect costs such as lost productivity add another $5 billion.[1]

- Prescription drugs represented the largest single direct medical expenditure related to asthma, over $6 billion.[1]

- In 2006, asthma prevalence was 20.1% higher in African Americans than in whites.[1]

- The prevalence of asthma in adult females was twenty three percent greater than the rate in males in 2006.[1]

- Approximately forty percent of children who have asthmatic parents will develop asthma.[4]

- In 2005, 8.9 percent of children in the United States currently had asthma.[8]

- Nine million US children under eighteen have been diagnosed with asthma at some point in their lifetime.[8]

- Nearly 4 million children have had an asthma attack in the previous year.[8]

- More than 12 million people in the United States report having an asthma attack in the past year.[7]

- Asthma accounts for 217,000 emergency room visits and 10.5 million physician office visits every year.[9]

- In 2006, almost 2.5 million people over the age of sixty five had asthma, and more than 1 million had an asthma attack or episode.[1]

- In a survey of US homes, approximately one-quarter had levels of dust mite allergens present in a bed at a level high enough to trigger asthma symptoms.[10]

- In 2007, twenty nine percent of children who had a food allergy also had asthma.[11]

- Asthma increases the odds of healthcare use in obese people by thirty three percent.[12]

- About 23 million people, including almost 7 million children, have asthma.[13]

- Approximately 2 million Hispanics in the US have asthma.[14]

- Asthma is the third-ranking cause of hospitalization among children under fifteen.[15]

- An average of one out of every ten school-aged child has asthma.[16]

- Annual expenditures for health and lost productivity due to asthma are estimated at over $20 billion, according to the National Heart, Lung and Blood Institute.[17]

- The latest data from Centers for Disease Control indicate an asthma prevalence rate of 8.4 percent in the United States.[18]

Sources:

1. American Lung Association. Epidemiology & Statistics Unit, Research and Program Services. Trends in Asthma Morbidity and Mortality, November 2007.
2. World Health Organization. Global surveillance, prevention and control of chronic respiratory diseases: a comprehensive approach, 2007.
3. Centers for Disease Control. Surveillance for Asthma—United States, 1960–1995, MMWR, 1998; 47 (SS-1).
4. Martinez FD, Wright AL, Taussig LM, et al. Asthma and wheezing in the first six years of life, *N Engl J Med,* 1995; 332:133–138.
5. Akinbami, L. Asthma prevalence, health care use and mortality: United States 2003–05, CDC National Center for Health Statistics, 2006.
6. American Lung Association, Epidemiology and Statistics Unit, Research and Program Services. Trends in Asthma Morbidity and Mortality, November 2007. (ALA age group analysis of NHIS through 2005.
7. Summary Health Statistics for US Children: National Health Interview Survey, 2008.
8. Akinbami LJ. The state of childhood asthma, United States, 1980–2005. Advance data from vital and health statistics; no 381, Hyattsville, MD: National Center for Health Statistics. 2006.
9. Pitts SR, Niska RW, Xu J, Burt CW. National Hospital Ambulatory Medical Care Survey: 2006 emergency department summary. National health statistics reports; no 7. Hyattsville, MD: National Center for Health Statistics.
10. Arbes SJ, et al. House dust mite allergen in US beds: Results from the first national survey of lead and allergens in housing. *J Allergy Clin Immunol,* 2003; 111:408–414.
11. Branum AM, Lukacs SL. Food allergy among US children: Trends in prevalence and hospitalizations. NCHS data brief, no 10. Hyattsville, MD: National Center for Health Statistics, 2008.
12. Pronk NP, Tan AW, O'Connor P. Obesity, fitness, willingness to communicate and health care costs. *Med Sci Sports Exerc,* 1999; 31:1535–1543.
13. Summary Health Statistics for US Adults: National Health Interview Survey, 2008 and Summary Health Statistics for US Children: National Health Interview Survey, 2008.
14. Akinbami L. Asthma Prevalence, Heath Care Use and Mortality; United States 2003–2005.
15. DeFrances CJ, Cullen KA, Kozak LJ. National Hospital Discharge Survey: 2005 Annual Summary with Detailed Diagnosis and Procedure Data. National Center for Health Statistics. Vital Health Statistics 12 (165); 2007.

16. American Lung Association, Epidemiology and Statistics Unit, Research and Program Services. Trends in Asthma Morbidity and Mortality, November 2007.
17. National Heart, Lung and Blood Institute Chartbook on Cardiovascular, Lung and Blood Diseases, US Department of Health and Human Services, National Institute of Health, 2009.
18. Centers for Disease Control, 2011.

Obesity and Asthma

Childhood asthma risk may depend on weight and age

Asthma and obesity are both major public health concerns that often begin in childhood and share some common risk factors. Both conditions have increased in prevalence in the last twenty years, raising speculation that they may be related. Early childhood is a dynamic period for growth as well as disease development, therefore it is important to examine the associations between asthma and obesity, beginning at birth.

Zhang and colleagues studied weight status from birth to five years of age to determine its relationship to the occurrence of asthma at ages six to eight. The authors used data from the Childhood Origin of Asthma (COAST) project, analyzing data on 285 full-term babies who were genetically at high risk of developing asthma due to parental history of asthma or respiratory allergies. The data included the children's history of respiratory illnesses, symptoms, medication, lung function, weight and height, environmental exposures and family histories of allergy and asthma.

The authors found that in the first year of life, being overweight was associated with a decreased risk of asthma and better lung function at ages six and eight. Beyond age one, being overweight was no longer protective for asthma and could even confer a higher risk for asthma. If a child became overweight later in childhood, i.e., overweight at age five but not at age one, there was a higher risk for developing asthma at age six or eight. Asthma, therefore, was found to be associated with being overweight in early childhood, but not in infancy. The authors recommend that nutrition during infancy should be optimized to promote lung growth and development, but after age one, attention should be focused on balanced nutrition to prevent overweight and obesity, which may be a potential risk factor for asthma. This study appeared in the *JACI, volume 126, Issue 6, pp. 1157–1162, December 2010.*

Body mass index and asthma incidence in the Black Women's Health Study

In recent years, asthma has risen to epidemic proportions in the United States, with many cases developing as adult-onset asthma. Several factors have been implicated in the development of adult-onset asthma, such as current smoking, socioeconomic status, household allergens and childhood or prenatal exposures—with the most consistent link being obesity. Higher incidences of current asthma, asthma-related emergency room visits, hospitalizations and deaths are seen in blacks than in whites and in women than men. Although black women have a high incidence of both obesity and asthma, there has been little research focused directly on that relationship in this ethnic group. In a study released by *The Journal of Allergy and Clinical Immunology, volume 123, Issue 1, pp.89–95, January 2009,* Coogan et al. report on their test of the hypothesis that a higher body mass index (BMI), the statistical comparison of body weight-to-height, would be associated with the incidence of adult-onset asthma in black women. Over a period of ten years, the authors followed a group of 46,000 subjects enrolled in the Black Women's Health Study, collecting data on new asthma diagnoses and use of asthma medication. The authors found that among this group of women as BMI increased, the risk of asthma also increased. They also noticed that incidence of asthma was higher among those women who reported a weight gain since age eighteen. The authors' findings showed a positive association between BMI and asthma risk in black women despite age, level of energy expenditure, smoking history, sleep apnea, or parental history of asthma. This finding has great public health importance given the high prevalence of obesity among black women.

Gender and Asthma

The effect of sex on asthma control from the National Asthma Survey

James Temprano, MD, MHA and David Mannino, MD

In a study from *The Journal of Allergy & Clinical Immunology, volume 123, Issue 4, pages 854–860, April 2009,* Temprano and Mannino took a new look at male and female differences in asthma control. Using data from four states (Alabama, California, Illinois and Texas) participating in the National Asthma Survey, the authors compared levels of asthma control between the genders based on short-term measures (recent symptoms, asthma attacks and albuterol use) and long-term measures (asthma attacks, work days lost, urgent care visits and hospitalizations in the previous year).

They found that, based on any of the measures, women were more likely than men to have poor short-term and long-term asthma control, even though women reported higher use of inhaled corticosteroid and routine asthma care visits. These differences persisted even after considering factors such as age, race, socioeconomic status, education, health insurance, weight-to-height ratio, and smoking status.

Further research is needed to determine whether these findings can be attributed to differences in health reporting or to the differences in male and female physiologic responses to the disease. Health care providers should be aware that there are differences in asthma control between men and women, and that women may benefit from improved asthma education, monitoring or treatment.

Asthma and Allergies in Women 2009/2010—AAAAI
Website report

Dessislava Ianakieva and Richard W Honsinger, MD, MACP, FAAAAI reported that recent studies indicate that women's menstrual cycles can play a role in asthma symptoms. Prior to puberty, asthma and hospitalizations for asthma are more common in boys than in girls. At the time of puberty, asthma occurs equally in boys and girls. By age twenty four, more women are affected than men[1]. Overall, women are thirty percent more likely to have asthma and have a forty percent higher asthma death rate than men.[4] Premenstrual asthma (PMA) is a condition in which asthma symptoms and lung function worsen a few days before menstruation.[2] According to one study, fifty seven percent of women with asthma, experience worsening of symptoms and increased medication use and fourteen percent had a significant decrease in lung function before their menstruation.[1] During days twenty two through twenty eight of the menstrual cycle, the hormones progesterone and estrogen decrease, reaching their lowest levels at day twenty eight. Progesterone and/or estrogen affect the airways or the cells of the immune system, making an asthma attack more likely.[1] Also, blood vessels in the lungs are found to form and disappear in rhythm with a woman's hormones, leading to increasing and decreasing ability of the lungs to take in oxygen. During the first two weeks of menstruation, estrogen levels increase and signal the formation of new blood vessels in the uterus and in the lungs. As estrogen levels decrease dramatically before menstruation, the decrease in blood vessels can also help explain the worsening of asthma symptoms experienced in PMA.[4] However, hormones by themselves do not explain the entire reasoning of PMA. The use of oral contraceptives does not prevent PMA and use of hormone replacement therapy (synthetic estrogen) in postmenopausal women increases the risk of developing adult onset asthma.[3] If you have PMA, keep a diary of asthma symptoms in relation to your menstrual period. Also, talk to your doctor about increasing preventative medication before menstruation.

Allergic Rhinitis

Allergic rhinitis is the inflammation of nasal mucous membranes. Symptoms include sneezing, itchy nose and roof of the mouth, throat, eyes and ears, runny nose, congestion and watery eyes. These symptoms are thought to be hormonally induced during pregnancy and menstrual cycles. Studies have shown that symptoms of allergic rhinitis increased in one-third of pregnant patients because of increased sinus congestion from the blood vessels in the nose expanding and increased blood volume. Pregnancy rhinitis occurs without an infection, allergic, or medication-related cause. The condition starts before the last six weeks of pregnancy (corresponding to thirty four weeks gestation), continues until delivery and clears up within two weeks after delivery. There may also be an association of nasal congestion with ovulation and the rise of estrogen during the menstrual cycle in some women.

Sources:

1. Murphy V and Gibson P. Premenstrual Asthma: Prevalence, Cycle-to-Cycle Variability and Relationship to Oral contraceptive use and Menstrual Symptoms. *Journal of Asthma*, Vol. 45, Issue 8, pp. 696–704, 2008.
2. Tan KS. Premenstrual Asthma: Epidemiology, Pathogenesis and Treatment. *Drugs*, 2001; 61 (14): 2079–2086.
3. Chhabra SK. Premenstrual Asthma. *Indian J Chest Dis Allied Sci* 2005; 47: 109–116.
4. Farha S et al. Effects of the Menstrual Cycle on Lung Function Variables in Women with Asthma. *American Journal of Respiratory and Critical Care Medicine* Vol 180. pp. 304–310, (2009).
5. Wallace DV, MD and Dykewicz MS, MD et al. The diagnosis and management of rhinitis: An updated practice parameter. *J Allergy Clin Immunol*, August 2008.

Vitamin D Deficiency and Asthma

Do low levels of vitamin D mean higher asthma risk?

Asthma is the most common cause of childhood emergency department visits, hospitalizations, and missed school days in the United States. According to the National Health Interview Survey, as of 2007, 8 million children between the ages of five and seventeen have been diagnosed with asthma. Oral corticosteroids are often used to treat patients with severe asthma who cannot control their symptoms with a combination of inhaled corticosteroids and long-acting β-agonists. While inhaled corticosteroids (ICS) effectively manage asthma symptoms, higher ICS doses increase the potential for side effects including reduced bone density, increased fracture risk, and adrenal suppression. It has been argued that different factors associated with westernization have led to lower vitamin D levels and increasing allergy, which in turn has resulted in higher rates of asthma.

In *The Journal of Allergy and Clinical Immunology, volume 125, Issue 5, pp. 995–1000, May 2010,* Searing and colleagues investigated the prevalence of vitamin D insufficiency in children with asthma. Data was collected between April 1, 2008 and October 31, 2009 on one hundred children between the ages of zero and eighteen with asthma who were referred to National Jewish Health. The patients were primarily from higher northern latitudes (above 35 degrees N). They found that forty seven percent of the patients had vitamin D levels that are considered insufficient and seventeen percent of the patients were found to be vitamin D deficient. The patients with low vitamin D levels were found to have higher levels of IgE, a marker of allergy, and had more positive reactions to allergens.

The authors also tested lung function and found that low vitamin D correlated with low FEV1, the amount of air a person can exhale in one second. In addition, lower vitamin D levels were associated with inhaled or oral corticosteroid use. When the authors tested different amounts of vitamin D on the function of corticosteroids, they found that vitamin D enhanced the anti-inflammatory effect of the corticosteroids. These data suggest that low vitamin D levels may be associated with increased asthma severity. Further studies are needed to determine whether increasing vitamin D levels into the normal range will help control asthma in children with low vitamin D levels.

Summary

The recent reports above about atopic diseases seem to point to growing allergy problems in women and obesity and estrogens are hinted at as possible culprits. As an allergist who sees manifestation of allergic diseases in pediatric and adult patients, I have come to conclude that the growing atopy in American adults is due to the estrogen epidemic. The next chapter will look at atopic diseases as windows to the whole body and point out the estrogen connection to many of the atopic diseases treated by all allergists.

ESTROGENS AND ADULT-ONSET ALLERGIES

The studies reported in previous sections increasingly point to the high levels of adult-onset asthma and allergic rhinitis in women than men. Some of these studies as shown above have hinted that female hormone imbalance plays a major role in these atopic diseases after puberty.

Recently, research conducted by professor Midoro-Horiuti and colleagues at the University of Texas Medical Branch (UTMB) in Galveston, Texas, demonstrated that estradiol activates mast cells via a non-genomic estrogen receptor-alpha(ER-α) and calcium influx. The research that appeared in *Molecular Immunology* volume 44 in 2007 demonstrated that estradiol alone induced partial release of the preformed, granular protein β-hexosaminidase from RBL-2H3, BMMC, and HMC-1, but not from BMMC derived from estrogen receptor-α knock-out mice. The newly synthesized LTC4 was also released from RBL-2H3. Estradiol also enhanced IgE-induced degranulation and potentiated LTC4 production. Intracellular Ca2+ concentration increased prior to and in parallel with mediator release. Estrogen receptor antagonists or Ca2+ chelation inhibited these estrogenic effects.

They concluded that binding of physiological concentrations of estradiol to a membrane estrogen receptor-α initiates a rapid onset and progressive influx of extracellular Ca2+, which supports the synthesis and release of allergic mediators. Estradiol also enhances IgE-dependent mast cell activation, resulting in a shift of the allergen dose response.

The same research group examined the effects of lipophilic pollutants that have estrogen-like activities and are termed environmental estrogens in allergic diseases. These pollutants tend to degrade slowly in the environment and to bioaccumulate and bioconcentrate in the food chain; they also have long biological half-lives.

The goal in this study was to identify possible pathogenic roles for environmental estrogens in the development of allergic diseases. They screened a number of environmental estrogens for their ability to modulate the release of allergic mediators from mast cells. They incubated a human mast cell line and primary mast cell cultures derived from bone marrow of wild type and estrogen receptor-α(ER-α)-deficient mice with environmental estrogens with and without estradiol or IgE and allergens. They then assessed degranulation of mast cells by quantifying the release of beta-hexosaminidase.

The results showed that all the environmental estrogens tested caused rapid, dose-related release of beta-hexosaminidase from mast cells and enhanced IgE-mediated release. The combination of physiologic concentrations of 17-β-estradiol and several concentrations of environmental estrogens had additive effects on mast cell degranulation. Comparison of bone marrow mast cells from ER-α-sufficient and ER-α-deficient mice indicated that much of the effect of environmental estrogens was mediated by ER-α. They concluded that their findings suggest that estrogenic environmental pollutants might promote allergic diseases by inducing and enhancing mast cell degranulation by physiologic estrogens and exposure to allergens.

This study appeared in *Environmental Health Perspectives* 115:48–52, (2007).

Evidence on Allergic Diseases

Allergic diseases are multiple and include:
- Allergic rhinitis
- Asthma
- Atopic dermatitis (eczema)
- Food allergy and anaphylaxis
- Drug allergy and anaphylaxis
- Urticaria and angioedema
- Sinusitis which is a consequence of allergic and non-allergic rhinitis
- Allergic Conjunctivitis

The following tables present discharges for these allergic conditions. The reported statistics seek to tease out the prevalence of atopic diseases in women compared to men. Once the evidence is established then a discussion will follow to explain the findings.

TABLE 115

2008 National statistics—first-listed diagnosis only

Patient and hospital characteristics for ICD-9-CM first-listed diagnosis code 477.0 Rhinitis Due To Pollen

		All ED visits (those that resulted in admission to the hospital and those that did not)	Only hospital visits that originated in the ED	Only ED visits that ended in discharge (no hospital admission)	Standard errors		
					All ED Visits	Admitted to the hospital from the ED	Discharged from the ED
All discharges		7,067 (100.00%)	*	7,027 (100.00%)	703	*	702
Age (mean)		27.42	43.62	27.32	0.75	0.75	0.75
Age group	<1	153 (2.16%)	*	153 (100.00%)	44	*	44 (0.00%)
	1–17	2,364 (33.45%)	*	2,355 (99.64%)	297	*	297 (0.26%)
	18–44	3,179 (44.98%)	*	3,167 (99.64%)	347	*	346 (0.21%)
	45–64	1,098 (15.53%)	*	1,090 (99.31%)	123	*	123 (0.51%)
	65–84	257 (3.63%)	*	243 (94.85%)	40	*	39 (2.95%)
	85+	*	*	*	*	*	*
Sex	Male	3,076 (43.53%)	*	3,059 (99.46%)	316	*	315 (0.27%)
	Female	3,991 (56.47%)	*	3,967 (99.40%)	414	*	414 (0.28%)
Median income for zip code	Low	2,425 (34.32%)	*	2,408 (99.29%)	323	*	322 (0.45%)
	Not low	4,493 (63.58%)	*	4,480 (99.70%)	508	*	507 (0.17%)
	Missing	149 (2.10%)	*	139 (93.24%)	33	*	32 (4.73%)
Region	Northeast	2,039 (28.86%)	*	2,021 (99.07%)	411	*	411 (0.50%)
	Midwest	1,177 (16.65%)	*	1,172 (99.59%)	189	*	187 (0.38%)
	South	2,391 (33.84%)	*	2,374 (99.29%)	314	*	312 (0.44%)
	West	1,460 (20.66%)	*	1,460 (100.00%)	438	*	438 (0.00%)

* Denotes missing values

Allergic rhinitis due to pollen is more prevalent in females at 56.5%, and is seen more in the prime-age group, ages (18–44), at 45%, followed by the young, ages (1–17) at 33.5%, and then older adults ages 45–64 at 15.5%, and finally ages 65–84 at 3.6%.

TABLE 116

Patient and hospital characteristics for ICD-9-CM first-listed diagnosis code 477.8 Allergic Rhinitis Nec

		All ED visits (those that resulted in admission to the hospital and those that did not)	Only hospital visits that originated in the ED	Only ED visits that ended in discharge (no hospital admission)	Standard errors		
					All ED Visits	Admitted to the hospital from the ED	Discharged from the ED
All discharges		3,971 (100.00%)	*	3,941 (100.00%)	243	*	242
Age (mean)		29.59	29.56	29.59	0.74	0.74	0.74
Age group	<1	*	*	*	*	*	*
	1–17	1,216 (30.63%)	*	1,211 (99.55%)	106	*	106 (0.45%)
	18–44	1,847 (46.51%)	*	1,831 (99.15%)	128	*	128 (0.43%)
	45–64	648 (16.31%)	*	639 (98.72%)	74	*	74 (0.92%)
	65–84	219 (5.51%)	*	219 (100.00%)	32	*	32 (0.00%)
	85+	*	*	*	*	*	*
Sex	Male	1,490 (37.53%)	*	1,475 (98.95%)	114	*	114 (0.54%)
	Female	2,480 (62.47%)	*	2,467 (99.45%)	164	*	163 (0.32%)
Median income for zip code	Low	1,361 (34.26%)	*	1,352 (99.34%)	133	*	133 (0.47%)
	Not low	2,501 (62.99%)	*	2,486 (99.40%)	178	*	178 (0.30%)
	Missing	109 (2.75%)	*	104 (95.04%)	27	*	26 (4.87%)
Region	Northeast	911 (22.95%)	*	897 (98.39%)	133	*	133 (1.20%)
	Midwest	842 (21.20%)	*	842 (100.00%)	124		124 (0.00%)
	South	1,556 (39.20%)	*	1,542 (99.05%)	139	*	138 (0.46%)
	West	661 (16.65%)	*	661 (100.00%)	80	*	80 (0.00%)

* Denotes missing values

Allergic rhinitis Nec is more prevalent in females at 62.5%, and males have 37.5% but is seen more in the prime-age group, ages 18–44, at 46.5%, followed by the young, ages (1–17) at 30.6%, and then older adults ages 45–64 at 16.3% and then in ages 65–84 at 5.5%. The South leads with 39.2% followed by the Northeast at 23%, the Midwest at 21.2% and the West at 16.7%.

TABLE 117

Patient and hospital characteristics for
ICD-9-CM first-listed diagnosis code
477.9 Allergic Rhinitis Nos

		All ED visits (those that resulted in admission to the hospital and those that did not)	Only hospital visits that originated in the ED	Only ED visits that ended in discharge (no hospital admission)	Standard errors		
					All ED Visits	Admitted to the hospital from the ED	Discharged from the ED
All discharges		74,898 (100.00%)	159 (100.00%)	74,739 (100.00%)	3,814	33	3,812
Age (mean)		26.58	53.41	26.52	0.52	0.52	0.52
Age group	<1	2,343 (3.13%)	*	2,343 (100.00%)	179	*	179 (0.00%)
	1–17	27,083 (36.16%)	*	27,072 (99.96%)	1,814	*	1,814 (0.02%)
	18–44	30,824 (41.15%)	*	30,786 (99.88%)	1,651	*	1,651 (0.05%)
	45–64	10,800 (14.42%)	65 (0.61%)	10,735 (99.39%)	803	19 (0.18%)	803 (0.18%)
	65–84	3,549 (4.74%)	*	3,507 (98.82%)	227	*	226 (0.36%)
	85+	299 (0.40%)	*	296 (99.00%)	39	*	39 (1.00%)
Sex	Male	33,163 (44.28%)	75 (0.23%)	33,088 (99.77%)	1,713	20 (0.06%)	1,711 (0.06%)
	Female	41,730 (55.72%)	84 (0.20%)	41,646 (99.80%)	2,177	23 (0.06%)	2,177 (0.06%)
	Missing	*	*	*	*	*	*
Median income for zip code	Low	30,119 (40.21%)	*	30,056 (99.79%)	2,346	*	2,346 (0.08%)
	Not low	43,152 (57.61%)	86 (0.20%)	43,065 (99.80%)	2,201	22 (0.05%)	2,199 (0.05%)
	Missing	1,627 (2.17%)	*	1,618 (99.42%)	142	*	141 (0.57%)
Region	Northeast	17,690 (23.62%)	*	17,644 (99.74%)	2,778	*	2,779 (0.12%)
	Midwest	15,742 (21.02%)	*	15,720 (99.86%)	1,550	*	1,549 (0.08%)
	South	31,556 (42.13%)	*	31,482 (99.76%)	1,871	*	1,869 (0.07%)
	West	9,910 (13.23%)	*	9,893 (99.83%)	960	*	959 (0.09%)

* Denotes missing values

Allergic rhinitis Nos is more prevalent in females at 55.7%,
males have 44.3% and is seen more in the prime-age group, ages
18–44, at 41.2%, followed by the young, ages 1–17, at 36.2%
and then older adults ages 45–64 at 14.4% and then ages 65–84
at 4.7%. The South leads with 42.1% followed by the Northeast
with 23.6%, the Midwest with 21% and the West with 13.2%.

TABLE 118

2008 National statistics—first-listed diagnosis only

Patient and hospital characteristics for
ICD-9-CM first-listed diagnosis code
472.0 Chronic Rhinitis

	All ED visits (those that resulted in admission to the hospital and those that did not)	Only hospital visits that originated in the ED	Only ED visits that ended in discharge (no hospital admission)	Standard errors		
				All ED Visits	Admitted to the hospital from the ED	Discharged from the ED
All discharges	19,230 (100.00%)	*	19,173 (100.00%)	2,460	*	2,459
Age (mean)	16.86	49.66	16.76	1.03	1.03	1.03
Age group <1	4,803 (24.97%)	*	4,790 (99.74%)	726	*	726 (0.16%)
1–17	7,665 (39.86%)	*	7,665 (100.00%)	1,296	*	1,296 (0.00%)
18–44	3,926 (20.42%)	*	3,916 (99.74%)	348	*	348 (0.15%)
45–64	1,836 (9.55%)	*	1,825 (99.37%)	188	*	187 (0.37%)
65–84	816 (4.25%)	*	806 (98.73%)	81	*	80 (0.74%)
85+	183 (0.95%)	*	171 (93.25%)	31	*	29 (4.76%)
Sex Male	9,156 (47.61%)	*	9,133 (99.75%)	1,216	*	1,216 (0.13%)
Female	10,074 (52.39%)	*	10,040 (99.67%)	1,264	*	1,264 (0.12%)
Median income for zip code Low	8,267 (42.99%)	*	8,240 (99.67%)	1,443	*	1,442 (0.15%)
Not low	10,625 (55.25%)	*	10,595 (99.72%)	1,255	*	1,255 (0.12%)
Missing	338 (1.76%)	*	338 (100.00%)	57	*	57 (0.00%)
Region Northeast	2,022 (10.52%)	*	2,014 (99.59%)	283	*	281 (0.28%)
Midwest	4,362 (22.68%)	*	4,353 (99.80%)	603	*	601 (0.20%)
South	11,304 (58.78%)	*	11,269 (99.69%)	2,362	*	2,362 (0.13%)
West	1,542 (8.02%)	*	1,537 (99.68%)	175	*	175 (0.32%)

* Denotes missing values

Chronic rhinitis is more prevalent in females at 52.4%, and is found more in the young, ages 1–17 at 39.9%, followed by children less than one year old with 25%, the prime-age, ages 18–44, at 20.4%, then older adults ages 45–64 with 9.56% and finally the very old ages 65–84, at 4.25%. Chronic rhinitis is more prevalent in the South at 58.8% and the Midwest at 22.7%, followed by the Northeast at 10.5% and the West at 8%.

TABLE 119

2008 National statistics—first-listed diagnosis only

Patient and hospital characteristics for
ICD-9-CM first-listed diagnosis code
461.0 Ac Maxillary Sinusitis

		All ED visits (those that resulted in admission to the hospital and those that did not)	Only hospital visits that originated in the ED	Only ED visits that ended in discharge (no hospital admission)	Standard errors		
					All ED Visits	Admitted to the hospital from the ED	Discharged from the ED
All discharges		35,242 (100.00%)	1,707 (100.00%)	33,535 (100.00%)	3,061	112	3,057
Age (mean)		37.58	52.59	36.82	0.33	0.33	0.33
Age group	<1	*	*	*	*	*	*
	1–17	2,851 (8.09%)	121 (4.24%)	2,730 (95.76%)	286	25 (0.91%)	284 (0.91%)
	18–44	21,338 (60.55%)	429 (2.01%)	20,910 (97.99%)	2,064	50 (0.30%)	2,063 (0.30%)
	45–64	8,448 (23.97%)	542 (6.41%)	7,906 (93.59%)	709	63 (0.86%)	703 (0.86%)
	65–84	2,232 (6.33%)	473 (21.17%)	1,759 (78.83%)	167	48 (2.23%)	159 (2.23%)
	85+	322 (0.91%)	124 (38.51%)	198 (61.49%)	41	25 (5.94%)	32 (5.94%)
Sex	Male	12,367 (35.09%)	783 (6.33%)	11,584 (93.67%)	986	69 (0.72%)	983 (0.72%)
	Female	22,871 (64.90%)	923 (4.04%)	21,948 (95.96%)	2,110	82 (0.50%)	2,106 (0.50%)
	Missing	*	*	*	*	*	*
Median income for zip code	Low	11,449 (32.49%)	545 (4.76%)	10,904 (95.24%)	1,341	64 (0.76%)	1,338 (0.76%)
	Not low	23,058 (65.43%)	1,090 (4.73%)	21,968 (95.27%)	2,098	82 (0.53%)	2,093 (0.53%)
	Missing	734 (2.08%)	*	663 (90.27%)	88	*	84 (3.27%)
Region	Northeast	6,799 (19.29%)	358 (5.27%)	6,440 (94.73%)	1,671	51 (1.38%)	1,663 (1.38%)
	Midwest	8,462 (24.01%)	283 (3.34%)	8,179 (96.66%)	1,339	40 (0.72%)	1,341 (0.72%)
	South	16,373 (46.46%)	764 (4.67%)	15,609 (95.33%)	2,147	77 (0.76%)	2,146 (0.76%)
	West	3,609 (10.24%)	302 (8.37%)	3,307 (91.63%)	418	48 (1.59%)	417 (1.59%)

* Denotes missing values

Acute maxillary sinusitis is more prevalent in females at 64.9%, and in the prime-age group, ages 18–44, at 60.6%, followed by older adults, ages 45–64, at 24% and then the young, ages 1–17, at 8.1% and in ages 65–84, at 6.33%. Acute maxillary sinusitis is more prevalent in the South at 46.5% and the Midwest at 24%, followed by the Northeast at 19.3% and the West at 10.2%.

TABLE 120

Patient and hospital characteristics for ICD-9-CM first-listed diagnosis code 461.1 Acute Frontal Sinusitis

		All ED visits (those that resulted in admission to the hospital and those that did not)	Only hospital visits that originated in the ED	Only ED visits that ended in discharge (no hospital admission)	Standard errors		
					All ED Visits	Admitted to the hospital from the ED	Discharged from the ED
All discharges		12,716 (100.00%)	249 (100.00%)	12,467 (100.00%)	1,516	37	1,511
Age (mean)		34.96	41.22	34.83	0.42	0.42	0.42
Age group	<1	*	*	*	*	*	*
	1–17	1,526 (12.00%)	*	1,501 (98.34%)	203	*	203 (0.73%)
	18–44	7,784 (61.21%)	132 (1.69%)	7,652 (98.31%)	983	25 (0.34%)	978 (0.34%)
	45–64	2,750 (21.63%)	*	2,694 (97.96%)	338	*	337 (0.64%)
	65–84	600 (4.72%)	*	573 (95.45%)	79	*	78 (2.15%)
	85+	*	*	*	*	*	*
Sex	Male	4,698 (36.95%)	110 (2.33%)	4,588 (97.67%)	535	22 (0.52%)	533 (0.52%)
	Female	8,018 (63.05%)	140 (1.74%)	7,878 (98.26%)	1,000	26 (0.36%)	996 (0.36%)
Median income for zip code	Low	4,661 (36.65%)	56 (1.21%)	4,604 (98.79%)	772	16 (0.38%)	771 (0.38%)
	Not low	7,698 (60.54%)	150 (1.95%)	7,547 (98.05%)	925	26 (0.40%)	924 (0.40%)
	Missing	358 (2.81%)	*	315 (88.13%)	61	*	55 (4.93%)
Region	Northeast	3,056 (24.03%)	*	2,990 (97.85%)	881	*	874 (0.90%)
	Midwest	2,254 (17.72%)	71 (3.14%)	2,183 (96.86%)	481	17 (0.93%)	479 (0.93%)
	South	6,281 (49.40%)	67 (1.06%)	6,214 (98.94%)	1,113	16 (0.30%)	1,112 (0.30%)
	West	1,125 (8.85%)	46 (4.08%)	1,079 (95.92%)	229	14 (1.47%)	230 (1.47%)

* Denotes missing values

TABLE 121

Patient and hospital characteristics for ICD-9-CM first-listed diagnosis code 461.2 Acute Ethmoidal Sinusitis

| | | All ED visits (those that resulted in admission to the hospital and those that did not) | Only hospital visits that originated in the ED | Only ED visits that ended in discharge (no hospital admission) | Standard errors | | |
					All ED Visits	Admitted to the hospital from the ED	Discharged from the ED
All discharges		3,372 (100.00%)	573 (100.00%)	2,799 (100.00%)	220	65	211
Age (mean)		39.64	46.46	38.25	0.74	0.74	0.74
Age group	<1	*	*	*	*	*	*
	1–17	429 (12.72%)	94 (21.83%)	335 (78.17%)	53	21 (4.29%)	46 (4.29%)
	18–44	1,593 (47.25%)	160 (10.05%)	1,433 (89.95%)	119	28 (1.76%)	116 (1.76%)
	45–64	904 (26.81%)	143 (15.77%)	761 (84.23%)	85	27 (2.90%)	81 (2.90%)
	65–84	389 (11.53%)	136 (34.96%)	253 (65.04%)	43	39 (8.98%)	44 (8.98%)
	85+	*	*	*	*	*	*
Sex	Male	1,548 (45.92%)	289 (18.65%)	1,260 (81.35%)	122	49 (2.82%)	109 (2.82%)
	Female	1,819 (53.95%)	284 (15.60%)	1,535 (84.40%)	141	39 (2.14%)	135 (2.14%)
	Missing	*	*	*	*	*	*
Median income for zip code	Low	1,039 (30.80%)	182 (17.53%)	857 (82.47%)	111	41 (4.12%)	112 (4.12%)
	Not low	2,206 (65.42%)	366 (16.61%)	1,840 (83.39%)	156	51 (2.10%)	143 (2.10%)
	Missing	127 (3.77%)	*	103 (80.94%)	27	*	25 (7.71%)
Region	Northeast	632 (18.76%)	134 (21.19%)	498 (78.81%)	116	32 (5.11%)	108 (5.11%)
	Midwest	815 (24.18%)	116 (14.22%)	700 (85.78%)	94	26 (2.90%)	86 (2.90%)
	South	1,372 (40.69%)	226 (16.45%)	1,146 (83.55%)	146	35 (2.75%)	142 (2.75%)
	West	552 (16.37%)	*	455 (82.42%)	69	*	72 (6.59%)

* Denotes missing values

TABLE 122

Patient and hospital characteristics for ICD-9-CM first-listed diagnosis code 461.3 Acute Sphenoidal Sinusitis

		All ED visits (those that resulted in admission to the hospital and those that did not)	Only hospital visits that originated in the ED	Only ED visits that ended in discharge (no hospital admission)	Standard errors		
					All ED Visits	Admitted to the hospital from the ED	Discharged from the ED
All discharges		1,410 (100.00%)	238 (100.00%)	1,172 (100.00%)	110	34	101
Age (mean)		45.23	59.92	42.24	1.60	1.60	1.60
Age group	1–17	160 (11.34%)	*	155 (96.92%)	28	*	28 (3.04%)
	18–44	595 (42.19%)	62 (10.50%)	532 (89.50%)	63	16 (2.73%)	62 (2.73%)
	45–64	295 (20.91%)	*	251 (85.04%)	38	*	36 (4.46%)
	65–84	276 (19.54%)	106 (38.38%)	170 (61.62%)	47	24 (7.59%)	39 (7.59%)
	85+	85 (6.01%)	*	*	21	*	*
Sex	Male	434 (30.76%)	77 (17.75%)	357 (82.25%)	52	19 (3.91%)	47 (3.91%)
	Female	976 (69.24%)	161 (16.52%)	815 (83.48%)	86	27 (2.62%)	80 (2.62%)
Median income for zip code	Low	303 (21.46%)	*	258 (85.40%)	45	*	43 (4.30%)
	Not low	1,048 (74.34%)	175 (16.66%)	874 (83.34%)	91	29 (2.51%)	83 (2.51%)
	Missing	59 (4.20%)	*	*	16	*	*
Region	Northeast	187 (13.27%)	*	136 (72.87%)	32	*	30 (7.90%)
	Midwest	283 (20.05%)	57 (20.20%)	226 (79.80%)	45	16 (5.22%)	41 (5.22%)
	South	630 (44.71%)	102 (16.25%)	528 (83.75%)	79	22 (3.16%)	72 (3.16%)
	West	310 (21.97%)	*	282 (90.99%)	52	*	49 (3.49%)

* Denotes missing values

TABLE 123

Patient and hospital characteristics for ICD-9-CM first-listed diagnosis code 461.8 Other Acute Sinusitis

		All ED visits (those that resulted in admission to the hospital and those that did not)	Only hospital visits that originated in the ED	Only ED visits that ended in discharge (no hospital admission)	Standard errors		
					All ED Visits	Admitted to the hospital from the ED	Discharged from the ED
All discharges		10,999 (100.00%)	974 (100.00%)	10,025 (100.00%)	1,893	104	1,881
Age (mean)		34.92	43.99	34.03	0.79	0.79	0.79
Age group	<1	*	*	*	*	*	*
	1–17	1,563 (14.21%)	181 (11.61%)	1,382 (88.39%)	334	38 (3.09%)	328 (3.09%)
	18–44	6,395 (58.14%)	327 (5.11%)	6,068 (94.89%)	1,164	61 (1.29%)	1,162 (1.29%)
	45–64	2,172 (19.75%)	210 (9.66%)	1,962 (90.34%)	374	34 (1.99%)	367 (1.99%)
	65–84	719 (6.54%)	213 (29.64%)	506 (70.36%)	100	34 (5.06%)	93 (5.06%)
	85+	65 (0.59%)	*	*	17	*	*
Sex	Male	4,051 (36.83%)	418 (10.31%)	3,634 (89.69%)	662	55 (1.98%)	655 (1.98%)
	Female	6,948 (63.17%)	557 (8.01%)	6,391 (91.99%)	1,248	69 (1.64%)	1,241 (1.64%)
Median income for zip code	Low	3,210 (29.18%)	186 (5.80%)	3,023 (94.20%)	818	36 (1.76%)	815 (1.76%)
	Not low	7,432 (67.57%)	715 (9.62%)	6,717 (90.38%)	1,433	75 (1.98%)	1,425 (1.98%)
	Missing	358 (3.25%)	*	284 (79.47%)	81	*	75 (7.04%)
Region	Northeast	*	289 (8.92%)	*	*	72 (3.44%)	*
	Midwest	900 (8.19%)	186 (20.71%)	714 (79.29%)	134	30 (3.70%)	127 (3.70%)
	South	6,113 (55.58%)	365 (5.97%)	5,748 (94.03%)	1,578	58 (1.62%)	1,566 (1.62%)
	West	743 (6.75%)	134 (17.98%)	609 (82.02%)	162	38 (5.83%)	159 (5.83%)

* Denotes missing values

TABLE 124

Patient and hospital characteristics for
ICD-9-CM first-listed diagnosis code
461.9 Acute Sinusitis Nos

		All ED visits (those that resulted in admission to the hospital and those that did not)	Only hospital visits that originated in the ED	Only ED visits that ended in discharge (no hospital admission)	Standard errors		
					All ED Visits	Admitted to the hospital from the ED	Discharged from the ED
All discharges		348,238 (100.00%)	2,203 (100.00%)	346,034 (100.00%)	19,179	153	19,165
Age (mean)		34.28	51.71	34.17	0.23	0.23	0.23
Age group	<1	3,421 (0.98%)	*	3,397 (99.30%)	418	*	416 (0.28%)
	1–17	52,527 (15.08%)	256 (0.49%)	52,271 (99.51%)	3,556	37 (0.08%)	3,552 (0.08%)
	18–44	196,773 (56.51%)	499 (0.25%)	196,274 (99.75%)	10,720	67 (0.04%)	10,716 (0.04%)
	45–64	74,691 (21.45%)	630 (0.84%)	74,061 (99.16%)	4,349	63 (0.09%)	4,342 (0.09%)
	65–84	18,867 (5.42%)	637 (3.37%)	18,231 (96.63%)	1,113	61 (0.36%)	1,106 (0.36%)
	85+	1,958 (0.56%)	157 (8.00%)	1,801 (92.00%)	135	26 (1.29%)	131 (1.29%)
Sex	Male	127,162 (36.52%)	968 (0.76%)	126,194 (99.24%)	7,172	88 (0.08%)	7,165 (0.08%)
	Female	221,045 (63.48%)	1,236 (0.56%)	219,809 (99.44%)	12,094	92 (0.05%)	12,087 (0.05%)
	Missing	*	*	*	*	*	*
Median income for zip code	Low	121,933 (35.01%)	670 (0.55%)	121,263 (99.45%)	8,990	85 (0.08%)	8,984 (0.08%)
	Not low	218,496 (62.74%)	1,441 (0.66%)	217,055 (99.34%)	13,078	107 (0.06%)	13,055 (0.06%)
	Missing	7,809 (2.24%)	*	7,716 (98.81%)	582	*	581 (0.37%)
Region	Northeast	52,339 (15.03%)	459 (0.88%)	51,880 (99.12%)	5,257	100 (0.21%)	5,255 (0.21%)
	Midwest	100,758 (28.93%)	516 (0.51%)	100,242 (99.49%)	15,648	59 (0.09%)	15,641 (0.09%)
	South	162,959 (46.80%)	989 (0.61%)	161,970 (99.39%)	9,415	88 (0.06%)	9,400 (0.06%)
	West	32,182 (9.24%)	240 (0.75%)	31,942 (99.25%)	2,586	44 (0.14%)	2,582 (0.14%)

* Denotes missing values

Acute sinusitis Nos is more prevalent in females at 63.5%, and also more in the prime-age group, ages 18–44, at 56.5%, followed by older adults, ages 45–64, at 21.5%, then the young, ages 1–17, at 15.1% and finally ages 65–84 at 5.42%. Acute sinusitis nos is more prevalent in the South with 46.8% and the Midwest with 28.9%, followed by the Northeast with 15.0% and the West with 9.2%.

TABLE 125

2008 National statistics—first-listed diagnosis only

Patient and hospital characteristics for
ICD-9-CM first-listed diagnosis code
473.0 Chr Maxillary Sinusitis

		All ED visits (those that resulted in admission to the hospital and those that did not)	Only hospital visits that originated in the ED	Only ED visits that ended in discharge (no hospital admission)	Standard errors		
					All ED Visits	Admitted to the hospital from the ED	Discharged from the ED
All discharges		17,573 (100.00%)	1,084 (100.00%)	16,489 (100.00%)	896	79	875
Age (mean)		38.46	47.41	37.87	0.49	0.49	0.49
Age group	<1	*	*	*	*	*	*
	1–17	2,111 (12.01%)	200 (9.46%)	1,912 (90.54%)	223	38 (1.54%)	206 (1.54%)
	18–44	9,334 (53.11%)	237 (2.54%)	9,097 (97.46%)	538	35 (0.39%)	535 (0.39%)
	45–64	4,324 (24.61%)	301 (6.96%)	4,023 (93.04%)	238	38 (0.89%)	233 (0.89%)
	65–84	1,503 (8.55%)	223 (14.83%)	1,280 (85.17%)	105	31 (1.97%)	99 (1.97%)
	85+	268 (1.52%)	100 (37.13%)	168 (62.87%)	40	25 (7.07%)	30 (7.07%)
Sex	Male	6,947 (39.53%)	494 (7.12%)	6,453 (92.88%)	375	52 (0.73%)	363 (0.73%)
	Female	10,622 (60.44%)	590 (5.55%)	10,032 (94.45%)	576	54 (0.52%)	564 (0.52%)
	Missing	*	*	*	*	*	*
Median income for zip code	Low	5,961 (33.92%)	317 (5.31%)	5,644 (94.69%)	502	49 (0.80%)	487 (0.80%)
	Not low	11,120 (63.28%)	727 (6.54%)	10,392 (93.46%)	581	61 (0.56%)	567 (0.56%)
	Missing	493 (2.80%)	*	452 (91.81%)	66	*	63 (3.09%)
Region	Northeast	2,656 (15.12%)	228 (8.59%)	2,428 (91.41%)	400	31 (1.64%)	398 (1.64%)
	Midwest	4,819 (27.42%)	241 (5.00%)	4,578 (95.00%)	441	35 (0.74%)	433 (0.74%)
	South	7,266 (41.35%)	482 (6.63%)	6,784 (93.37%)	600	58 (0.73%)	576 (0.73%)
	West	2,832 (16.12%)	134 (4.72%)	2,698 (95.28%)	295	27 (1.04%)	296 (1.04%)

* Denotes missing values

TABLE 126
Patient and hospital characteristics for ICD-9-CM first-listed diagnosis code 473.1 Chr Frontal Sinusitis

		All ED visits (those that resulted in admission to the hospital and those that did not)	Only hospital visits that originated in the ED	Only ED visits that ended in discharge (no hospital admission)	Standard errors		
					All ED Visits	Admitted to the hospital from the ED	Discharged from the ED
All discharges		4,085 (100.00%)	169 (100.00%)	3,916 (100.00%)	328	29	326
Age (mean)		35.34	52.46	34.60	0.76	0.76	0.76
Age group	1–17	559 (13.68%)	*	546 (97.68%)	84	*	83 (1.37%)
	18–44	2,380 (58.27%)	54 (2.29%)	2,326 (97.71%)	210	15 (0.63%)	208 (0.63%)
	45–64	816 (19.96%)	*	771 (94.49%)	85	*	83 (1.76%)
	65–84	310 (7.58%)	*	262 (84.51%)	42	*	39 (4.71%)
	85+	*	*	*	*	*	*
Sex	Male	1,777 (43.49%)	95 (5.34%)	1,682 (94.66%)	141	20 (1.13%)	139 (1.13%)
	Female	2,308 (56.51%)	74 (3.22%)	2,234 (96.78%)	217	18 (0.79%)	215 (0.79%)
Median income for zip code	Low	1,510 (36.96%)	*	1,460 (96.71%)	184	*	182 (1.10%)
	Not low	2,460 (60.21%)	115 (4.67%)	2,345 (95.33%)	205	24 (1.00%)	203 (1.00%)
	Missing	115 (2.83%)	*	111 (95.99%)	30	*	30 (3.99%)
Region	Northeast	788 (19.28%)	*	740 (93.93%)	176	*	176 (2.36%)
	Midwest	981 (24.02%)	*	939 (95.64%)	157	*	156 (1.70%)
	South	1,537 (37.63%)	*	1,497 (97.39%)	192	*	191 (0.91%)
	West	779 (19.07%)	*	741 (95.06%)	124	*	120 (1.50%)

* Denotes missing values

TABLE 127

Patient and hospital characteristics for ICD-9-CM first-listed diagnosis code 473.2 Chr Ethmoidal Sinusitis

		All ED visits (those that resulted in admission to the hospital and those that did not)	Only hospital visits that originated in the ED	Only ED visits that ended in discharge (no hospital admission)	Standard errors		
					All ED Visits	Admitted to the hospital from the ED	Discharged from the ED
All discharges		4,969 (100.00%)	485 (100.00%)	4,484 (100.00%)	298	50	285
Age (mean)		39.06	43.32	38.60	0.67	0.67	0.67
Age group	<1	*	*	*	*	*	*
	1–17	675 (13.58%)	104 (15.39%)	571 (84.61%)	70	24 (3.13%)	62 (3.13%)
	18–44	2,409 (48.49%)	121 (5.01%)	2,289 (94.99%)	171	24 (0.98%)	168 (0.98%)
	45–64	1,286 (25.88%)	136 (10.61%)	1,150 (89.39%)	99	23 (1.76%)	95 (1.76%)
	65–84	514 (10.34%)	106 (20.69%)	407 (79.31%)	60	23 (3.79%)	52 (3.79%)
	85+	72 (1.45%)	*	60 (82.98%)	18	*	16 (9.07%)
Sex	Male	2,426 (48.81%)	226 (9.32%)	2,200 (90.68%)	171	31 (1.27%)	166 (1.27%)
	Female	2,539 (51.10%)	259 (10.20%)	2,280 (89.80%)	167	36 (1.33%)	158 (1.33%)
	Missing	*	*	*	*	*	*
Median income for zip code	Low	1,512 (30.44%)	164 (10.84%)	1,348 (89.16%)	150	28 (1.87%)	144 (1.87%)
	Not low	3,374 (67.90%)	294 (8.72%)	3,080 (91.28%)	227	41 (1.14%)	217 (1.14%)
	Missing	82 (1.66%)	*	*	24	*	*
Region	Northeast	698 (14.05%)	132 (18.97%)	566 (81.03%)	98	29 (4.20%)	94 (4.20%)
	Midwest	1,237 (24.89%)	86 (6.97%)	1,150 (93.03%)	161	21 (1.63%)	156 (1.63%)
	South	2,364 (47.58%)	211 (8.95%)	2,153 (91.05%)	210	32 (1.23%)	199 (1.23%)
	West	670 (13.49%)	55 (8.18%)	615 (91.82%)	93	15 (2.36%)	92 (2.36%)

* Denotes missing values

TABLE 128

Patient and hospital characteristics for ICD-9-CM first-listed diagnosis code 473.3 Chr Sphenoidal Sinusitis

		All ED visits (those that resulted in admission to the hospital and those that did not)	Only hospital visits that originated in the ED	Only ED visits that ended in discharge (no hospital admission)	Standard errors		
					All ED Visits	Admitted to the hospital from the ED	Discharged from the ED
All discharges		1,966 (100.00%)	281 (100.00%)	1,685 (100.00%)	125	39	117
Age (mean)		43.75	57.85	41.39	1.15	1.15	1.15
Age group	1–17	224 (11.41%)	*	203 (90.46%)	35	*	32 (4.78%)
	18–44	872 (44.37%)	65 (7.47%)	807 (92.53%)	77	19 (2.03%)	73 (2.03%)
	45–64	439 (22.34%)	*	387 (88.18%)	50	*	47 (3.53%)
	65–84	369 (18.77%)	115 (31.24%)	254 (68.76%)	43	21 (4.87%)	36 (4.87%)
	85+	61 (3.11%)	*	*	17	*	*
Sex	Male	585 (29.75%)	81 (13.84%)	504 (86.16%)	57	22 (3.42%)	52 (3.42%)
	Female	1,381 (70.25%)	201 (14.52%)	1,181 (85.48%)	99	32 (2.18%)	92 (2.18%)
Median income for zip code	Low	484 (24.62%)	78 (16.11%)	406 (83.89%)	54	22 (4.22%)	50 (4.22%)
	Not low	1,452 (73.84%)	196 (13.48%)	1,256 (86.52%)	109	33 (2.11%)	101 (2.11%)
	Missing	*	*	*	*	*	*
Region	Northeast	226 (11.47%)	*	189 (83.60%)	44	*	41 (6.29%)
	Midwest	487 (24.79%)	56 (11.53%)	431 (88.47%)	60	16 (3.24%)	57 (3.24%)
	South	987 (50.19%)	157 (15.91%)	830 (84.09%)	90	28 (2.67%)	84 (2.67%)
	West	267 (13.55%)	*	235 (88.25%)	46	*	42 (5.26%)

* Denotes missing values

TABLE 129

Patient and hospital characteristics for ICD-9-CM first-listed diagnosis code 473.8 Chronic Sinusitis Nec

		All ED visits (those that resulted in admission to the hospital and those that did not)	Only hospital visits that originated in the ED	Only ED visits that ended in discharge (no hospital admission)	Standard errors		
					All ED Visits	Admitted to the hospital from the ED	Discharged from the ED
All discharges		7,886 (100.00%)	757 (100.00%)	7,129 (100.00%)	1,274	112	1,258
Age (mean)		33.30	38.49	32.74	2.05	2.05	2.05
Age group	<1	*	*	*	*	*	*
	1–17	*	259 (13.63%)	*	*	76 (5.13%)	*
	18–44	3,573 (45.31%)	168 (4.69%)	3,406 (95.31%)	548	31 (1.03%)	544 (1.03%)
	45–64	1,700 (21.55%)	170 (10.01%)	1,529 (89.99%)	209	40 (2.43%)	204 (2.43%)
	65–84	538 (6.82%)	129 (23.95%)	409 (76.05%)	62	25 (4.58%)	58 (4.58%)
	85+	102 (1.30%)	*	71 (68.96%)	21	*	18 (10.05%)
Sex	Male	3,393 (43.03%)	388 (11.43%)	3,005 (88.57%)	533	76 (2.54%)	521 (2.54%)
	Female	4,493 (56.97%)	369 (8.22%)	4,124 (91.78%)	762	50 (1.66%)	756 (1.66%)
Median income for zip code	Low	2,935 (37.21%)	192 (6.56%)	2,742 (93.44%)	670	50 (1.96%)	659 (1.96%)
	Not low	4,759 (60.35%)	544 (11.43%)	4,216 (88.57%)	645	76 (2.02%)	637 (2.02%)
	Missing	192 (2.44%)	*	*	53	*	*
Region	Northeast	*	117 (7.70%)	*	*	31 (3.07%)	*
	Midwest	1,409 (17.86%)	106 (7.53%)	1,302 (92.47%)	212	23 (1.79%)	208 (1.79%)
	South	3,907 (49.54%)	410 (10.50%)	*	1,131	98 (3.52%)	*
	West	1,054 (13.36%)	*	930 (88.25%)	282	*	277 (4.27%)

* Denotes missing values

TABLE 130
Patient and hospital characteristics for ICD-9-CM first-listed diagnosis code 473.9 Chronic Sinusitis Nos

		All ED visits (those that resulted in admission to the hospital and those that did not)	Only hospital visits that originated in the ED	Only ED visits that ended in discharge (no hospital admission)	Standard errors		
					All ED Visits	Admitted to the hospital from the ED	Discharged from the ED
All discharges		332,400 (100.00%)	2,219 (100.00%)	330,181 (100.00%)	23,712	190	23,675
Age (mean)		33.58	45.03	33.51	0.26	0.26	0.26
Age group	<1	3,736 (1.12%)	*	3,689 (98.73%)	298	*	297 (0.46%)
	1–17	60,812 (18.29%)	494 (0.81%)	60,319 (99.19%)	5,273	109 (0.18%)	5,252 (0.18%)
	18–44	176,437 (53.08%)	423 (0.24%)	176,014 (99.76%)	12,548	55 (0.03%)	12,538 (0.03%)
	45–64	70,869 (21.32%)	643 (0.91%)	70,226 (99.09%)	5,120	72 (0.11%)	5,109 (0.11%)
	65–84	18,401 (5.54%)	466 (2.53%)	17,935 (97.47%)	1,163	46 (0.28%)	1,158 (0.28%)
	85+	2,134 (0.64%)	145 (6.78%)	1,989 (93.22%)	151	27 (1.26%)	148 (1.26%)
	Missing	*	*	*	*	*	*
Sex	Male	124,544 (37.47%)	973 (0.78%)	123,571 (99.22%)	8,549	104 (0.09%)	8,529 (0.09%)
	Female	207,830 (62.52%)	1,245 (0.60%)	206,584 (99.40%)	15,230	119 (0.07%)	15,211 (0.07%)
	Missing	*	*	*	*	*	*
Median income for zip code	Low	121,643 (36.60%)	640 (0.53%)	121,004 (99.47%)	11,570	91 (0.08%)	11,556 (0.08%)
	Not low	202,786 (61.01%)	1,494 (0.74%)	201,292 (99.26%)	13,418	138 (0.07%)	13,386 (0.07%)
	Missing	7,970 (2.40%)	85 (1.07%)	7,885 (98.93%)	675	23 (0.28%)	671 (0.28%)
Region	Northeast	44,269 (13.32%)	520 (1.17%)	43,750 (98.83%)	4,399	95 (0.23%)	4,387 (0.23%)
	Midwest	110,316 (33.19%)	481 (0.44%)	109,834 (99.56%)	21,732	78 (0.10%)	21,712 (0.10%)
	South	141,566 (42.59%)	999 (0.71%)	140,567 (99.29%)	7,912	139 (0.09%)	7,861 (0.09%)
	West	36,249 (10.91%)	219 (0.60%)	36,030 (99.40%)	2,841	42 (0.12%)	2,834 (0.12%)

* Denotes missing values

Chronic sinusitis Nos is more prevalent in females at 62.5%, and is also seen more in the prime-age group, ages 18–44, at 53.1%, followed by older adults, ages 45–64, at 21.3% and then the young, ages 1–17, at 18.3% and ages 65–84, at 5.5%. Chronic sinusitis is more prevalent in the South and the Midwest followed by the Northeast and the West.

TABLE 131

Patient and hospital characteristics for ICD-9-CM first-listed diagnosis code 471.9 Nasal Polyp Nos

		All ED visits (those that resulted in admission to the hospital and those that did not)	Only hospital visits that originated in the ED	Only ED visits that ended in discharge (no hospital admission)	Standard errors		
					All ED Visits	Admitted to the hospital from the ED	Discharged from the ED
All discharges		1,146 (100.00%)	*	1,129 (100.00%)	87	*	87
Age (mean)		36.42	75.54	35.83	1.58	1.58	1.58
Age group	<1	*	*	*	*	*	*
	1–17	270 (23.59%)	*	270 (100.00%)	41	*	41 (0.00%)
	18–44	422 (36.79%)	*	422 (100.00%)	47	*	47 (0.00%)
	45–64	327 (28.57%)	*	327 (100.00%)	46	*	46 (0.00%)
	65–84	93 (8.10%)	*	79 (85.53%)	20	*	19 (6.98%)
	85+	*	*	*	*	*	*
Sex	Male	574 (50.07%)	*	561 (97.81%)	63	*	62 (1.09%)
	Female	572 (49.93%)	*	568 (99.21%)	54	*	54 (0.79%)
Median income for zip code	Low	428 (37.32%)	*	420 (98.25%)	52	*	52 (1.26%)
	Not low	690 (60.19%)	*	680 (98.61%)	62	*	62 (0.80%)
	Missing	*	*	*	*	*	*
Region	Northeast	286 (24.98%)	*	286 (100.00%)	44	*	44 (0.00%)
	Midwest	198 (17.23%)	*	198 (100.00%)	36	*	36 (0.00%)
	South	470 (41.02%)	*	458 (97.32%)	52	*	51 (1.32%)
	West	192 (16.77%)	*	188 (97.65%)	42	*	42 (2.39%)

* Denotes missing values

TABLE 132

2008 National statistics—first-listed diagnosis only

Patient and hospital characteristics for
ICD-9-CM first-listed diagnosis code
708.0 Allergic Urticaria

		All ED visits (those that resulted in admission to the hospital and those that did not)	Only hospital visits that originated in the ED	Only ED visits that ended in discharge (no hospital admission)	Standard errors		
					All ED Visits	Admitted to the hospital from the ED	Discharged from the ED
All discharges		166,216 (100.00%)	2,032 (100.00%)	164,184 (100.00%)	5,883	120	5,853
Age (mean)		29.79	43.34	29.62	0.27	0.27	0.27
Age group	<1	3,985 (2.40%)	*	3,947 (99.04%)	243	*	241 (0.32%)
	1–17	50,523 (30.40%)	344 (0.68%)	50,179 (99.32%)	2,223	44 (0.08%)	2,209 (0.08%)
	18–44	69,154 (41.60%)	621 (0.90%)	68,533 (99.10%)	2,542	60 (0.09%)	2,536 (0.09%)
	45–64	30,103 (18.11%)	545 (1.81%)	29,558 (98.19%)	1,088	54 (0.18%)	1,078 (0.18%)
	65–84	11,442 (6.88%)	406 (3.55%)	11,036 (96.45%)	486	44 (0.38%)	478 (0.38%)
	85+	1,009 (0.61%)	78 (7.75%)	931 (92.25%)	76	20 (1.92%)	74 (1.92%)
Sex	Male	66,274 (39.87%)	744 (1.12%)	65,530 (98.88%)	2,425	66 (0.10%)	2,406 (0.10%)
	Female	99,932 (60.12%)	1,288 (1.29%)	98,644 (98.71%)	3,559	86 (0.09%)	3,545 (0.09%)
	Missing	*	*	*	*	*	*
Median income for zip code	Low	42,678 (25.68%)	413 (0.97%)	42,265 (99.03%)	2,209	51 (0.12%)	2,203 (0.12%)
	Not low	119,684 (72.01%)	1,539 (1.29%)	118,146 (98.71%)	4,963	105 (0.09%)	4,932 (0.09%)
	Missing	3,854 (2.32%)	*	3,773 (97.91%)	370	*	367 (0.67%)
Region	Northeast	34,273 (20.62%)	560 (1.63%)	33,713 (98.37%)	2,970	66 (0.22%)	2,959 (0.22%)
	Midwest	29,756 (17.90%)	365 (1.23%)	29,391 (98.77%)	1,934	43 (0.16%)	1,929 (0.16%)
	South	68,657 (41.31%)	799 (1.16%)	67,858 (98.84%)	3,879	79 (0.11%)	3,851 (0.11%)
	West	33,530 (20.17%)	308 (0.92%)	33,222 (99.08%)	2,647	44 (0.13%)	2,636 (0.13%)

* Denotes missing values

Allergic urticaria was more prevalent in females at 60.1%, and is also found more in the prime-age group, ages 18–44, at 41.6%, followed by the young and older adults, ages 1–17 and 45–64, at 30.4% and 18.1% respectively, and older adults, ages 65–84, at 6.9%. Allergic urticaria in 2008 was more prevalent in the South with 41.3%, and the Northeast with 20.6%, the West with 20.2%, and the Midwest with 17.9%.

TABLE 133

Patient and hospital characteristics for ICD-9-CM first-listed diagnosis code 708.1 Idiopathic Urticaria

		All ED visits (those that resulted in admission to the hospital and those that did not)	Only hospital visits that originated in the ED	Only ED visits that ended in discharge (no hospital admission)	Standard errors		
					All ED Visits	Admitted to the hospital from the ED	Discharged from the ED
All discharges		5,202 (100.00%)	92 (100.00%)	5,110 (100.00%)	561	21	561
Age (mean)		26.60	38.00	26.39	1.32	1.32	1.32
Age group	<1	121 (2.33%)	*	118 (96.97%)	30	*	29 (3.03%)
	1–17	1,928 (37.06%)	*	1,922 (99.71%)	333	*	333 (0.30%)
	18–44	2,022 (38.88%)	*	1,981 (97.94%)	198	*	197 (0.69%)
	45–64	883 (16.98%)	*	842 (95.32%)	100	*	98 (1.70%)
	65–84	206 (3.97%)	*	206 (100.00%)	33	*	33 (0.00%)
	85+	*	*	*	*	*	*
Sex	Male	2,182 (41.94%)	*	2,148 (98.46%)	263	*	263 (0.62%)
	Female	3,020 (58.06%)	59 (1.94%)	2,962 (98.06%)	320	18 (0.61%)	319 (0.61%)
Median income for zip code	Low	1,392 (26.77%)	*	1,367 (98.15%)	210	*	210 (0.86%)
	Not low	3,721 (71.53%)	66 (1.78%)	3,655 (98.22%)	464	18 (0.53%)	463 (0.53%)
	Missing	88 (1.70%)	*	88 (100.00%)	23	*	23 (0.00%)
Region	Northeast	1,422 (27.33%)	*	1,378 (96.93%)	380	*	380 (1.39%)
	Midwest	1,386 (26.64%)	*	1,376 (99.27%)	236	*	236 (0.54%)
	South	1,271 (24.43%)	*	1,238 (97.37%)	213	*	212 (1.01%)
	West	1,123 (21.59%)	*	1,118 (99.56%)	264	*	264 (0.45%)

* Denotes missing values

TABLE 134

Patient and hospital characteristics for ICD-9-CM first-listed diagnosis code 708.8 Urticaria Nec

		All ED visits (those that resulted in admission to the hospital and those that did not)	Only hospital visits that originated in the ED	Only ED visits that ended in discharge (no hospital admission)	Standard errors		
					All ED Visits	Admitted to the hospital from the ED	Discharged from the ED
All discharges		14,330 (100.00%)	193 (100.00%)	14,136 (100.00%)	1,336	31	1,335
Age (mean)		26.08	27.98	26.05	0.68	0.68	0.68
Age group	<1	394 (2.75%)	*	385 (97.76%)	64	*	65 (1.67%)
	1–17	5,453 (38.05%)	77 (1.40%)	5,376 (98.60%)	600	21 (0.39%)	598 (0.39%)
	18–44	5,569 (38.86%)	55 (0.98%)	5,515 (99.02%)	508	15 (0.28%)	508 (0.28%)
	45–64	2,054 (14.33%)	*	2,016 (98.19%)	214	*	212 (0.61%)
	65–84	782 (5.46%)	*	770 (98.48%)	89	*	89 (0.89%)
	85+	78 (0.54%)	*	74 (94.62%)	23	*	22 (5.03%)
Sex	Male	6,116 (42.68%)	77 (1.26%)	6,039 (98.74%)	573	20 (0.34%)	572 (0.34%)
	Female	8,213 (57.32%)	116 (1.42%)	8,097 (98.58%)	795	23 (0.30%)	793 (0.30%)
Median income for zip code	Low	4,652 (32.46%)	49 (1.06%)	4,602 (98.94%)	624	14 (0.33%)	624 (0.33%)
	Not low	9,355 (65.29%)	144 (1.54%)	9,211 (98.46%)	946	26 (0.31%)	945 (0.31%)
	Missing	323 (2.25%)	*	323 (100.00%)	48	*	48 (0.00%)
Region	Northeast	4,338 (30.28%)	*	4,298 (99.06%)	1,084	*	1,084 (0.40%)
	Midwest	3,231 (22.55%)	*	3,193 (98.83%)	565	*	563 (0.43%)
	South	4,665 (32.56%)	86 (1.84%)	4,579 (98.16%)	481	22 (0.48%)	478 (0.48%)
	West	2,095 (14.62%)	*	2,066 (98.62%)	247	*	246 (0.53%)

* Denotes missing values

TABLE 135
Patient and hospital characteristics for ICD-9-CM first-listed diagnosis code 708.9 Urticaria Nos

| | | All ED visits (those that resulted in admission to the hospital and those that did not) | Only hospital visits that originated in the ED | Only ED visits that ended in discharge (no hospital admission) | Standard errors | | |
					All ED Visits	Admitted to the hospital from the ED	Discharged from the ED
All discharges		262,970 (100.00%)	687 (100.00%)	262,283 (100.00%)	7,784	65	7,773
Age (mean)		25.40	34.24	25.38	0.38	0.38	0.38
Age group	<1	7,866 (2.99%)	*	7,851 (99.81%)	510	*	507 (0.10%)
	1–17	104,945 (39.91%)	236 (0.22%)	104,710 (99.78%)	4,616	37 (0.04%)	4,609 (0.04%)
	18–44	97,638 (37.13%)	181 (0.19%)	97,457 (99.81%)	2,978	32 (0.03%)	2,973 (0.03%)
	45–64	37,093 (14.11%)	150 (0.41%)	36,942 (99.59%)	1,090	27 (0.07%)	1,088 (0.07%)
	65–84	13,985 (5.32%)	93 (0.67%)	13,892 (99.33%)	468	22 (0.15%)	465 (0.15%)
	85+	1,438 (0.55%)	*	1,427 (99.21%)	94	*	94 (0.57%)
	Missing	*	*	*	*	*	*
Sex	Male	108,376 (41.21%)	236 (0.22%)	108,140 (99.78%)	3,529	37 (0.03%)	3,523 (0.03%)
	Female	154,580 (58.78%)	451 (0.29%)	154,129 (99.71%)	4,424	48 (0.03%)	4,419 (0.03%)
	Missing	*	*	*	*	*	*
Median income for zip code	Low	80,474 (30.60%)	227 (0.28%)	80,247 (99.72%)	3,819	38 (0.05%)	3,811 (0.05%)
	Not low	176,916 (67.28%)	451 (0.25%)	176,465 (99.75%)	5,931	51 (0.03%)	5,920 (0.03%)
	Missing	5,580 (2.12%)	*	5,571 (99.83%)	409	*	409 (0.12%)
Region	Northeast	45,233 (17.20%)	142 (0.31%)	45,092 (99.69%)	3,276	37 (0.08%)	3,273 (0.08%)
	Midwest	72,318 (27.50%)	161 (0.22%)	72,157 (99.78%)	3,860	31 (0.04%)	3,853 (0.04%)
	South	91,957 (34.97%)	267 (0.29%)	91,690 (99.71%)	4,684	37 (0.04%)	4,677 (0.04%)
	West	53,462 (20.33%)	117 (0.22%)	53,345 (99.78%)	3,608	23 (0.04%)	3,605 (0.04%)

* Denotes missing values

Urticaria Nos was more prevalent in females at 58.9%, and in the young, ages 1–17, at 39.9%, followed by the prime-age, 18–44, 37.1%, and older adults, ages 45–64, at14.1%, and then ages 65–84 at 5.3%. Urticaria Nos in 2008 was more prevalent in the South with 35% and the Midwest with 27.5%, followed by the West with 20.3% and the Northeast with 17.2%.

TABLE 136

2008 National statistics—first-listed diagnosis only

Patient and hospital characteristics for
ICD-9-CM first-listed diagnosis code
995.0 Anaphylactic Shock

	All ED visits (those that resulted in admission to the hospital and those that did not)	Only hospital visits that originated in the ED	Only ED visits that ended in discharge (no hospital admission)	Standard errors		
				All ED Visits	Admitted to the hospital from the ED	Discharged from the ED
All discharges	14,071 (100.00%)	3,835 (100.00%)	10,236 (100.00%)	568	180	490
Age (mean)	40.99	51.11	37.20	0.62	0.62	0.62
Age group <1	65 (0.46%)	*	61 (94.31%)	17	*	17 (5.61%)
1–17	2,237 (15.90%)	301 (13.47%)	1,936 (86.53%)	200	46 (1.85%)	184 (1.85%)
18–44	5,136 (36.50%)	945 (18.41%)	4,190 (81.59%)	262	78 (1.40%)	240 (1.40%)
45–64	4,804 (34.14%)	1,530 (31.84%)	3,274 (68.16%)	238	101 (1.67%)	193 (1.67%)
65–84	1,671 (11.88%)	961 (57.52%)	710 (42.48%)	103	73 (2.58%)	61 (2.58%)
85+	158 (1.12%)	94 (59.22%)	65 (40.78%)	28	22 (8.51%)	18 (8.51%)
Sex Male	5,829 (41.42%)	1,507 (25.85%)	4,322 (74.15%)	255	88 (1.44%)	231 (1.44%)
Female	8,234 (58.51%)	2,328 (28.28%)	5,905 (71.72%)	366	137 (1.38%)	307 (1.38%)
Missing	*	*	*	*	*	*
Median income for zip code Low	3,415 (24.27%)	944 (27.63%)	2,471 (72.37%)	235	85 (1.88%)	190 (1.88%)
Not low	10,319 (73.33%)	2,783 (26.97%)	7,535 (73.03%)	482	154 (1.28%)	413 (1.28%)
Missing	338 (2.40%)	109 (32.16%)	229 (67.84%)	56	26 (6.80%)	48 (6.80%)
Region Northeast	2,765 (19.65%)	873 (31.57%)	1,892 (68.43%)	329	83 (3.54%)	299 (3.54%)
Midwest	3,589 (25.51%)	872 (24.28%)	2,718 (75.72%)	250	88 (1.74%)	199 (1.74%)
South	4,901 (34.83%)	1,338 (27.31%)	3,563 (72.69%)	303	103 (1.81%)	260 (1.81%)
West	2,815 (20.01%)	752 (26.73%)	2,063 (73.27%)	244	84 (2.54%)	208 (2.54%)

* Denotes missing values

Anaphylactic shock was more prevalent in females at 58.5%, and is found more in the prime-age group, ages 18–44, at 36.5%, followed by the 45–64 age group at 34.1%, then the young, ages 1–17, at 15.9%, and older adults, ages 65–84, at 11.9%. Anaphylactic shock in 2008 was more prevalent in the South with 34.8%, and the Midwest with 25.5%, the West with 20.0% and the Northeast with 19.7%.

TABLE 137

Patient and hospital characteristics for ICD-9-CM first-listed diagnosis code 995.1 Angioneurotic Edema

		All ED visits (those that resulted in admission to the hospital and those that did not)	Only hospital visits that originated in the ED	Only ED visits that ended in discharge (no hospital admission)	Standard errors		
					All ED Visits	Admitted to the hospital from the ED	Discharged from the ED
All discharges		97,085 (100.00%)	13,705 (100.00%)	83,380 (100.00%)	2,595	567	2,309
Age (mean)		48.90	59.62	47.14	0.29	0.29	0.29
Age group	<1	229 (0.24%)	*	211 (92.09%)	39	*	39 (4.00%)
	1–17	10,019 (10.32%)	263 (2.63%)	9,756 (97.37%)	486	41 (0.39%)	476 (0.39%)
	18–44	26,985 (27.80%)	2,088 (7.74%)	24,898 (92.26%)	856	132 (0.45%)	811 (0.45%)
	45–64	33,830 (34.85%)	5,659 (16.73%)	28,170 (83.27%)	997	273 (0.64%)	858 (0.64%)
	65–84	22,995 (23.68%)	4,763 (20.72%)	18,231 (79.28%)	710	231 (0.79%)	596 (0.79%)
	85+	3,027 (3.12%)	913 (30.16%)	2,114 (69.84%)	151	73 (1.98%)	124 (1.98%)
Sex	Male	42,246 (43.51%)	5,725 (13.55%)	36,520 (86.45%)	1,164	266 (0.53%)	1,042 (0.53%)
	Female	54,826 (56.47%)	7,979 (14.55%)	46,846 (85.45%)	1,535	365 (0.55%)	1,363 (0.55%)
	Missing	*	*	*	*	*	*
Median income for zip code	Low	29,830 (30.73%)	4,616 (15.47%)	25,214 (84.53%)	1,261	295 (0.71%)	1,076 (0.71%)
	Not low	65,258 (67.22%)	8,675 (13.29%)	56,583 (86.71%)	2,185	444 (0.54%)	1,950 (0.54%)
	Missing	1,997 (2.06%)	414 (20.75%)	1,583 (79.25%)	181	89 (3.77%)	152 (3.77%)
Region	Northeast	14,381 (14.81%)	2,830 (19.68%)	11,551 (80.32%)	971	283 (1.72%)	861 (1.72%)
	Midwest	21,599 (22.25%)	3,016 (13.96%)	18,583 (86.04%)	1,074	219 (0.85%)	968 (0.85%)
	South	44,990 (46.34%)	6,127 (13.62%)	38,864 (86.38%)	1,928	415 (0.70%)	1,686 (0.70%)
	West	16,115 (16.60%)	1,732 (10.75%)	14,383 (89.25%)	959	147 (0.83%)	900 (0.83%)

* Denotes missing values

Angioneurotic edema was more prevalent in females at 56.5%, and was found more in the 45–64 age group at 34.9%, then the prime-age group, ages 18–44, at 27.8%, followed by the older adults, ages 65–84, at 23.7%, and the young, ages 1–17, at 10.3%. Angioneurotic edema in 2008 was more prevalent in the South with 46.3%, and the Midwest with 22.3%, the West with 16.6% and the Northeast with 14.8%.

TABLE 138

Patient and hospital characteristics for
ICD-9-CM first-listed diagnosis code
995.27 Drug Allergy Nec

		All ED visits (those that resulted in admission to the hospital and those that did not)	Only hospital visits that originated in the ED	Only ED visits that ended in discharge (no hospital admission)	Standard errors		
					All ED Visits	Admitted to the hospital from the ED	Discharged from the ED
All discharges		26,882 (100.00%)	400 (100.00%)	26,483 (100.00%)	1,576	61	1,573
Age (mean)		38.87	55.31	38.62	0.38	0.38	0.38
Age group	<1	644 (2.39%)	*	644 (100.00%)	74	*	74 (0.00%)
	1–17	3,772 (14.03%)	*	3,745 (99.29%)	290	*	290 (0.30%)
	18–44	11,780 (43.82%)	95 (0.81%)	11,685 (99.19%)	742	28 (0.24%)	742 (0.24%)
	45–64	6,932 (25.79%)	121 (1.75%)	6,810 (98.25%)	420	26 (0.38%)	417 (0.38%)
	65–84	3,331 (12.39%)	126 (3.77%)	3,205 (96.23%)	220	28 (0.85%)	219 (0.85%)
	85+	425 (1.58%)	*	394 (92.68%)	54	*	52 (2.74%)
Sex	Male	8,591 (31.96%)	129 (1.50%)	8,462 (98.50%)	546	29 (0.34%)	543 (0.34%)
	Female	18,289 (68.03%)	271 (1.48%)	18,018 (98.52%)	1,063	45 (0.26%)	1,064 (0.26%)
	Missing	*	*	*	*	*	*
Median income for zip code	Low	8,109 (30.17%)	119 (1.47%)	7,990 (98.53%)	622	26 (0.32%)	619 (0.32%)
	Not low	18,144 (67.49%)	272 (1.50%)	17,872 (98.50%)	1,275	47 (0.28%)	1,274 (0.28%)
	Missing	629 (2.34%)	*	620 (98.56%)	114	*	114 (1.04%)
Region	Northeast	4,184 (15.56%)	*	4,036 (96.46%)	455	*	455 (1.21%)
	Midwest	6,965 (25.91%)	*	6,910 (99.20%)	827	*	825 (0.31%)
	South	11,214 (41.72%)	155 (1.38%)	11,059 (98.62%)	1,001	27 (0.26%)	998 (0.26%)
	West	4,519 (16.81%)	*	4,478 (99.09%)	768	*	768 (0.34%)

* Denotes missing values

Drug allergy was more prevalent in females at 68.0%, and is found more in the prime-age group, ages 18–44, at 43.8%, followed by the 45–64 age group at 25.8%, then the young, ages 1–17, at 14.0%, and older adults, ages 65–84, at 12.4%. Drug allergy in 2008 was more prevalent in the South with 41.7%, and the Midwest with 25.9%, the West with 16.8% and the Northeast with 15.6%.

TABLE 139

Patient and hospital characteristics for
ICD-9-CM first-listed diagnosis code
995.3 Allergy, Unspecified

		All ED visits (those that resulted in admission to the hospital and those that did not)	Only hospital visits that originated in the ED	Only ED visits that ended in discharge (no hospital admission)	Standard errors		
					All ED Visits	Admitted to the hospital from the ED	Discharged from the ED
All discharges		301,927 (100.00%)	752 (100.00%)	301,175 (100.00%)	10,681	77	10,671
Age (mean)		31.77	42.08	31.74	0.26	0.26	0.26
Age group	<1	6,158 (2.04%)	*	6,148 (99.85%)	346	*	346 (0.11%)
	1–17	80,225 (26.57%)	114 (0.14%)	80,111 (99.86%)	3,399	24 (0.03%)	3,393 (0.03%)
	18–44	129,108 (42.76%)	272 (0.21%)	128,835 (99.79%)	4,827	45 (0.04%)	4,825 (0.04%)
	45–64	63,074 (20.89%)	241 (0.38%)	62,833 (99.62%)	2,242	35 (0.06%)	2,239 (0.06%)
	65–84	21,284 (7.05%)	93 (0.43%)	21,191 (99.57%)	871	20 (0.09%)	871 (0.09%)
	85+	2,071 (0.69%)	*	2,048 (98.90%)	124	*	124 (0.45%)
	Missing	*	*	*	*	*	*
Sex	Male	116,283 (38.51%)	303 (0.26%)	115,980 (99.74%)	4,194	41 (0.04%)	4,187 (0.04%)
	Female	185,586 (61.47%)	450 (0.24%)	185,137 (99.76%)	6,589	55 (0.03%)	6,586 (0.03%)
	Missing	*	*	*	*	*	*
Median income for zip code	Low	86,107 (28.52%)	204 (0.24%)	85,902 (99.76%)	4,389	33 (0.04%)	4,381 (0.04%)
	Not low	208,189 (68.95%)	540 (0.26%)	207,649 (99.74%)	8,651	66 (0.03%)	8,646 (0.03%)
	Missing	7,632 (2.53%)	*	7,624 (99.90%)	948	*	947 (0.07%)
Region	Northeast	63,949 (21.18%)	244 (0.38%)	63,705 (99.62%)	5,388	54 (0.09%)	5,387 (0.09%)
	Midwest	50,971 (16.88%)	113 (0.22%)	50,858 (99.78%)	3,249	24 (0.05%)	3,243 (0.05%)
	South	138,654 (45.92%)	276 (0.20%)	138,378 (99.80%)	8,020	41 (0.03%)	8,013 (0.03%)
	West	48,353 (16.01%)	119 (0.25%)	48,234 (99.75%)	3,189	28 (0.06%)	3,182 (0.06%)

* Denotes missing values

TABLE 140

Patient and hospital characteristics for ICD-9-CM first-listed diagnosis code 995.61 Anaphylactic Shock Peanuts

| | | All ED visits (those that resulted in admission to the hospital and those that did not) | Only hospital visits that originated in the ED | Only ED visits that ended in discharge (no hospital admission) | Standard errors | | |
					All ED Visits	Admitted to the hospital from the ED	Discharged from the ED
All discharges		3,064 (100.00%)	431 (100.00%)	2,633 (100.00%)	214	49	204
Age (mean)		18.05	25.46	16.84	0.88	0.88	0.88
Age group	<1	*	*	*	*	*	*
	1–17	1,785 (58.26%)	202 (11.34%)	1,582 (88.66%)	163	33 (1.82%)	156 (1.82%)
	18–44	831 (27.11%)	94 (11.30%)	737 (88.70%)	75	21 (2.46%)	73 (2.46%)
	45–64	305 (9.95%)	90 (29.62%)	215 (70.38%)	40	23 (6.27%)	34 (6.27%)
	65–84	59 (1.93%)	*	*	16	*	*
	85+	*	*	*	*	*	*
Sex	Male	1,742 (56.88%)	234 (13.46%)	1,508 (86.54%)	132	32 (1.91%)	129 (1.91%)
	Female	1,317 (43.00%)	196 (14.92%)	1,121 (85.08%)	115	32 (2.25%)	107 (2.25%)
	Missing	*	*	*	*	*	*
Median income for zip code	Low	603 (19.68%)	89 (14.78%)	514 (85.22%)	82	21 (3.11%)	75 (3.11%)
	Not low	2,403 (78.45%)	324 (13.50%)	2,079 (86.50%)	189	44 (1.77%)	179 (1.77%)
	Missing	*	*	*	*	*	*
Region	Northeast	793 (25.88%)	153 (19.32%)	640 (80.68%)	114	30 (4.17%)	111 (4.17%)
	Midwest	790 (25.80%)	68 (8.60%)	722 (91.40%)	107	17 (2.07%)	102 (2.07%)
	South	953 (31.10%)	144 (15.12%)	809 (84.88%)	129	28 (3.00%)	123 (3.00%)
	West	528 (17.23%)	66 (12.47%)	462 (87.53%)	67	20 (3.34%)	61 (3.34%)

* Denotes missing values

TABLE 141

Patient and hospital characteristics for ICD-9-CM first-listed diagnosis code 995.64 Anaphylactic Shock Tree Nuts and Seeds

		All ED visits (those that resulted in admission to the hospital and those that did not)	Only hospital visits that originated in the ED	Only ED visits that ended in discharge (no hospital admission)	Standard errors		
					All ED Visits	Admitted to the hospital from the ED	Discharged from the ED
All discharges		1,557 (100.00%)	185 (100.00%)	1,372 (100.00%)	130	31	124
Age (mean)		23.27	36.55	21.47	1.33	1.33	1.33
Age group	<1	*	*	*	*	*	*
	1–17	789 (50.68%)	*	740 (93.77%)	90	*	87 (1.88%)
	18–44	483 (31.01%)	*	422 (87.38%)	62	*	58 (3.70%)
	45–64	189 (12.15%)	52 (27.26%)	138 (72.74%)	30	15 (6.72%)	26 (6.72%)
	65–84	72 (4.60%)	*	*	20	*	*
	85+	*	*	*	*	*	*
Sex	Male	820 (52.66%)	114 (13.91%)	706 (86.09%)	82	22 (2.59%)	78 (2.59%)
	Female	733 (47.09%)	71 (9.72%)	662 (90.28%)	73	20 (2.69%)	71 (2.69%)
	Missing	*	*	*	*	*	*
Median income for zip code	Low	184 (11.81%)	*	150 (81.84%)	33	*	29 (5.81%)
	Not low	1,313 (84.33%)	141 (10.74%)	1,172 (89.26%)	119	27 (1.98%)	113 (1.98%)
	Missing	*	*	*	*	*	*
Region	Northeast	489 (31.38%)	65 (13.36%)	423 (86.64%)	77	18 (3.89%)	75 (3.89%)
	Midwest	483 (31.00%)	*	445 (92.21%)	73	*	67 (3.21%)
	South	279 (17.90%)	48 (17.06%)	231 (82.94%)	48	14 (4.50%)	43 (4.50%)
	West	307 (19.72%)	*	272 (88.64%)	59	*	59 (4.21%)

* Denotes missing values

TABLE 142

Patient and hospital characteristics for
ICD-9-CM first-listed diagnosis code
995.62 Anaphylactic Shock Crustacians

		All ED visits (those that resulted in admission to the hospital and those that did not)	Only hospital visits that originated in the ED	Only ED visits that ended in discharge (no hospital admission)	Standard errors		
					All ED Visits	Admitted to the hospital from the ED	Discharged from the ED
All discharges		984 (100.00%)	157 (100.00%)	827 (100.00%)	107	29	99
Age (mean)		33.89	40.11	32.71	1.07	1.07	1.07
Age group	<1	*	*	*	*	*	*
	1–17	166 (16.86%)	*	157 (94.50%)	37	*	37 (3.88%)
	18–44	573 (58.20%)	91 (15.92%)	482 (84.08%)	68	23 (3.87%)	64 (3.87%)
	45–64	182 (18.50%)	*	150 (82.18%)	29	*	26 (6.00%)
	65–84	*	*	*	*	*	*
	85+	*	*	*	*	*	*
Sex	Male	411 (41.74%)	61 (14.92%)	350 (85.08%)	57	17 (3.82%)	53 (3.82%)
	Female	573 (58.26%)	96 (16.70%)	478 (83.30%)	75	24 (3.74%)	68 (3.74%)
Median income for zip code	Low	251 (25.48%)	*	203 (80.95%)	44	*	40 (6.12%)
	Not low	706 (71.70%)	94 (13.35%)	612 (86.65%)	85	22 (2.89%)	79 (2.89%)
	Missing	*	*	*	*	*	*
Region	Northeast	299 (30.37%)	*	252 (84.29%)	72	*	65 (5.10%)
	Midwest	216 (21.98%)	*	*	54	*	*
	South	292 (29.67%)	*	246 (84.20%)	46	*	40 (4.55%)
	West	177 (17.99%)	*	161 (90.82%)	36	*	35 (4.65%)

* Denotes missing values

TABLE 143

Patient and hospital characteristics for ICD-9-CM first-listed diagnosis code 995.63 Anaphylactic Shock Fruits and Vegetables

		All ED visits (those that resulted in admission to the hospital and those that did not)	Only hospital visits that originated in the ED	Only ED visits that ended in discharge (no hospital admission)	Standard errors		
					All ED Visits	Admitted to the hospital from the ED	Discharged from the ED
All discharges		691 (100.00%)	147 (100.00%)	544 (100.00%)	72	27	68
Age (mean)			31.61	40.94	29.07	1.99	1.99	1.99
Age group	<1	*	*	*	*	*	*
	1–17	189 (27.35%)	*	169 (89.59%)	34	*	33 (5.13%)
	18–44	318 (46.02%)	59 (18.49%)	259 (81.51%)	40	15 (4.62%)	38 (4.62%)
	45–64	129 (18.71%)	*	*	36	*	*
	65–84	*	*	*	*	*	*
	85+	*	*	*	*	*	*
Sex	Male	280 (40.45%)	65 (23.26%)	215 (76.74%)	49	19 (6.11%)	44 (6.11%)
	Female	411 (59.55%)	82 (20.03%)	329 (79.97%)	47	19 (4.40%)	44 (4.40%)
Median income for zip code	Low	160 (23.10%)	*	*	44	*	*
	Not low	511 (74.02%)	110 (21.56%)	401 (78.44%)	55	23 (4.19%)	50 (4.19%)
	Missing	*	*	*	*	*	*
Region	Northeast	228 (33.03%)	*	187 (81.81%)	42	*	42 (6.14%)
	Midwest	116 (16.79%)	*	77 (66.15%)	24	*	20 (9.38%)
	South	179 (25.97%)	*	145 (80.96%)	34	*	29 (5.27%)
	West	167 (24.21%)	*	135 (80.60%)	41	*	40 (9.12%)

* Denotes missing values

TABLE 144

Patient and hospital characteristics for ICD-9-CM first-listed diagnosis code 995.65 Anaphylactic Shock to Fish

		All ED visits (those that resulted in admission to the hospital and those that did not)	Only hospital visits that originated in the ED	Only ED visits that ended in discharge (no hospital admission)	Standard errors		
					All ED Visits	Admitted to the hospital from the ED	Discharged from the ED
All discharges		1,477 (100.00%)	247 (100.00%)	1,230 (100.00%)	136	38	131
Age (mean)		33.88	38.97	32.86	1.16	1.16	1.16
Age group	<1	*	*	*	*	*	*
	1–17	315 (21.35%)	*	261 (82.90%)	49	*	42 (4.75%)
	18–44	734 (49.70%)	76 (10.35%)	658 (89.65%)	91	18 (2.59%)	89 (2.59%)
	45–64	323 (21.88%)	85 (26.19%)	238 (73.81%)	45	20 (5.56%)	40 (5.56%)
	65–84	96 (6.53%)	*	64 (66.43%)	21	*	16 (9.57%)
	85+	*	*	*	*	*	*
Sex	Male	570 (38.61%)	117 (20.50%)	453 (79.50%)	68	25 (3.95%)	60 (3.95%)
	Female	907 (61.39%)	130 (14.33%)	777 (85.67%)	96	26 (2.89%)	94 (2.89%)
Median income for zip code	Low	400 (27.07%)	60 (15.06%)	340 (84.94%)	78	17 (4.62%)	76 (4.62%)
	Not low	1,060 (71.79%)	183 (17.26%)	877 (82.74%)	95	34 (3.02%)	88 (3.02%)
	Missing	*	*	*	*	*	*
Region	Northeast	376 (25.44%)	107 (28.35%)	269 (71.65%)	83	29 (8.52%)	81 (8.52%)
	Midwest	250 (16.93%)	*	232 (92.85%)	47	*	44 (3.28%)
	South	507 (34.34%)	89 (17.51%)	418 (82.49%)	80	21 (4.37%)	78 (4.37%)
	West	344 (23.29%)	*	310 (90.22%)	54	*	51 (3.26%)

* Denotes missing values

TABLE 145

Patient and hospital characteristics for
ICD-9-CM first-listed diagnosis code
995.69 Anaphylactic Shock Due to Other Specified Food

		All ED visits (those that resulted in admission to the hospital and those that did not)	Only hospital visits that originated in the ED	Only ED visits that ended in discharge (no hospital admission)	Standard errors		
					All ED Visits	Admitted to the hospital from the ED	Discharged from the ED
All discharges		2,346 (100.00%)	430 (100.00%)	1,916 (100.00%)	169	53	148
Age (mean)		29.76	38.99	27.69	1.07	1.07	1.07
Age group	<1	*	*	*	*	*	*
	1–17	777 (33.10%)	87 (11.18%)	690 (88.82%)	94	22 (2.66%)	89 (2.66%)
	18–44	896 (38.20%)	119 (13.29%)	777 (86.71%)	76	24 (2.46%)	71 (2.46%)
	45–64	502 (21.41%)	144 (28.60%)	359 (71.40%)	52	25 (4.23%)	44 (4.23%)
	65–84	102 (4.36%)	59 (58.21%)	*	21	17 (10.15%)	*
	85+	*	*	*	*	*	*
Sex	Male	1,135 (48.40%)	239 (21.01%)	897 (78.99%)	107	40 (2.86%)	90 (2.86%)
	Female	1,211 (51.60%)	191 (15.80%)	1,019 (84.20%)	93	31 (2.32%)	84 (2.32%)
Median income for zip code	Low	509 (21.69%)	81 (15.91%)	428 (84.09%)	76	21 (4.06%)	72 (4.06%)
	Not low	1,775 (75.66%)	311 (17.54%)	1,463 (82.46%)	138	49 (2.36%)	119 (2.36%)
	Missing	*	*	*	*	*	*
Region	Northeast	688 (29.32%)	199 (28.92%)	489 (71.08%)	105	40 (4.16%)	82 (4.16%)
	Midwest	511 (21.78%)	87 (16.98%)	424 (83.02%)	72	25 (4.14%)	62 (4.14%)
	South	729 (31.09%)	102 (13.99%)	627 (86.01%)	90	21 (2.84%)	85 (2.84%)
	West	418 (17.81%)	*	376 (89.91%)	65	*	62 (3.44%)

* Denotes missing values

TABLE 146

Patient and hospital characteristics for ICD-9-CM first-listed diagnosis code 995.7 Adverse Food Reaction Nec

		All ED visits (those that resulted in admission to the hospital and those that did not)	Only hospital visits that originated in the ED	Only ED visits that ended in discharge (no hospital admission)	Standard errors		
					All ED Visits	Admitted to the hospital from the ED	Discharged from the ED
All discharges		26,610 (100.00%)	569 (100.00%)	26,041 (100.00%)	1,262	59	1,253
Age (mean)		27.86	48.45	27.41	0.45	0.45	0.45
Age group	<1	877 (3.29%)	*	871 (99.40%)	89	*	89 (0.49%)
	1–17	8,470 (31.83%)	*	8,401 (99.19%)	516	*	517 (0.28%)
	18–44	11,339 (42.61%)	147 (1.30%)	11,192 (98.70%)	563	25 (0.23%)	562 (0.23%)
	45–64	4,471 (16.80%)	199 (4.45%)	4,271 (95.55%)	258	31 (0.65%)	250 (0.65%)
	65–84	1,344 (5.05%)	125 (9.27%)	1,220 (90.73%)	102	22 (1.53%)	96 (1.53%)
	85+	105 (0.39%)	*	80 (76.57%)	22	*	20 (8.41%)
	Missing	*	*	*	*	*	*
Sex	Male	11,503 (43.23%)	227 (1.98%)	11,276 (98.02%)	590	35 (0.30%)	586 (0.30%)
	Female	15,102 (56.75%)	342 (2.26%)	14,760 (97.74%)	740	43 (0.29%)	735 (0.29%)
	Missing	*	*	*	*	*	*
Median income for zip code	Low	5,922 (22.26%)	153 (2.58%)	5,770 (97.42%)	369	35 (0.59%)	365 (0.59%)
	Not low	19,922 (74.86%)	390 (1.96%)	19,531 (98.04%)	1,097	45 (0.23%)	1,088 (0.23%)
	Missing	766 (2.88%)	*	740 (96.57%)	96	*	95 (1.52%)
Region	Northeast	6,513 (24.48%)	169 (2.59%)	6,344 (97.41%)	827	39 (0.66%)	825 (0.66%)
	Midwest	5,325 (20.01%)	*	5,273 (99.03%)	414	*	408 (0.31%)
	South	9,022 (33.90%)	229 (2.54%)	8,793 (97.46%)	637	32 (0.34%)	626 (0.34%)
	West	5,750 (21.61%)	120 (2.08%)	5,631 (97.92%)	576	25 (0.47%)	575 (0.47%)

* Denotes missing values

TABLE 147

National statistics—first-listed diagnosis only

Patient and hospital characteristics for ICD-9-CM first-listed diagnosis code 493.00 Ext Ast W/O Stat Ast Nos (after Oct 1, 2001)

		All ED visits (those that resulted in admission to the hospital and those that did not)	Only hospital visits that originated in the ED	Only ED visits that ended in discharge (no hospital admission)	Standard errors		
					All ED Visits	Admitted to the hospital from the ED	Discharged from the ED
All discharges		26,356 (100.00%)	1,147 (100.00%)	25,209 (100.00%)	5,838	313	5,662
Age (mean)		13.73	16.07	13.62	2.33	2.33	2.33
Age group	<1	*	*	*	*	*	*
	1–17	17,319 (65.71%)	*	16,721 (96.55%)	4,726	*	4,605 (0.89%)
	18–44	4,436 (16.83%)	54 (1.23%)	4,382 (98.77%)	711	15 (0.37%)	709 (0.37%)
	45–64	1,758 (6.67%)	124 (7.03%)	1,635 (92.97%)	447	25 (2.26%)	447 (2.26%)
	65–84	422 (1.60%)	88 (20.77%)	*	103	20 (6.01%)	*
	85+	*	*	*	*	*	*
Sex	Male	14,626 (55.49%)	580 (3.96%)	14,046 (96.04%)	3,517	162 (0.88%)	3,414 (0.88%)
	Female	11,730 (44.51%)	567 (4.84%)	11,163 (95.16%)	2,342	158 (1.20%)	2,268 (1.20%)
Median income for zip code	Low	11,555 (43.84%)	*	11,061 (95.72%)	3,245	*	3,159 (1.34%)
	Not low	14,393 (54.61%)	621 (4.32%)	13,772 (95.68%)	3,149	149 (0.90%)	3,064 (0.90%)
	Missing	408 (1.55%)	*	377 (92.39%)	83	*	78 (3.02%)
Region	Northeast	*	*	*	*	*	*
	Midwest	*	*	*	*	*	*
	South	3,559 (13.50%)	222 (6.25%)	3,337 (93.75%)	533	45 (1.30%)	519 (1.30%)
	West	*	*	*	*	*	*

* Denotes missing values

TABLE 148

2006 Hospital stays for children only—principal only

Outcomes by patient and hospital characteristics for
ICD-9-CM principal diagnosis code
493.00 Ext Ast W/O Stat Ast Nos (after Oct 1, 2001)

		Total number of discharges	LOS (length of stay), days (median)	Charges, $ (median)	Costs, $ (median)	Aggregate costs
All discharges		1,133 (100.00%)	2.0	6,265	2,153	3,204,048
Age group	<1	288 (25.42%)	2.0	7,300	2,593	940,938
	1–4	599 (52.90%)	1.0	5,792	2,007	1,566,091
	5–9	161 (14.23%)	2.0	6,404	2,336	433,916
	10–14	73 (6.41%)	2.0	7,100	2,261	237,927
	15–17	*	*	*	*	*
Sex	Male	667 (58.85%)	2.0	6,142	2,148	1,853,849
	Female	436 (38.51%)	2.0	6,346	2,174	1,268,778
	Missing	30 (2.64%)	2.0	7,781	2,328	81,421
Median income for zip code	Low	355 (31.30%)	2.0	5,954	2,044	907,659
	Not low	745 (65.77%)	2.0	6,519	2,261	2,196,701
	Missing	33 (2.93%)	1.0	3,533	1,755	99,688
Region	Northeast	117 (10.30%)	2.0	6,632	2,446	398,773
	Midwest	*	2.0	5,238	2,089	726,960
	South	292 (25.73%)	2.0	5,481	1,941	691,775
	West	433 (38.23%)	1.0	7,125	2,348	1,386,540

* Denotes missing values

TABLE 149

Outcomes by patient and hospital characteristics for
ICD-9-CM principal diagnosis code
493.01 Extrinsic Asthma with Status Asthmaticus

		Total number of discharges	LOS (length of stay), days (median)	Charges, $ (median)	Costs, $ (median)	Aggregate costs
All discharges		8,038 (100.00%)	2.0	9,074	3,561	40,713,506
Age group	<1	*	2.0	8,270	3,217	1,257,495
	1–4	3,049 (37.93%)	2.0	7,896	3,174	12,932,996
	5–9	2,722 (33.86%)	2.0	9,215	3,587	14,121,233
	10–14	1,530 (19.03%)	3.0	11,620	4,476	9,847,342
	15–17	436 (5.43%)	3.0	12,079	4,050	2,554,440
Sex	Male	4,990 (62.08%)	2.0	8,670	3,474	24,254,156
	Female	2,923 (36.37%)	2.0	9,624	3,705	16,043,440
	Missing	125 (1.55%)	2.0	8,894	2,755	415,909
Median income for zip code	Low	2,622 (32.62%)	2.0	9,918	3,669	13,145,561
	Not low	5,133 (63.86%)	2.0	8,802	3,434	25,749,859
	Missing	*	2.0	5,982	5,628	1,818,086
Region	Northeast	926 (11.52%)	2.0	10,261	4,819	5,341,754
	Midwest	1,033 (12.85%)	2.0	8,267	3,623	5,587,541
	South	*	2.0	9,674	3,552	16,841,033
	West	*	2.0	8,376	3,345	12,943,178

* Denotes missing values

TABLE 150

Outcomes by patient and hospital characteristics for
ICD-9-CM principal diagnosis code
493.02 Extrinsic Asthma with Acute Exacerbation

		Total number of discharges	LOS (length of stay), days (median)	Charges, $ (median)	Costs, $ (median)	Aggregate costs
All discharges		10,968 (100.00%)	2.0	6,835	2,556	36,339,127
Age group	<1	948 (8.65%)	2.0	8,064	2,925	3,894,310
	1–4	4,979 (45.40%)	2.0	6,537	2,419	14,991,979
	5–9	3,113 (28.38%)	2.0	6,908	2,545	10,222,682
	10–14	1,487 (13.55%)	2.0	7,271	2,901	5,602,069
	15–17	441 (4.02%)	2.0	7,172	2,928	1,628,087
Sex	Male	6,872 (62.66%)	2.0	6,681	2,492	22,205,572
	Female	3,872 (35.30%)	2.0	7,124	2,615	13,370,601
	Missing	224 (2.04%)	2.0	10,587	3,151	762,954
Median income for zip code	Low	4,197 (38.26%)	2.0	7,162	2,497	13,433,915
	Not low	6,378 (58.16%)	2.0	6,739	2,526	21,010,325
	Missing	*	2.0	5,269	4,149	1,894,886
Region	Northeast	*	2.0	8,291	2,733	7,429,152
	Midwest	2,233 (20.36%)	2.0	5,623	2,465	6,920,114
	South	2,663 (24.28%)	2.0	5,963	2,220	7,342,770
	West	4,012 (36.58%)	2.0	8,127	2,781	14,647,091

* Denotes missing values

TABLE 151

Patient and hospital characteristics for
ICD-9-CM first-listed diagnosis code
493.02 Extrinsic Asthma with Acute Exacerbation

		All ED visits (those that resulted in admission to the hospital and those that did not)	Only hospital visits that originated in the ED	Only ED visits that ended in discharge (no hospital admission)	Standard errors		
					All ED Visits	Admitted to the hospital from the ED	Discharged from the ED
All discharges		49,897 (100.00%)	15,033 (100.00%)	*	12,903	3,576	*
Age (mean)	12.32	16.68	10.45	1.79	1.79	1.79	*
Age group	<1	*	*	*	*	*	*
	1–17	*	*	*	*	*	*
	18–44	5,868 (11.76%)	2,598 (44.28%)	3,270 (55.72%)	632	288 (3.19%)	444 (3.19%)
	45–64	2,779 (5.57%)	1,546 (55.63%)	1,233 (44.37%)	383	156 (5.25%)	290 (5.25%)
	65–84	630 (1.26%)	458 (72.71%)	*	88	59 (6.18%)	*
	85+	45 (0.09%)	*	*	13	*	*
	Missing	*	*	*	*	*	
Sex	Male	29,170 (58.46%)	7,813 (26.78%)	*	8,239	2,207 (5.83%)	*
	Female	20,726 (41.54%)	7,220 (34.84%)	13,506 (65.16%)	4,712	1,397 (5.72%)	3,853 (5.72%)
Median income for zip code	Low	*	*	*	*	*	*
	Not low	26,317 (52.74%)	8,361 (31.77%)	*	6,864	1,789 (5.07%)	*
	Missing	*	*	316 (29.33%)	*	*	89 (8.50%)
Region	Northeast	*	*	*	*	*	*
	Midwest	*	*	*	*	*	*
	South	5,375 (10.77%)	2,009 (37.37%)	3,367 (62.63%)	952	267 (3.92%)	753 (3.92%)
	West	*	*	*	*	*	*

* Denotes missing values

TABLE 152

Patient and hospital characteristics for ICD-9-CM first-listed diagnosis code 493.20 Chronic Obstr Asthma W/O Status As Nos (after Oct 1, 2001)

		All ED visits (those that resulted in admission to the hospital and those that did not)	Only hospital visits that originated in the ED	Only ED visits that ended in discharge (no hospital admission)	Standard errors		
					All ED Visits	Admitted to the hospital from the ED	Discharged from the ED
All discharges		19,350 (100.00%)	4,442 (100.00%)	14,908 (100.00%)	875	248	804
Age (mean)		56.46	64.56	54.05	0.40	0.40	0.40
Age group	<1	*	*	*	*	*	*
	1–17	481 (2.48%)	*	466 (96.95%)	54	*	53 (1.77%)
	18–44	3,680 (19.02%)	401 (10.89%)	3,279 (89.11%)	251	53 (1.32%)	234 (1.32%)
	45–64	8,814 (45.55%)	1,797 (20.39%)	7,017 (79.61%)	470	126 (1.49%)	445 (1.49%)
	65–84	5,370 (27.75%)	1,732 (32.26%)	3,638 (67.74%)	265	114 (1.90%)	229 (1.90%)
	85+	973 (5.03%)	493 (50.61%)	481 (49.39%)	79	59 (3.97%)	52 (3.97%)
Sex	Male	6,832 (35.31%)	1,439 (21.06%)	5,393 (78.94%)	319	112 (1.56%)	296 (1.56%)
	Female	12,517 (64.69%)	3,003 (23.99%)	9,514 (76.01%)	626	171 (1.36%)	571 (1.36%)
Median income for zip code	Low	7,209 (37.25%)	1,640 (22.74%)	5,569 (77.26%)	479	156 (1.96%)	427 (1.96%)
	Not low	11,594 (59.92%)	2,703 (23.32%)	8,891 (76.68%)	609	166 (1.39%)	553 (1.39%)
	Missing	547 (2.83%)	99 (18.12%)	448 (81.88%)	57	23 (3.80%)	51 (3.80%)
Region	Northeast	2,940 (15.19%)	728 (24.78%)	2,212 (75.22%)	328	98 (3.13%)	294 (3.13%)
	Midwest	4,273 (22.08%)	944 (22.08%)	3,330 (77.92%)	377	97 (2.41%)	355 (2.41%)
	South	8,347 (43.14%)	2,098 (25.14%)	6,248 (74.86%)	514	191 (2.09%)	460 (2.09%)
	West	3,790 (19.58%)	672 (17.73%)	3,118 (82.27%)	501	80 (2.38%)	472 (2.38%)

* Denotes missing values

TABLE 153

Patient and hospital characteristics for ICD-9-CM first-listed diagnosis code 493.21 Chronic Obstr Asthma W Status Asth (after Oct 1, 2001)

		All ED visits (those that resulted in admission to the hospital and those that did not)	Only hospital visits that originated in the ED	Only ED visits that ended in discharge (no hospital admission)	Standard errors		
					All ED Visits	Admitted to the hospital from the ED	Discharged from the ED
All discharges		6,635 (100.00%)	5,341 (100.00%)	1,294 (100.00%)	369	317	147
Age (mean)			56.64	57.96	51.20	0.62	0.62	0.62
Age group	<1	*	*	*	*	*	*
	1–17	187 (2.82%)	86 (46.15%)	101 (53.85%)	38	24 (9.95%)	30 (9.95%)
	18–44	1,208 (18.20%)	905 (74.93%)	303 (25.07%)	99	81 (3.69%)	54 (3.69%)
	45–64	3,055 (46.04%)	2,534 (82.97%)	520 (17.03%)	209	180 (2.21%)	80 (2.21%)
	65–84	1,850 (27.88%)	1,516 (81.98%)	333 (18.02%)	137	127 (3.19%)	64 (3.19%)
	85+	332 (5.01%)	299 (89.91%)	*	47	44 (4.39%)	*
Sex	Male	1,856 (27.98%)	1,347 (72.56%)	509 (27.44%)	132	105 (3.03%)	71 (3.03%)
	Female	4,779 (72.02%)	3,994 (83.57%)	785 (16.43%)	277	251 (1.89%)	100 (1.89%)
Median income for zip code	Low	2,048 (30.87%)	1,618 (79.00%)	430 (21.00%)	170	138 (3.09%)	78 (3.09%)
	Not low	4,354 (65.62%)	3,513 (80.68%)	841 (19.32%)	290	246 (2.28%)	119 (2.28%)
	Missing	233 (3.50%)	209 (90.05%)	*	52	50 (4.21%)	*
Region	Northeast	1,395 (21.02%)	1,174 (84.19%)	*	185	158 (4.14%)	*
	Midwest	1,066 (16.06%)	867 (81.34%)	199 (18.66%)	119	106 (3.54%)	42 (3.54%)
	South	2,844 (42.86%)	2,263 (79.58%)	581 (20.42%)	236	210 (3.11%)	99 (3.11%)
	West	1,331 (20.05%)	1,036 (77.89%)	294 (22.11%)	179	142 (4.09%)	72 (4.09%)

* Denotes missing values

TABLE 154

Patient and hospital characteristics for
ICD-9-CM first-listed diagnosis code
493.22 Chronic Obstr Asth W Acute Exacerbation (after Oct 1, 2001)

		All ED visits (those that resulted in admission to the hospital and those that did not)	Only hospital visits that originated in the ED	Only ED visits that ended in discharge (no hospital admission)	Standard errors		
					All ED Visits	Admitted to the hospital from the ED	Discharged from the ED
All discharges		164,054 (100.00%)	125,303 (100.00%)	38,751 (100.00%)	6,145	5,264	1,801
Age (mean)		61.25	62.86	56.03	0.20	0.20	0.20
Age group	<1	48 (0.03%)	*	*	14	*	*
	1–17	987 (0.60%)	280 (28.32%)	708 (71.68%)	94	46 (4.08%)	82 (4.08%)
	18–44	20,152 (12.28%)	13,112 (65.06%)	7,040 (34.94%)	897	632 (1.32%)	419 (1.32%)
	45–64	73,686 (44.92%)	54,179 (73.53%)	19,507 (26.47%)	2,945	2,417 (1.03%)	986 (1.03%)
	65–84	58,187 (35.47%)	47,979 (82.46%)	10,208 (17.54%)	2,320	2,131 (0.91%)	564 (0.91%)
	85+	10,989 (6.70%)	9,714 (88.40%)	1,275 (11.60%)	507	480 (0.88%)	100 (0.88%)
	Missing	*	*	*	*	*	*
Sex	Male	52,608 (32.07%)	38,329 (72.86%)	14,279 (27.14%)	2,107	1,741 (1.13%)	750 (1.13%)
	Female	111,428 (67.92%)	86,969 (78.05%)	24,459 (21.95%)	4,171	3,626 (0.87%)	1,149 (0.87%)
	Missing	*	*	*	*	*	*
Median income for zip code	Low	58,276 (35.52%)	43,027 (73.83%)	15,249 (26.17%)	3,724	3,143 (1.52%)	1,091 (1.52%)
	Not low	99,778 (60.82%)	77,246 (77.42%)	22,533 (22.58%)	3,689	3,082 (0.82%)	1,081 (0.82%)
	Missing	6,000 (3.66%)	5,031 (83.85%)	969 (16.15%)	947	937 (2.79%)	96 (2.79%)
Region	Northeast	34,780 (21.20%)	30,640 (88.10%)	4,140 (11.90%)	3,735	3,625 (1.50%)	439 (1.50%)
	Midwest	33,688 (20.54%)	24,234 (71.93%)	9,455 (28.07%)	2,848	2,130 (1.50%)	929 (1.50%)
	South	66,756 (40.69%)	50,346 (75.42%)	16,410 (24.58%)	3,257	2,713 (1.41%)	1,177 (1.41%)
	West	28,829 (17.57%)	20,084 (69.66%)	8,745 (30.34%)	2,257	1,634 (1.88%)	897 (1.88%)

* Denotes missing values

TABLE 155

Patient and hospital characteristics for ICD-9-CM first-listed diagnosis code 493.81 Exercse Induced Bronchospasm

		All ED visits (those that resulted in admission to the hospital and those that did not)	Only hospital visits that originated in the ED	Only ED visits that ended in discharge (no hospital admission)	Standard errors		
					All ED Visits	Admitted to the hospital from the ED	Discharged from the ED
All discharges		2,180 (100.00%)	78 (100.00%)	2,102 (100.00%)	137	20	135
Age (mean)		16.02	31.61	15.44	0.49	0.49	0.49
Age group	<1	*	*	*	*	*	*
	1–17	1,670 (76.60%)	*	1,643 (98.41%)	121	*	121 (0.73%)
	18–44	435 (19.96%)	*	411 (94.54%)	48	*	47 (2.21%)
	45–64	*	*	*	*	*	*
	65–84	*	*	*	*	*	*
	85+	*	*	*	*	*	*
Sex	Male	962 (44.12%)	*	932 (96.87%)	76	*	74 (1.30%)
	Female	1,218 (55.88%)	*	1,171 (96.11%)	94	*	93 (1.31%)
Median income for zip code	Low	574 (26.32%)	*	549 (95.71%)	65	*	64 (1.98%)
	Not low	1,582 (72.55%)	*	1,529 (96.66%)	110	*	108 (1.05%)
	Missing	*	*	*	*	*	*
Region	Northeast	525 (24.10%)	*	512 (97.46%)	59	*	59 (1.47%)
	Midwest	523 (23.97%)	*	513 (98.17%)	70	*	69 (1.27%)
	South	663 (30.44%)	*	627 (94.43%)	78	*	75 (1.96%)
	West	469 (21.49%)	*	451 (96.24%)	66	*	67 (2.45%)

* Denotes missing values

TABLE 156

Patient and hospital characteristics for ICD-9-CM first-listed diagnosis code 493.82 Cough Variant Asthma

		All ED visits (those that resulted in admission to the hospital and those that did not)	Only hospital visits that originated in the ED	Only ED visits that ended in discharge (no hospital admission)	Standard errors		
					All ED Visits	Admitted to the hospital from the ED	Discharged from the ED
All discharges		3,427 (100.00%)	131 (100.00%)	3,296 (100.00%)	507	27	506
Age (mean)		15.21	44.30	14.05	1.31	1.31	1.31
Age group	<1	*	*	*	*	*	*
	1–17	2,442 (71.24%)	*	2,417 (98.98%)	429	*	427 (0.43%)
	18–44	586 (17.10%)	*	545 (93.00%)	104	*	103 (2.73%)
	45–64	242 (7.05%)	*	205 (84.94%)	45	*	43 (5.29%)
	65–84	86 (2.51%)	*	67 (78.15%)	20	*	18 (9.76%)
	85+	*	*	*	*	*	
Sex	Male	1,703 (49.69%)	*	1,671 (98.10%)	284	*	284 (0.77%)
	Female	1,724 (50.31%)	99 (5.73%)	1,625 (94.27%)	240	23 (1.49%)	239 (1.49%)
Median income for zip code	Low	1,284 (37.46%)	*	1,263 (98.40%)	283	*	283 (0.81%)
	Not low	2,079 (60.66%)	96 (4.60%)	1,983 (95.40%)	323	23 (1.23%)	321 (1.23%)
	Missing	*	*	*	*	*	*
Region	Northeast	1,596 (46.57%)	*	1,551 (97.21%)	409	*	412 (1.21%)
	Midwest	559 (16.31%)	*	540 (96.66%)	153	*	154 (1.87%)
	South	810 (23.64%)	*	755 (93.16%)	206	*	199 (2.26%)
	West	*	*	*	*	*	*

* Denotes missing values

TABLE 157

Patient and hospital characteristics for
ICD-9-CM first-listed diagnosis code
493.90 Asth W/O Status Asthmaticus Nos (after Oct 1, 2001) 2008

		All ED visits (those that resulted in admission to the hospital and those that did not)	Only hospital visits that originated in the ED	Only ED visits that ended in discharge (no hospital admission)	Standard errors		
					All ED Visits	Admitted to the hospital from the ED	Discharged from the ED
All discharges		545,269 (100.00%)	15,109 (100.00%)	530,160 (100.00%)	20,003	765	19,723
Age (mean)		26.28	38.88	25.92	0.44	0.44	0.44
Age group	<1	20,242 (3.71%)	1,256 (6.20%)	18,986 (93.80%)	1,534	129 (0.64%)	1,493 (0.64%)
	1–17	201,292 (36.92%)	4,134 (2.05%)	197,158 (97.95%)	10,567	355 (0.17%)	10,458 (0.17%)
	18–44	207,009 (37.96%)	2,615 (1.26%)	204,395 (98.74%)	7,656	179 (0.09%)	7,607 (0.09%)
	45–64	89,548 (16.42%)	3,128 (3.49%)	86,420 (96.51%)	3,490	179 (0.21%)	3,442 (0.21%)
	65–84	23,367 (4.29%)	2,793 (11.95%)	20,574 (88.05%)	881	198 (0.74%)	805 (0.74%)
	85+	3,806 (0.70%)	1,184 (31.11%)	2,622 (68.89%)	245	124 (2.18%)	172 (2.18%)
	Missing	*	*	*	*	*	*
Sex	Male	248,923 (45.65%)	6,315 (2.54%)	242,608 (97.46%)	10,016	369 (0.15%)	9,894 (0.15%)
	Female	296,269 (54.33%)	8,794 (2.97%)	287,476 (97.03%)	10,362	452 (0.15%)	10,198 (0.15%)
	Missing	*	*	*	*	*	*
Median income for zip code	Low	181,991 (33.38%)	4,975 (2.73%)	177,016 (97.27%)	9,890	389 (0.21%)	9,741 (0.21%)
	Not low	350,802 (64.34%)	9,754 (2.78%)	341,048 (97.22%)	14,967	591 (0.16%)	14,724 (0.16%)
	Missing	12,476 (2.29%)	380 (3.05%)	12,096 (96.95%)	941	59 (0.47%)	927 (0.47%)
Region	Northeast	135,327 (24.82%)	3,409 (2.52%)	131,919 (97.48%)	12,158	382 (0.29%)	12,025 (0.29%)
	Midwest	106,469 (19.53%)	2,651 (2.49%)	103,817 (97.51%)	6,786	297 (0.27%)	6,699 (0.27%)
	South	212,634 (39.00%)	7,190 (3.38%)	205,444 (96.62%)	12,582	562 (0.26%)	12,356 (0.26%)
	West	90,839 (16.66%)	1,859 (2.05%)	88,980 (97.95%)	6,923	187 (0.20%)	6,844 (0.20%)

* Denotes missing values

TABLE 158

Outcomes by patient and hospital characteristics for
ICD-9-CM principal diagnosis code
493.90 Asthma W/O Status Asthma Nos (after Oct 1, 2001)

		Total number of discharges	LOS (length of stay), days (median)	Charges, $ (median)	Costs, $ (median)	Aggregate costs
All discharges		12,989 (100.00%)	2.0	5,235	1,952	31,646,629
Age group	<1	3,060 (23.56%)	2.0	5,399	2,001	7,956,130
	1–4	6,813 (52.45%)	2.0	5,044	1,867	15,707,982
	5–9	2,042 (15.72%)	2.0	5,354	1,991	4,980,520
	10–14	766 (5.90%)	2.0	5,636	2,220	2,003,741
	15–17	308 (2.37%)	2.0	6,339	2,461	998,257
Sex	Male	7,843 (60.39%)	2.0	5,096	1,895	18,620,235
	Female	5,004 (38.53%)	2.0	5,406	2,045	12,614,879
	Missing	141 (1.09%)	1.0	8,816	2,145	411,515
Median income for zip code	Low	4,984 (38.37%)	2.0	5,089	1,947	12,021,891
	Not low	7,606 (58.56%)	2.0	5,358	1,946	18,421,988
	Missing	398 (3.07%)	2.0	4,362	2,418	1,202,750
Region	Northeast	2,391 (18.41%)	2.0	5,650	2,059	6,164,762
	Midwest	2,343 (18.04%)	2.0	4,380	1,908	5,540,232
	South	6,316 (48.62%)	2.0	5,001	1,875	14,389,188
	West	1,939 (14.92%)	2.0	7,099	2,239	5,552,446

HCUP 2006-CHILDREN

* Denotes missing values

TABLE 159

Patient and hospital characteristics for
ICD-9-CM first-listed diagnosis code
493.90 Asth W/O Stat Asthm Nos (after Oct 1, 2001) 2006

		All ED visits (those that resulted in admission to the hospital and those that did not)	Only hospital visits that originated in the ED	Only ED visits that ended in discharge (no hospital admission)	Standard errors		
					All ED Visits	Admitted to the hospital from the ED	Discharged from the ED
All discharges		526,868 (100.00%)	16,811 (100.00%)	510,057 (100.00%)	20,975	798	20,687
Age (mean)		25.67	36.73	25.30	0.63	0.63	0.63
Age group	<1	20,380 (3.87%)	1,516 (7.44%)	18,864 (92.56%)	1,500	167 (0.79%)	1,443 (0.79%)
	1–17	202,729 (38.48%)	5,051 (2.49%)	197,678 (97.51%)	14,016	404 (0.19%)	13,836 (0.19%)
	18–44	197,550 (37.50%)	2,729 (1.38%)	194,821 (98.62%)	7,650	168 (0.09%)	7,608 (0.09%)
	45–64	79,917 (15.17%)	3,512 (4.39%)	76,405 (95.61%)	3,054	180 (0.24%)	3,008 (0.24%)
	65–84	22,737 (4.32%)	2,904 (12.77%)	19,832 (87.23%)	883	182 (0.75%)	825 (0.75%)
	85+	3,542 (0.67%)	1,089 (30.73%)	2,454 (69.27%)	206	105 (2.22%)	157 (2.22%)
	Missing	*	*	*	*	*	*
Sex	Male	243,661 (46.25%)	7,135 (2.93%)	236,526 (97.07%)	10,957	426 (0.18%)	10,813 (0.18%)
	Female	283,187 (53.75%)	9,676 (3.42%)	273,511 (96.58%)	10,424	445 (0.16%)	10,274 (0.16%)
	Missing	*	*	*	*	*	*
Median income for zip code	Low	182,220 (34.59%)	5,476 (3.01%)	176,744 (96.99%)	10,722	407 (0.22%)	10,559 (0.22%)
	Not low	333,923 (63.38%)	11,029 (3.30%)	322,894 (96.70%)	15,498	587 (0.17%)	15,227 (0.17%)
	Missing	10,725 (2.04%)	305 (2.84%)	10,420 (97.16%)	661	39 (0.36%)	652 (0.36%)
Region	Northeast	121,313 (23.03%)	3,492 (2.88%)	117,820 (97.12%)	12,010	331 (0.29%)	11,860 (0.29%)
	Midwest	113,787 (21.60%)	3,055 (2.69%)	110,731 (97.31%)	10,482	310 (0.30%)	10,381 (0.30%)
	South	195,080 (37.03%)	7,724 (3.96%)	187,356 (96.04%)	11,707	588 (0.31%)	11,517 (0.31%)
	West	96,688 (18.35%)	2,539 (2.63%)	94,149 (97.37%)	6,984	292 (0.27%)	6,848 (0.27%)

* Denotes missing values

TABLE 160
Patient and hospital characteristics for ICD-9-CM first-listed diagnosis code 493.91 Asthma W Status Asthmaticus 2008

		All ED visits (those that resulted in admission to the hospital and those that did not)	Only hospital visits that originated in the ED	Only ED visits that ended in discharge (no hospital admission)	Standard errors		
					All ED Visits	Admitted to the hospital from the ED	Discharged from the ED
All discharges		45,171 (100.00%)	30,670 (100.00%)	14,502 (100.00%)	3,182	2,585	1,150
Age (mean)		19.88	19.27	21.18	0.93	0.93	0.93
Age group	<1	1,096 (2.43%)	721 (65.73%)	376 (34.27%)	164	129 (4.76%)	68 (4.76%)
	1–17	26,509 (58.68%)	18,819 (70.99%)	7,689 (29.01%)	2,712	2,224 (2.68%)	906 (2.68%)
	18–44	10,605 (23.48%)	6,448 (60.80%)	4,157 (39.20%)	551	387 (2.12%)	326 (2.12%)
	45–64	5,386 (11.92%)	3,606 (66.96%)	1,779 (33.04%)	286	220 (2.23%)	157 (2.23%)
	65–84	1,381 (3.06%)	935 (67.70%)	446 (32.30%)	141	88 (3.94%)	84 (3.94%)
	85+	191 (0.42%)	137 (71.69%)	*	25	38 (16.64%)	*
	Missing	*	*	*	*	*	*
Sex	Male	22,807 (50.49%)	15,359 (67.34%)	7,449 (32.66%)	1,879	1,555 (2.42%)	659 (2.42%)
	Female	22,356 (49.49%)	15,311 (68.49%)	7,045 (31.51%)	1,363	1,082 (1.81%)	534 (1.81%)
	Missing	*	*	*	*	*	*
Median income for zip code	Low	14,925 (33.04%)	10,177 (68.18%)	4,749 (31.82%)	1,609	1,324 (3.04%)	554 (3.04%)
	Not low	28,525 (63.15%)	19,091 (66.93%)	9,435 (33.07%)	1,922	1,465 (2.05%)	819 (2.05%)
	Missing	*	*	318 (18.50%)	*	*	50 (8.76%)
Region	Northeast	11,607 (25.70%)	8,702 (74.97%)	2,905 (25.03%)	1,782	1,627 (4.47%)	520 (4.47%)
	Midwest	8,430 (18.66%)	5,670 (67.25%)	2,761 (32.75%)	1,638	1,216 (3.91%)	566 (3.91%)
	South	18,791 (41.60%)	12,302 (65.47%)	6,489 (34.53%)	1,977	1,537 (3.23%)	815 (3.23%)
	West	6,343 (14.04%)	3,996 (63.00%)	2,347 (37.00%)	602	440 (2.76%)	263 (2.76%)

* Denotes missing values

TABLE 161

Outcomes by patient and hospital characteristics for ICD-9-CM principal diagnosis code 493.91 Asthma W Status Asthmaticus

		Total number of discharges	LOS (length of stay), days (median)	Charges, $ (median)	Costs, $ (median)	Aggregate costs
All discharges		34,694 (100.00%)	2.0	7,635	2,933	145,062,964
Age group	<1	1,631 (4.70%)	2.0	7,351	2,776	6,445,960
	1–4	14,279 (41.16%)	2.0	6,900	2,695	53,984,097
	5–9	10,840 (31.24%)	2.0	8,027	3,016	46,144,858
	10–14	5,943 (17.13%)	2.0	8,716	3,363	28,628,498
	15–17	2,001 (5.77%)	2.0	8,620	3,454	9,859,552
Sex	Male	21,324 (61.46%)	2.0	7,522	2,876	87,153,716
	Female	13,035 (37.57%)	2.0	7,719	3,022	56,489,136
	Missing	335 (0.97%)	2.0	12,531	3,388	1,420,112
Median income for zip code	Low	12,327 (35.53%)	2.0	7,675	2,888	50,834,377
	Not low	21,000 (60.53%)	2.0	7,736	2,881	86,039,851
	Missing	*	2.0	5,914	5,330	8,188,736
Region	Northeast	8,465 (24.40%)	2.0	8,579	3,580	43,582,191
	Midwest	7,627 (21.98%)	2.0	5,749	2,649	27,479,624
	South	15,142 (43.64%)	2.0	7,745	2,702	58,331,577
	West	3,460 (9.97%)	2.0	10,588	3,255	15,669,572

HCUP 2006—CHILDREN

* Denotes missing values

TABLE 162
Patient and hospital characteristics for ICD-9-CM first-listed diagnosis code 493.91 Asthma W Status Asthmaticus

| | | All ED visits (those that resulted in admission to the hospital and those that did not) | Only hospital visits that originated in the ED | Only ED visits that ended in discharge (no hospital admission) | Standard errors | | |
					All ED Visits	Admitted to the hospital from the ED	Discharged from the ED
All discharges		59,103 (100.00%)	40,423 (100.00%)	18,680 (100.00%)	6,626	4,742	2,975
Age (mean)		17.31	17.16	17.66	1.34	1.34	1.34
Age group	<1	1,695 (2.87%)	1,215 (71.71%)	479 (28.29%)	311	269 (4.49%)	83 (4.49%)
	1–17	38,303 (64.81%)	26,630 (69.52%)	11,673 (30.48%)	6,188	4,391 (4.67%)	2,798 (4.67%)
	18–44	12,031 (20.36%)	7,537 (62.65%)	4,494 (37.35%)	682	415 (1.86%)	388 (1.86%)
	45–64	5,672 (9.60%)	4,016 (70.80%)	1,656 (29.20%)	349	230 (2.25%)	192 (2.25%)
	65–84	1,187 (2.01%)	868 (73.10%)	319 (26.90%)	100	82 (3.30%)	48 (3.30%)
	85+	178 (0.30%)	124 (69.81%)	54 (30.19%)	31	26 (6.92%)	15 (6.92%)
	Missing	*	*	*	*	*	*
Sex	Male	30,279 (51.23%)	20,467 (67.60%)	9,812 (32.40%)	3,913	2,841 (3.70%)	1,718 (3.70%)
	Female	28,824 (48.77%)	19,956 (69.23%)	8,868 (30.77%)	2,765	1,939 (2.85%)	1,286 (2.85%)
Median income for zip code	Low	19,623 (33.20%)	13,842 (70.54%)	5,781 (29.46%)	2,681	2,391 (4.18%)	826 (4.18%)
	Not low	38,764 (65.59%)	26,022 (67.13%)	12,743 (32.87%)	4,837	3,048 (3.04%)	2,282 (3.04%)
	Missing	715 (1.21%)	559 (78.11%)	157 (21.89%)	110	86 (3.68%)	39 (3.68%)
Region	Northeast	16,498 (27.91%)	11,378 (68.97%)	*	4,381	2,398 (8.84%)	*
	Midwest	12,816 (21.68%)	*	3,746 (29.23%)	3,360	*	896 (7.67%)
	South	23,455 (39.68%)	15,839 (67.53%)	7,615 (32.47%)	3,607	2,678 (2.92%)	1,213 (2.92%)
	West	6,335 (10.72%)	4,136 (65.29%)	2,198 (34.71%)	640	448 (3.79%)	352 (3.79%)

HCUP 2006

* Denotes missing values

TABLE 163

Patient and hospital characteristics for
ICD-9-CM first-listed diagnosis code
493.92 Asthma W Acute Exacerbation

		All ED visits (those that resulted in admission to the hospital and those that did not)	Only hospital visits that originated in the ED	Only ED visits that ended in discharge (no hospital admission)	Standard errors		
					All ED Visits	Admitted to the hospital from the ED	Discharged from the ED
All discharges		967,449 (100.00%)	129,311 (100.00%)	838,137 (100.00%)	34,702	7,146	30,777
Age (mean)		28.01	34.63	26.98	0.43	0.43	0.43
Age group	<1	12,762 (1.32%)	2,898 (22.71%)	9,864 (77.29%)	1,107	288 (1.63%)	925 (1.63%)
	1–17	339,980 (35.14%)	36,308 (10.68%)	303,671 (89.32%)	18,356	3,310 (0.73%)	16,362 (0.73%)
	18–44	393,010 (40.62%)	41,842 (10.65%)	351,168 (89.35%)	13,659	2,213 (0.44%)	12,388 (0.44%)
	45–64	175,852 (18.18%)	33,467 (19.03%)	142,385 (80.97%)	6,906	2,008 (0.91%)	5,910 (0.91%)
	65–84	40,385 (4.17%)	12,165 (30.12%)	28,220 (69.88%)	1,652	784 (1.43%)	1,261 (1.43%)
	85+	5,446 (0.56%)	2,617 (48.05%)	2,829 (51.95%)	260	180 (2.02%)	160 (2.02%)
	Missing	*	*	*	*	*	*
Sex	Male	429,861 (44.43%)	48,123 (11.19%)	381,738 (88.81%)	16,903	2,923 (0.53%)	15,232 (0.53%)
	Female	537,410 (55.55%)	81,189 (15.11%)	456,221 (84.89%)	18,403	4,497 (0.66%)	16,006 (0.66%)
	Missing	*	*	*	*	*	*
Median income for zip code	Low	343,389 (35.49%)	44,964 (13.09%)	298,426 (86.91%)	21,612	4,658 (1.05%)	19,006 (1.05%)
	Not low	599,134 (61.93%)	78,053 (13.03%)	521,081 (86.97%)	22,012	3,939 (0.47%)	19,473 (0.47%)
	Missing	24,925 (2.58%)	6,294 (25.25%)	18,631 (74.75%)	2,283	1,635 (4.84%)	1,322 (4.84%)
Region	Northeast	252,237 (26.07%)	42,494 (16.85%)	209,742 (83.15%)	22,022	5,674 (1.93%)	19,614 (1.93%)
	Midwest	197,666 (20.43%)	22,664 (11.47%)	175,003 (88.53%)	12,124	1,589 (0.58%)	11,056 (0.58%)
	South	352,264 (36.41%)	45,295 (12.86%)	306,969 (87.14%)	21,913	3,471 (0.57%)	19,190 (0.57%)
	West	165,282 (17.08%)	18,859 (11.41%)	146,423 (88.59%)	9,598	2,073 (1.00%)	8,487 (1.00%)

* Denotes missing values

TABLE 164

Outcomes by patient and hospital characteristics for ICD-9-CM principal diagnosis code 493.92 Asthma W Acute Exacerbation

		Total number of discharges	LOS (length of stay), days (median)	Charges, $ (median)	Costs, $ (median)	Aggregate costs
All discharges		68,434 (100.00%)	2.0	5,800	2,225	196,877,714
Age group	<1	5,386 (7.87%)	2.0	5,889	2,193	16,846,176
	1–4	32,285 (47.18%)	2.0	5,469	2,096	87,467,751
	5–9	18,670 (27.28%)	2.0	6,029	2,290	53,387,302
	10–14	8,717 (12.74%)	2.0	6,322	2,482	27,786,605
	15–17	3,377 (4.93%)	2.0	6,411	2,572	11,389,880
Sex	Male	42,368 (61.91%)	2.0	5,684	2,179	119,625,020
	Female	25,259 (36.91%)	2.0	5,927	2,291	74,480,496
	Missing	808 (1.18%)	2.0	10,505	2,863	2,772,197
Median income for zip code	Low	25,246 (36.89%)	2.0	5,749	2,172	70,033,621
	Not low	41,036 (59.96%)	2.0	5,863	2,215	116,530,284
	Missing	2,152 (3.14%)	2.0	5,439	3,219	10,313,809
Region	Northeast	19,181 (28.03%)	2.0	6,029	2,393	60,441,332
	Midwest	14,082 (20.58%)	2.0	5,105	2,181	38,123,586
	South	23,816 (34.80%)	2.0	5,459	2,011	59,258,028
	West	11,356 (16.59%)	2.0	7,563	2,578	39,054,768

HCUP 2006—CHILDREN

* Denotes missing values

TABLE 165
Patient and hospital characteristics for ICD-9-CM first-listed diagnosis code
493.92 Asthma W Acute Exacerbation 2006

		All ED visits (those that resulted in admission to the hospital and those that did not)	Only hospital visits that originated in the ED	Only ED visits that ended in discharge (no hospital admission)	Standard errors		
					All ED Visits	Admitted to the hospital from the ED	Discharged from the ED
All discharges		972,293 (100.00%)	121,935 (100.00%)	850,358 (100.00%)	35,940	4,847	32,933
Age (mean)		27.08	33.55	26.15	0.55	0.55	0.55
Age group	<1	15,392 (1.58%)	2,852 (18.53%)	12,541 (81.47%)	1,369	263 (1.47%)	1,225 (1.47%)
	1–17	364,308 (37.47%)	36,219 (9.94%)	328,089 (90.06%)	23,543	3,515 (0.77%)	21,608 (0.77%)
	18–44	384,999 (39.60%)	40,370 (10.49%)	344,629 (89.51%)	13,464	1,584 (0.26%)	12,273 (0.26%)
	45–64	162,574 (16.72%)	29,278 (18.01%)	133,296 (81.99%)	5,653	1,091 (0.48%)	4,921 (0.48%)
	65–84	39,777 (4.09%)	10,986 (27.62%)	28,791 (72.38%)	1,227	448 (0.85%)	987 (0.85%)
	85+	5,212 (0.54%)	2,205 (42.31%)	3,007 (57.69%)	231	132 (1.71%)	160 (1.71%)
	Missing	*	*	*	*	*	*
Sex	Male	439,936 (45.25%)	46,648 (10.60%)	393,288 (89.40%)	19,258	2,568 (0.48%)	17,832 (0.48%)
	Female	532,287 (54.75%)	75,281 (14.14%)	457,006 (85.86%)	17,389	2,566 (0.36%)	15,676 (0.36%)
	Missing	*	*	*	*	*	*
Median income for zip code	Low	342,652 (35.24%)	42,646 (12.45%)	300,006 (87.55%)	21,978	2,628 (0.47%)	19,871 (0.47%)
	Not low	612,219 (62.97%)	77,386 (12.64%)	534,833 (87.36%)	24,055	3,510 (0.45%)	21,938 (0.45%)
	Missing	17,421 (1.79%)	1,902 (10.92%)	15,519 (89.08%)	801	131 (0.68%)	748 (0.68%)
Region	Northeast	243,263 (25.02%)	33,944 (13.95%)	209,319 (86.05%)	21,553	2,986 (1.12%)	19,944 (1.12%)
	Midwest	202,834 (20.86%)	22,086 (10.89%)	180,748 (89.11%)	16,590	1,495 (0.72%)	15,707 (0.72%)
	South	352,444 (36.25%)	44,380 (12.59%)	308,064 (87.41%)	19,719	2,555 (0.52%)	17,931 (0.52%)
	West	173,751 (17.87%)	21,525 (12.39%)	152,227 (87.61%)	12,771	2,412 (0.83%)	10,888 (0.83%)

* Denotes missing values

TABLE 166

2008 National statistics—first-listed diagnosis only

Patient and hospital characteristics for ICD-9-CM
first-listed diagnosis code
372.00 Acute Conjunctivitis Nos

		All ED visits (those that resulted in admission to the hospital and those that did not)	Only hospital visits that originated in the ED	Only ED visits that ended in discharge (no hospital admission)	Standard errors		
					All ED Visits	Admitted to the hospital from the ED	Discharged from the ED
All discharges		101,249 (100.00%)	114 (100.00%)	101,134 (100.00%)	6,327	26	6,330
Age (mean)		20.90	26.70	20.89	0.64	0.64	0.64
Age group	<1	9,843 (9.72%)	*	9,800 (99.57%)	837	*	841 (0.20%)
	1–17	41,166 (40.66%)	*	41,144 (99.95%)	3,432	*	3,432 (0.02%)
	18–44	35,365 (34.93%)	*	35,354 (99.97%)	2,168	*	2,168 (0.02%)
	45–64	11,515 (11.37%)	*	11,487 (99.76%)	727	*	726 (0.10%)
	65–84	2,958 (2.92%)	*	2,954 (99.89%)	206	*	206 (0.11%)
	85+	402 (0.40%)	*	395 (98.22%)	47	*	47 (1.27%)
Sex	Male	46,980 (46.40%)	48 (0.10%)	46,932 (99.90%)	3,081	14 (0.03%)	3,083 (0.03%)
	Female	54,257 (53.59%)	66 (0.12%)	54,190 (99.88%)	3,306	19 (0.04%)	3,307 (0.04%)
	Missing	*	*	*	*	*	*
Median income for zip code	Low	30,493 (30.12%)	*	30,459 (99.89%)	3,100	*	3,101 (0.04%)
	Not low	68,891 (68.04%)	*	68,821 (99.90%)	4,710	*	4,713 (0.03%)
	Missing	1,865 (1.84%)	*	1,855 (99.46%)	172	*	172 (0.38%)
Region	Northeast	30,960 (30.58%)	*	30,921 (99.87%)	4,074	*	4,078 (0.07%)
	Midwest	23,220 (22.93%)	*	23,202 (99.92%)	3,344	*	3,345 (0.04%)
	South	30,396 (30.02%)	*	30,353 (99.86%)	2,924	*	2,925 (0.05%)
	West	16,673 (16.47%)	*	16,658 (99.91%)	1,923	*	1,921 (0.05%)

* Denotes missing values

TABLE 167

Patient and hospital characteristics for ICD-9-CM
first-listed diagnosis code
372.30 Conjunctivitis Nos 2008

		All ED visits (those that resulted in admission to the hospital and those that did not)	Only hospital visits that originated in the ED	Only ED visits that ended in discharge (no hospital admission)	Standard errors		
					All ED Visits	Admitted to the hospital from the ED	Discharged from the ED
All discharges		377,933 (100.00%)	282 (100.00%)	377,651 (100.00%)	12,513	66	12,505
Age (mean)		21.68	31.01	21.67	0.35	0.35	0.35
Age group	<1	35,899 (9.50%)	*	35,834 (99.82%)	1,807	*	1,804 (0.06%)
	1–17	145,562 (38.52%)	56 (0.04%)	145,506 (99.96%)	6,349	16 (0.01%)	6,347 (0.01%)
	18–44	138,489 (36.64%)	*	138,425 (99.95%)	4,662	*	4,662 (0.03%)
	45–64	44,668 (11.82%)	*	44,626 (99.91%)	1,485	*	1,485 (0.03%)
	65–84	11,453 (3.03%)	*	11,411 (99.63%)	435	*	432 (0.11%)
	85+	1,858 (0.49%)	*	1,845 (99.29%)	105	*	104 (0.41%)
	Missing	*	*	*	*	*	*
Sex	Male	174,112 (46.07%)	*	174,006 (99.94%)	5,832	*	5,829 (0.02%)
	Female	203,792 (53.92%)	176 (0.09%)	203,616 (99.91%)	6,799	41 (0.02%)	6,795 (0.02%)
	Missing	*	*	*	*	*	*
Median income for zip code	Low	134,542 (35.60%)	*	134,396 (99.89%)	6,847	*	6,844 (0.04%)
	Not low	234,789 (62.12%)	132 (0.06%)	234,657 (99.94%)	8,705	26 (0.01%)	8,699 (0.01%)
	Missing	8,601 (2.28%)	*	8,598 (99.96%)	691	*	690 (0.04%)
Region	Northeast	69,312 (18.34%)	*	69,220 (99.87%)	5,634	*	5,630 (0.04%)
	Midwest	104,777 (27.72%)	*	104,752 (99.98%)	6,819	*	6,819 (0.01%)
	South	144,513 (38.24%)	*	144,371 (99.90%)	7,794	*	7,785 (0.04%)
	West	59,330 (15.70%)	*	59,308 (99.96%)	4,193	*	4,190 (0.02%)

* Denotes missing values

TABLE 168

Patient and hospital characteristics for ICD-9-CM first-listed diagnosis code
372.14 Chr Allrg Conjunctiv Nec 2008

		All ED visits (those that resulted in admission to the hospital and those that did not)	Only hospital visits that originated in the ED	Only ED visits that ended in discharge (no hospital admission)	Standard errors		
					All ED Visits	Admitted to the hospital from the ED	Discharged from the ED
All discharges		36,456 (100.00%)	*	36,433 (100.00%)	1,527	*	1,526
Age (mean)		24.78	*	24.77	0.55	*	0.55
Age group	<1	439 (1.20%)	*	439 (100.00%)	51	*	51 (0.00%)
	1–17	15,851 (43.48%)	*	15,841 (99.94%)	1,039	*	1,039 (0.05%)
	18–44	13,617 (37.35%)	*	13,617 (100.00%)	586	*	586 (0.00%)
	45–64	5,169 (14.18%)	*	5,166 (99.94%)	262	*	262 (0.06%)
	65–84	1,252 (3.44%)	*	1,247 (99.57%)	91	*	91 (0.43%)
	85+	128 (0.35%)	*	124 (96.68%)	25	*	25 (3.29%)
Sex	Male	17,526 (48.08%)	*	17,526 (100.00%)	814	*	814 (0.00%)
	Female	18,925 (51.91%)	*	18,902 (99.88%)	800	*	799 (0.05%)
	Missing	*	*	*	*		*
Median income for zip code	Low	12,980 (35.61%)	*	12,973 (99.94%)	932	*	932 (0.04%)
	Not low	22,876 (62.75%)	*	22,866 (99.96%)	1,037	*	1,037 (0.03%)
	Missing	599 (1.64%)	*	594 (99.10%)	71	*	72 (0.91%)
Region	Northeast	9,181 (25.19%)	*	9,166 (99.84%)	895	*	894 (0.09%)
	Midwest	8,745 (23.99%)	*	8,741 (99.95%)	661	*	660 (0.05%)
	South	13,287 (36.45%)	*	13,284 (99.98%)	952	*	952 (0.02%)
	West	5,242 (14.38%)	*	5,242 (100.00%)	431	*	431 (0.00%)

* Denotes missing values

Summary

Tables 115–168 summarize the findings of atopic diseases in women and men and by region. The three major atopic diseases are more prevalent in women than men. Urticaria is also more prevalent in women than men. Newly adult-onset atopic diseases are hormone related until proven otherwise and estrogen seems to be the culprit and that is the reason why women tend to have more than men. The next section will shed light on this adult-onset atopy

Pathophysiology of Atopic Diseases

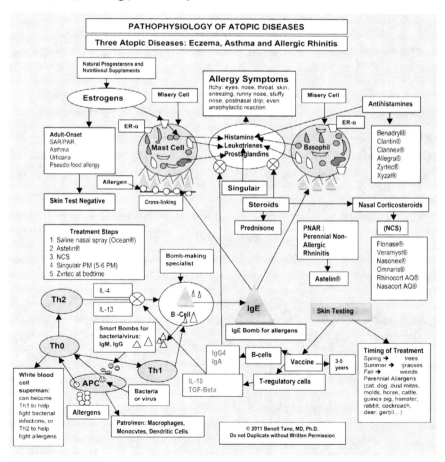

Allergic individuals inherit the genes from one of their parents or both. If one parent has allergies, the child has about a forty percent chance of developing allergies; if both parents have allergies, the child has about seventy percent to ninety percent chance of developing allergies. The allergy gene alone does not cause allergic reactions. To react, the individual has to have the gene and be in the right environment. Gene-environmental interactions lead to allergic reaction. The prevalence of allergic diseases in the developed world is partially explained by the hygiene hypothesis, which holds that allergies are due to too much cleanliness. In the developing countries, people's immune systems are busy fighting the widespread bacteria. However, in the developed world where individuals are not much exposed to bacteria, the immune system, looking for work, turns to fighting innocuous substances such as pollen and other allergens.

There are three diseases that go together and are known collectively as atopic diseases: atopic dermatitis (eczema), asthma, and allergic rhinitis. There is something called the atopic march in which children start with eczema around age four to five months, when they are first exposed to solids. If they get an upper respiratory infection such as respiratory syncytial virus (RSV) infection, they come down with their first wheeze that may continue until adulthood or may subside early in childhood. By age two, most children have developed their allergic rhinitis symptoms. Sometimes, the sequence is eczema-allergic rhinitis-asthma.

Food allergy is a fourth condition that may go along with these three atopic diseases. It often contributes to the exacerbations of atopic dermatitis, and when that is discovered, elimination of the food in the child's diet helps alleviate the atopic dermatitis problem.

Chronic sinusitis is a consequence of a poorly treated rhinitis. When the mucus does not drain from the sinuses, it becomes a breeding ground for bacteria that leads to a sinus infection called sinusitis. Acute sinusitis may be caused by a viral infection and therefore may not respond to antibiotics; but it may simply run its course. It is therefore important to observe an acute sinusitis for about seven days prior to initiating an antibiotic therapy.

In order to react to an allergen, the individual has to be sensitized. The process of sensitization starts with exposure of the allergen to an antigen-presenting cell (macrophages, monocytes, or dendritic cells). The APC then presents the allergen to Th0 cells that differentiate into Th2 cells instead of Th1. Th1 cells are specialized to stimulate B-cells to produce antibodies for fighting bacteria. Once the Th2 cells are formed, they produce IL-4 and IL-13 (interleukins) that stimulate the B-Cells to produce IgE. Once the IgE is formed, it circulates in the blood and finds its receptors on two white blood cells: mast cells that live in the skin and tissues, and basophils that live in the blood itself. These cells have the IgE FCεR1 (FC epsilon receptor 1) for IgE. Once the IgE finds its receptors, it binds them. At that point, these misery cells (as I call them, because they make millions of people miserable around the world) are armed and dangerous and waiting for the next encounter. When the individual is exposed to the same allergen again, the allergen goes through the nose, eventually makes its way to the blood system, and finds the IgEs that are already on the surface of the two cells and binds them. A cross-linking of the molecules occurs and that signals to the cells to pour out their preformed granules (degranulation). The first chemical granule that is released is histamine. Histamine is a nerve ending irritant and causes itching. The individual therefore experiences itchy eyes, itchy nose, itchy throat, sneezing, and runny nose.

To treat these symptoms, antihistamines such as Benadryl, Claritin, Clarinex, Allegra, Zyrtec or Xyzal are given. Zyrtec is one of the best antihistamines that became over-the-counter in January 2008.

The reason for discontinuing antihistamines for skin testing is that histamine is the positive control and saline the negative control. Antihistamines therefore will blunt the positive control and there will be no reactions (anergy).

If histamine had been the only chemical released by mast cells and basophils, the allergy solution would be simple. Use antihistamines and there will be no more symptoms. However, there are many other chemicals produced by the misery cells. Two of these chemicals, leukotrienes (LTC4) and prostaglandins tend to cause late-phase allergic reactions: stuffy nose, postnasal drip, coughing, and for asthmatics, constriction of the airways and, therefore, wheezing. Those symptoms tend to occur at night for most allergy and asthma sufferers because the leukotrienes are produced at night. To block the leukotrienes, montelukast (Singulair, the most popular LTRA)) and other Leukotriene receptor antagonists were conceived. Children and adults who have allergic rhinitis and asthma symptoms should therefore use a combination of a good antihistamine such as Zyrtec and a good LTRA such as Singulair.

The master blocker of all these chemicals released by the misery cells is steroids and that is why many physicians inject cortisone or give prednisone to their patients when they present with allergy symptoms. Systemic steroids however, have multiple undesirable effects in both adults and children and should be reserved only for short term bursts for brittle asthma or other severe atopic inflammation. For the treatment of allergic rhinitis, nasal corticosteroids that act locally are desirable and they are: Flonase, which is off patent and therefore Veramyst is now on the market. Nasonex, which has the same potency as Flonase, is most desirable for children and is approved for kids two years old and above. Flonase, Veramyst as well as Omnaris (Ceclosenide) are approved for children over four years of age. Budesonide (Rhinocort AQ) is also approved for pregnant women with allergies. Treatment for allergic diseases therefore requires a combination therapy: antihistamines to block the histamine released from mast cells and basophils, LTRA to block the leukotrienes, and nasal corticosteroids to block all the chemicals that participate in allergic reactions.

Estrogen Dominance and Adult-onset Allergies

As mentioned previously, allergies start in childhood. However, in my practice I am seeing more and more patients who present in adulthood, from age fifteen and beyond, with complaints of nasal symptoms, asthma symptoms, severe urticaria/angioedema, and even newly acquired food allergies such as to shellfish with Old Bay seasoning.

In reference to the UTMB studies, it is now well known that mast cells have a high affinity estrogen receptor-alpha and beta (ER-α, and ER-β) and progesterone receptors on their surface. Binding of endogenous estrogens and exogenous estrogens to these receptors cause mast cell degranulation with release of histamine and LTC4 that cause the allergy symptoms. I generally inform these patients that their allergy symptoms are not related to environmental allergens. To prove my point, I always offer a skin testing, and patients are always surprised to see that their skin testing results are negative. I couple the test with a measure of the endogenous hormones, and in most cases the estrogen is too high and the progesterone too low. I have been able to give low dose progesterone to these patients and their allergy symptoms improve. I have several patients who have responded beautifully, and the recalcitrant, steroid-dependent, estrogen-induced urticaria/angioedema have improved.

Xenoestrogens and phytoestrogens play a major role in this process, I therefore give the patients a list of xenoestrogens and phytoestrogens to avoid. I also recommend vitamins that help with their overall well-being. Many of these steroid-dependent allergic patients, suffering from steroid-dependent asthma or steroid-dependent dermatitis, also have important comorbidities: obesity, hypothyroidism, hyperlipidemia, hypertension, insulin resistance, and female menstrual disturbances such as menstrual irregularity, fibroid tumors with menorrhagia, metrorrhagia, metromenorrhagia, fibrocystic breast disease, ovarian cysts, and endometriosis. Often these patients have seen multiple physicians for these conditions. Some have had hysterectomies, while others have had breast biopsies that have revealed the presence of fibrocystic breast disease. Many of these women are on birth control pills to control their menstrual problems; many others are on antidepressants for depression, panic attacks, nervousness, and anxiety. Chronic chest pain due to anxiety is often seen in patients who have been evaluated by cardiologists, and in some cases cardiac catheterization has been performed without any findings. Many of these patients have high cholesterol. I have found these symptoms in patients as young as thirteen.

These patients most often have estrogen dominance. Estrogen dominance, by definition, is normal or high estrogen in the presence of deficient progesterone. The excess endogenous estrogen, coupled with xenoestrogens and phytoestrogens, cause allergic disease by stimulating the non-genomic estrogen receptors on the mast cells, and also by potentiating the effect of IgE antibody on the mast cells (and perhaps estrogen receptors on basophils), to release histamine and LTC4. The worst allergic reactions are the recurrent anaphylactic reactions with foods and also with allergen immunotherapy. When I was in allergy fellowship training at the Johns Hopkins Asthma and Allergy Center in Baltimore, we evaluated a patient who presented with the symptoms of anaphylaxis after ingesting crabs with Old Bay seasoning and drinking beer. I can remember this particular case because of its peculiarity. The women was around age sixty and presented with an episode of anaphylactic reaction after this particular meal. After evaluation, her skin testing was negative. She was scheduled to return to clinic with some crabs for a challenge in the office. She obviously passed the challenge with flying colors, because her reaction was not due to the shellfish itself, which she had always eaten and tolerated for years. The reaction was rather due to the Old Bay seasoning. I now realize that this lady had estrogen dominance. Old Bay seasoning contains five phytoestrogens: bay leaves, cinnamon, cloves, celery, and nutmeg. This patient also ingested beer, which contains hops, another phytoestrogen that helped release more estrogen. These phytoestrogens, coupled with her already high endogenous estrogens, caused an intense histamine and LTC4 release that led to the anaphylactic reaction. A food challenge that only contained the shellfish itself will therefore not cause the reaction.

The other situation that occurs most often is the anaphylactic reaction to allergen immunotherapy, which is also more common in women than men. I recently saw a woman who was on AIT and could not reach maintenance because of anaphylactic reactions. I reformulated her AIT extracts and started her on a slower injection schedule. She was able to go through the yellow vial, and on her second dose of the red vial she had another anaphylactic reaction. This time, instead of simply reformulating her AIT extracts or changing her injection schedule, I measured her hormones and, not surprisingly, her estrogen level was very high. I started her on progesterone and continued her on her AIT. She was also having unexplained syncope episodes and these symptoms resolved when she started on the progesterone therapy. In this case, the high endogenous estrogen caused a synergistic effect with the IgE on the mast cells that led to her recurrent anaphylactic reactions. Since this case, I have seen three more young women who had similar episodes. The most recent case of anaphylaxis occurred in my clinic in October 2010. The young woman was in day twelve or thirteen of her pre-ovulation phase, which is usually characterized by high estrogen level. She had an anaphylactic reaction to her AIT injection. I have since recommended that she skip her AIT injections in her pre-ovulatory phase. I have also started her on low-dose progesterone because her measured estrogen was elevated and her progesterone was low. She has not had any more episodes and she is tolerating her injections.

The case of skin test reactivity variation with the phases of the menstrual cycle and pre-menstrual asthma (late luteal phase asthma exacerbations in women are well documented in the allergy literature). However, allergists do not routinely take this into account in their practices when doing skin testing and when women react to allergen immunotherapy. In the case of pre-menstrual asthma, the authors of the publication that appeared in the *Journal of Asthma* recommended Singulair as a good treatment. It is clear that in the late luteal phase the progesterone falls below the estrogen and that transient estrogen dominance is responsible for making the mast cells highly responsive and for causing premenstrual asthma in young women. In these cases LTC4 is released in addition to histamine, and therefore a combination of antihistamines and LTRA will be optimal.

Allergists who are not aware of these estrogen reactions will do their usual standard workups for urticaria, and the results will be negative. The patient is then labeled as suffering from "idiopathic" urticaria, which means that the cause is unknown. The progression of treatment is usually something like this: antihistamines, and when the case is desperate, then steroids. To avoid any potential liability, patients are told to stop their AIT when they react to it. Allergists should therefore take into account estrogen dominance, phytoestrogens and xenoestrogens effects when evaluating patients suspected of adult-onset anaphylactic reactions and AIT-induced anaphylactic reactions. When the actual cause of the symptoms is discovered and treated, both the patient and the allergist are rewarded.

Since learning about hormones and their relationship to allergic reaction, I have been able to pinpoint the actual culprits in these so-called adult-onset food allergies. Recently, I saw a patient in my office who presented with urticaria. She was clear about the trigger: she and her husband had recently gone on a high protein diet, and she was eating a lot of soy protein. She then developed severe urticarial eruptions that improved when she stopped her soy protein diet. She then resumed and the urticaria returned. When she saw me, I confirmed with her that the soy protein was indeed causing her urticaria lesions by releasing too much estrogen. This patient already had important comorbidities: PCOS and menorrhagia, and she was status post hysterectomy for these symptoms. She was obese but started losing weight after her TAH/BSO. Another patient recently presented with similar episodes of urticaria after eating shrimp seasoned with thyme and rosemary, both phytoestrogens.

Another cause of adult-onset rhinitis independent of environmental allergens is perennial non-allergic rhinitis (PNAR) sometimes called vasomotor rhinitis. Patients most often will complain of irritants such as cigarette smoke, perfumes, scented candles, household cleaning agents, and sometimes flower scents such as rose and lily, scents that cause nasal symptoms. Although some respond to the usual rhinitis medications, most will respond best to Astelin, the only antihistamine nasal spray that, ironically, works well on non-allergic rhinitis. Astelin works because most of these PNAR cases are due to histamine release from mast cells secondary to non-genomic processes such as estrogen binding to its receptor-α on mast cells. Patients who present with allergy symptoms but who have negative skin tests should be evaluated for hormone imbalance; this will usually pay off. While measuring the hormones, do not forget to include vitamin D in the basic hormone panel. Vitamin D deficiency is rampant and is associated not only with heart disease but also with allergic diseases such as asthma.

Allergic diseases are on the rise and recent allergy literature indicates that adult onset asthma is more prevalent in women and the obese. Obesity, as shown in previous chapters, is highly associated with estrogen dominance, and women with increased estrogen dominance due to endogenous estrogen and progesterone imbalance with age therefore tend to have the highest rate of asthma and other atopic diseases as demonstrated by my HCUP data analysis.

Skin Testing and Allergy Vaccine

All the medications used in allergic rhinitis are palliatives and will not cure the rhinitis. In order to find out what is causing the nasal symptoms, skin testing is performed. The test has two purposes:

1. **Timing of medication treatment**
    - Spring symptoms are due to trees
    - Summer symptoms are due to grasses
    - Fall symptoms are due to weeds
    - Year-round (perennial) symptoms are due to cat, dog, dust mite, molds, cockroaches, horses, rabbits, guinea pigs, etc.

Patients with spring or fall allergies should pre-empt their season by starting the medication therapy two weeks prior to the beginning of the season instead of just reacting to it. Patients with year-round allergies should treat symptoms year-round.

2. **Allergy vaccine.**

The medications are only palliative and will not provide a long-term resolution of the allergy symptoms. The allergy vaccine is conceived as a long-term relief from allergens. The following will provide an in-depth discussion of allergen, immunotherapy, and immune cells response to the various forms of allergen vaccine.

Eosinophils and Atopic Diseases

Eosinophils are often seen at the site of allergic inflammation.

Activation of eosinophils leads to degranulation of toxic mediators, synthesis of other inflammatory mediators, and upregulation of FceR1/Fcg receptors to enhance effector functions.

Degranulation of toxic mediators by eosinophils is thought to mediate some of the tissue damage in allergic diseases.

Therapy for Atopic Diseases

Many types of inflammatory cells and mediators are involved in the chronic inflammatory response in atopic diseases.

Corticosteroids are highly effective in treating atopic diseases. They inhibit many mechanisms that contribute to chronic TH2-driven inflammation, inhibit cytokine production, and induce eosinophil death.

Inhibitors of the TH2 inflammatory response (blocking IL-4, IL-5, or leukotriene antagonists) are not as effective in atopic diseases as corticosteroids.

The symptoms of IgE-mediated allergic reactions (rhinitis, conjunctivitis, and asthma) can be ameliorated by temporary suppression of mediators and immune cells (by antihistamines, antileukotrienes, beta-adrenergic receptor antagonists, and corticosteroids).

However, a more long-term solution is allergen-specific immunotherapy that specifically restores a normal immunity against allergens. Allergen Specific Immunotherapy (SIT) is most efficiently used in allergy to insect venoms and allergic rhinitis.

Effects of Allergen-Specific Immunotherapy

Allergen-SIT is associated with: decrease in IL-4 and IL-5 production by CD4+ T cells.

A shift from Th2 cytokine pattern towards increased interferon-γ (IFN)-γ production.

A rise in allergen-blocking IgG antibodies particularly of the IgG4 class, which supposedly block allergen and IgE-facilitated antigen presentation.

Generation of IgE modulating CD8+ T cell and reduction in the number of mast cells and eosinophils, including the release of mediators.

Peripheral T-cell tolerance is characterized mainly by suppressed proliferative and cytokine responses against the major allergens and its T-cell recognition sites.

The T-cell tolerance is initiated by autocrine action of IL-10, which is increasingly produced by the antigen-specific T cells.

Tolerized T cells can be reactivated to produce either of the distinct Th1 or Th2 cytokine patterns depending on the cytokine present in the tissue microenvironment, and thus directing allergen-SIT towards successful or unsuccessful treatment.

The response to allergen immunotherapy is mostly mediated by T-regulatory cells and B-cells.

Effects of T-Regulatory Cell Cytokines

The IL-10 and TGF-B released by the T-regulatory cells:

- Decrease the IgE production by the B-cells and increase their production of IgA and IgG4
- Decrease the IgE-dependent activation of mast cells and basophils
- Decrease survival and activation of eosinophils
- Suppress mucus production by the epithelial cells and reduce airway hyper-reactivity
- Decrease the antigen presentation capacity of dendritic cells
- Decrease TH2 cytokine production and suppression of their proliferation

CHAPTER 7

OVERALL SUMMARY

Environmental pollution continues due to population pressures and the fight to feed a growing population.

- Farming for the masses uses synthetic chemicals that contaminate foods and water sources.
- The pollution leads to hypothyroidism, hyperestrogenism and hypoandrogenism that lead to obesity and its comorbidities.
- High estrogens lead to high insulin that in turn leads to craving for sugar-containing foods that quickly convert to glucose.
- The high blood glucose must be disposed to prevent damage to small vessels and organs; insulin takes care of this excess glucose by putting it into the adipocytes.
- When adipocytes are filled, they release leptin to signal to the hypothalamus that they have enough.
- The hypothalamus acts to reduce the appetite and cravings so as to allow the adipocytes to decompress.

- The decompression process is slow and the adipocytes do not see the results as expected. They therefore release more leptin to make their case but the plea falls on deaf ears, the message becoming "plenty but ineffective." This inefficiency is known as leptin resistance. When the hypothalamus does not respond, the adipocytes shield themselves, and the insulin, although plenty, has little capacity to push the glucose into the cells. This insulin incapacity is known as insulin resistance.

- Insulin resistance leads to a spill of glucose in the blood. This is known as type 2 diabetes.

- Leptin resistance leads to a decrease in serotonin, the "feel-good hormone."

- Decreased serotonin leads to nervousness, anxiety, panic attacks, depression, and mood swings in conditions like bipolar disorders.

- Nervousness, anxiety, panic attacks, depression, and mood swings lead to antidepressants and mood stabilizers that, in turn, cause more weight gain and perpetuate the vicious cycle.

- Treatment of diabetes uses three groups of medications: one group increases the amount of insulin produced by the pancreas, and they are called *sufonylureas;* the other group increases the capacity of the insulin to do its job better by putting more glucose into the adipocytes, and they are known as *thiazolinediones;* the other group suppresses new glucose formation in the liver, and the prototype is *metformin.* This group also has a second effect which is to help the insulin do its job better by putting more glucose into the adipocytes.

- Finally, when the pancreas is burned out and is unable to produce more insulin, insulin injections are given. All these medications lead to more obesity and increase the vicious cycle of increased insulin-obesity and insulin resistance and increased blood glucose. It is therefore of little surprise that diabetic patients never get better; eventually, they meet their demise in the form of end organ failure.

- Obesity has multiple comorbidities that lead to high morbidity and mortality.
- Obesity seems to strike young adults, especially prime age (18–44) women. This group is at increased risk because of the elevated levels of endogenous estrogens that couple with xenoestrogens and phytoestrogens to raise the insulin levels and contribute to hypothyroidism, both of which are major causes of obesity.
- High insulin levels also contribute to obesity-related comorbidities such as hypertension and hyperlipidemia that also require treatment.
- Hypertension medications such as beta-blockers lead to decreased thyroid function and cause more obesity, which perpetuates the vicious cycle.
- Treatment of hyperlipidemia often requires statin drugs that are effective in reducing total cholesterol and LDL cholesterol and remember that LDL is the starting material for sex hormones.
- Low cholesterol leads to low testosterone and even lower progesterone and, hence, makes the estrogen dominance worse (remember that estrogen is produced by adrenal glands, skin cells, and conversion of androgens such as testosterone to estrogen via aromatase which is produced in large quantities by adipocytes. This is in addition to ovarian production. In menopause, the ovarian function stops but the estrogen-making machine and estrogen production do not).
- Low testosterone leads to decreased libido, a source of marital discord and divorce but low testosterone also leads to obesity due to the increased insulin that follows.

- When testosterone gets converted to estrogens (estradiol and estrone), these estrogens couple with xenoestrogens and phytoestrogens to cause, in men, gynecomastia ("man boobs"), benign prostatic hypertrophy, and even prostate cancer.
- Too much estrogen in women also cause benign and malignant tumors.
- Treatment of estrogen-related tumors hardly ever involves measurement of estrogens.
- Many estrogen-induced conditions that lead to hysterectomies are accompanied by hormone replacement therapy with more estrogen. This exogenous estrogen, paired with the already high endogenous estrogen and xenoestrogens and phytoestrogens, lead to estrogen dominance symptoms that are hard to figure out since the estrogen dominance is never corrected.
- Estrogen dominance can be suspected if a patient has had a hysterectomy, a cholecystectomy, menstrual disturbances, tumors and cancers, infertility issues, and weight gain.
- Basic hormone panel and treatment of any hormone imbalance will be cost-effective.
- Start hormone evaluation at age thirty five for most women and men, or sooner if patients exhibit symptoms of progesterone deficiency, androgen deficiency or excess and estrogen dominance.

The following chapter will provide some solutions.

CHAPTER 8

OBESITY SOLUTIONS

To find viable solutions to the obesity epidemic, the variables affecting obesity should be analyzed one by one. Most recommendations for weight loss fail because they concentrate on one or two of these obesity determinants at a time and ignore all the other determinants. To understand my recommendations, I have brought equation (3) here in this chapter, so as to follow the effect of correcting each of the determinants.

$$\ln OBS = \ln A_0 + \alpha_1 \ln C + \alpha_2 \ln P + \alpha_3 \ln F + \alpha_4 \ln E + \alpha_5 \ln A + \alpha_6 \ln T + \alpha_7 \ln I + \varepsilon \qquad (3)$$

Many weight loss programs now recommend low carbohydrate diets, some focus on high protein diets and most recommend low fat diets. Few experts now incorporate balancing the hormones. The failure of most programs stems from not looking at all the determinants of the obesity equation.

Obesity Types

There are three body types in the obesity group and four body types in general today.

1. The lean body individuals (mostly young)
2. The abdominal obesity group often called "apple-shaped obesity"
3. The hips, thighs, and buttocks obesity group called "pear-shaped obesity"
4. The combination abdominal and hips/thighs/buttocks obesity group "apple/pear-obesity"

The abdominal obesity group has a protruding abdomen due to insulin resistance and leptin resistance. Most of these individuals have diabetes or will have diabetes. These future diabetics have been often told by their primary care physicians that they have a pre-diabetic condition. The second obesity group, the hips group for short, is more prevalent in women and is often associated with estrogen dominance. The HCUP data analysis confirmed that obesity and its comorbidities are more prevalent in women than men and more prevalent in the South and the Midwest.

When progesterone decreases, estrogen increases, and that leads to insulin increase. Initially, increased insulin causes hypoglycemia. Hospital discharges for hypoglycemia showed that hypoglycemia in 2008 was more prevalent in women and leading regions were the South and the Midwest, followed by the Northeast and by the West. This trend is the same for all estrogen-dominance related conditions and hypertension. When progesterone decreases, aldosterone decreases initially, and that leads to hypotension. I have seen several patients, especially women, who complain of hypotension. The low blood pressure causes the kidneys to release renin that converts angiotensinogen

I to angiotensin I; angiotensin I converts angiotensinogen II to angiotensin II using angiotensin converting enzyme (ACE). Angiotensin II then increases the aldosterone level. This increase in aldosterone often overshoots, and the blood pressure eventually increases and requires therapy. The low progesterone causes increase in estrogen that in turn increases the insulin. The high insulin causes salt retention in the renal tubules that ultimately leads to high blood pressure. These two mechanisms are the major reasons for increase in blood pressure, which is often called essential hypertension, meaning the cause is unknown. Women with chronic estrogen dominance have more hypertension than men as depicted in the HCUP data analysis. The South with its plethora of xenoestrogens has the highest rate of hypertension in the country, followed by the Midwest, the Northeast, and the West.

Adipocyte Biology

It is now well established that adipocytes (fat cells) produce immune substances known as adipokines. Some of these adipokines are responsible for inflammation, and therefore obese individuals experience several inflammatory processes such as athralgias, myalgias, asthma symptoms, and even rhinitis symptoms. Hospital discharges data on arthritis and fibromyalgia show that these condtions are also more prevalent in women than men. These conditions are due to the effects of low progesterone on cortisol disregulation, and the effects of TNF-α, IL-1, and IL-6. These cytokines produced by adipocytes perpetuate the low-grade inflammation with intermittent exacerbations when cytokine levels increase. It is well known that TNF-α and IL-6, for example, contribute to asthma and to rheumatoid arthritis flares. In both diseases there have been trials of TNF-α monoclonal antibodies that seem to relieve symptoms.

Since obesity has such dire consequences, most individuals who notice weight gain decide to lose the weight. The first thing often recommended by physicians and tried by patients is the unnatural and difficult route of dieting, which means restricting food intake. When the body senses the lack of food, it goes into a saving mode. Initially, the glucose-alanine cycle goes into gear to continue the supply of glucose. The glucose-alanine cycle converts muscle proteins to glucose and therefore muscle mass is lost. The body does everything possible to prevent its potential demise. The energy saving mode therefore causes loss of water and muscle mass but not fat. The individual therefore soon realizes that he or she is not losing any more weight. Out of desperation and discouragement, she resumes her normal diet. The body, a very smart machine, goes into a fast saving mode and tries to accumulate as much food in the form of fat as possible. The individual therefore gains even more weight than what he started with. This is the origin of what is known as the yo-yo diet.

In the quest to lose weight, there is often a total failure to take into account the hormones that started the weight gain cascade. To lose the weight, and keep it off, entails correcting the underlying hormone imbalance, eating from the right categories and in the right proportions of foods, and getting exercise. The solution is for the individual to eat for her hormone type.

Carbohydrate Recommendations

A patient with leptin resistance and/or insulin resistance should choose carbohydrates judiciously. All carbohydrates are not created equal. The carbohydrates high on the glycemic index and with high glycemic load should be avoided. To avoid insulin surge that leads to too much glucose being pushed into adipocytes, only low glycemic index carbohydrates should be consumed. The reduction in insulin that will ensue will reduce the high blood pressure. Many diet books and hormone books end their chapters with recipes. Considering that patients do not like the same foods, and that taste for food is as varied as taste for clothing and may depend on the culture and the region of patients' origin, I will not give any recipes in this book. I will recommend low glycemic index food choices so as to minimize the surge of glucose that tends to fuel the obesity problem, and ends with leptin resistance and insulin resistance that in turn are culprits in the bulk of the diseases treated by all physicians in the industrialized world. I frequently recommend Jennie Brand-Miller's *New Glucose Revolution Shopper's Guide* to my patients. The glycemic index (GI) is a measure of the power of foods (or, specifically, the carbohydrate in a food) to raise blood sugar (glucose) levels after being eaten. The GI values of foods must be measured using valid scientific methods. It cannot be guessed by looking at the composition of the food. Currently, only a few nutrition research groups around the world provide a legitimate testing service. Professor Brand-Miller of the Human Nutrition Unit at Sydney University has been at the forefront of glycemic index research for over a decade, and her research group has determined the GI values of more than 400 foods.

The GI value of a food is determined by feeding ten or more healthy people a portion of the food containing 50 grams of digestible (available) carbohydrate and then measuring the effect on their blood glucose levels over the next two hours. For each person, the area under their two-hour blood glucose response (glucose AUC) for this food is then measured. On another occasion, the same ten people consume an equal-carbohydrate portion of glucose sugar (the reference food) and their two-hour blood glucose response is also measured. A GI value for the test food is then calculated for each person by dividing their glucose AUC for the test food by their glucose AUC for the reference food. The final GI value for the test food is the average GI value for the ten people.

Foods with a high GI score contain rapidly digested carbohydrates, which produce a large rapid rise and fall in the level of blood glucose. In contrast, foods with a low GI score contain slowly digested carbohydrates, which produce a gradual, relatively low rise in the level of blood glucose.

Does a Low Carbohydrate Diet Always Work?

A low carbohydrate diet does not mean anything if you are eating a small amount of carbohydrates with high glycemic index. For example, dry dates have a glycemic index of 103; a few dates will transform more quickly into glucose than a bowl of Uncle Ben's converted rice that has a glycemic index of 44. Fruits and vegetables are highly recommended by nutritionists and doctors all over the world. However, ignoring the glycemic index of the fruits and vegetables can be a boomerang. For example, eating foods like grapes, ripe bananas, watermelon, dates, potatoes, or corn very often, can cause weight gain due to their high glycemic index and glycemic load. Hence, recommending fruits and vegetables can be counterproductive unless their glycemic index and glycemic load is taken into account.

Proteins Recommendations

Patients should also avoid eating proteins with high glucogenic amino acid content. A glucogenic amino acid is an amino acid that can be converted into glucose through gluconeogenesis. This is in contrast to ketogenic amino acids, which are converted into ketone bodies. The production of glucose from glucogenic amino acids involves these amino acids' being converted to alpha keto acids and then to glucose, with both processes occurring in the liver. This mechanism predominates during catabolysis, rising as fasting and starvation increase in severity.

Glucogenic Amino Acids

Glucogenic amino acids can be degraded to pyruvate or an intermediate in the Krebs cycle. They are named glucogenic because they can produce glucose under conditions of low glucose. This process is also known as gluconeogenesis, or the production of "new glucose." Amino acids form glucose through

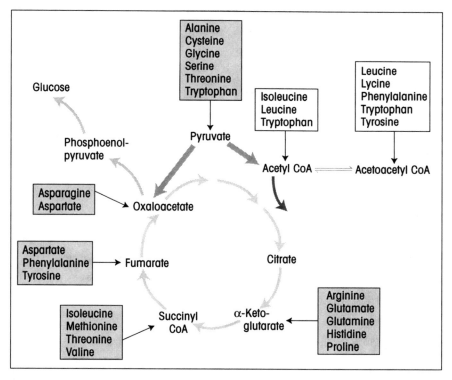

As shown in this diagram, the final product of glucose breakdown by our cells is pyruvate, which can be converted to oxaloacetate (OA), the main precursor for gluconeogenesis, or to Acetyl CoA, which can feed into the Krebs cycle and also make its way to oxaloacetate that will convert into new glucose. Notice that it will take acetyl CoA a longer time to reach its destination, whereas pyruvate converting to OA is a direct and quicker pathway. The following amino acids are glucogenic: alanine, cysteine, glycine, serine, threonine, tryptophan, asparagine, aspartate, phenylalanine, tyrosine, isoleucine, methionine, threonine, valine, arginine, glutamate, glutamine, histidine, and proline.

degradation to pyruvate or an intermediate in the Krebs cycle. Proteins rich in glucogenic amino acids, in the fed state, can also convert to pyruvate which in turn converts to oxaloacetate, and oxaloacetate converts back to glucose. Part of the pyruvate will convert to acetyl CoA, which is the starting material for cholesterol. Glucogenic amino acids convert readily into glucose and therefore will cause an insulin surge that in turn will push glucose into adipocytes and lead to worsening of obesity. This also causes salt retention that will lead to hypertension.

Ketogenic Amino Acids

In contrast, ketogenic amino acids can produce ketones when energy sources are low. Some of these amino acids are degraded directly to ketone bodies such as acetoacetate (see diagram above). They include leucine, lysine, phenylalanine, tryptophan, and tyrosine. The other ketogenic amino acids can be converted to acetyl CoA. Acetyl CoA has several different fates, one of which is the conversion to acetoacetate. Although not a preferential energy source, acetoacetate can be metabolized by the brain and muscle for energy when blood glucose is low. Acetoacetate cannot be used in gluconeogenesis, since acetyl CoA cannot be converted directly to oxaloacetate.

The Vegetables and Water Recommendations

For patients who have obesity problems, I often recommend what I call the Prophet Daniel's Diet that I present in the next section. Following this diet for a month will bring the weight down a bit and hence encourage the patient to follow the low glycemic index/load diet and the moderate to low protein diet. The Prophet Daniel's Diet will not work if patients love potatoes, and corn as vegetables and hate water. Patients should drink enough water a day for success in any diet.

The Prophet's Diet (Daniel 1: 1–18)

In the third year of the reign of Jehoiakim King of Judah, Nebuchadnezzar King of Babylon came to Jerusalem and besieged it. And the Lord gave Jehoiakim, King of Judah into his hand, with some of the articles of the house of the God, which he carried into the land of Shinar to the house of his god; and he brought the articles into the treasure house of his God.

Then the king instructed Ashpenaz, the master of his eunuchs, to bring some of the children of Israel and some of the king's descendants and some of the nobles, young men in whom there was no blemish, but good-looking, gifted in all wisdom, possessing knowledge and quick to understand, who had ability to serve in the king's palace, and whom they might teach the language and literature of the Chaldeans. And the king appointed for them a daily provision of the king's delicacies and of the wine which he drank, and three years of training for them, so that at the end of that time they might serve before the king. Now from among those of the sons of Judah were Daniel, Hananiah, Mishael, and Azariah. To them the chief of eunuchs gave names: Daniel the name Belteshazzar; to Hananiah, Shadrach; to Mishael, Meshach, and to Azariah, Abed-Nego.

But Daniel purposed in his heart that he would not defile himself with the portions of the king's delicacies, nor with the wine which he drank; therefore, he requested of the chief of eunuchs that he might not defile himself. Now God had brought Daniel into the favor and goodwill of the chief of the eunuchs. And the chief of the eunuchs said to Daniel, "I fear my lord the king, who has appointed your food and drink. For why should he see your faces looking worse than the young men who are your age? Then you would endanger my head before the king."

So Daniel said to the steward whom the chief of the eunuchs had set over Daniel, Hananiah, Mishael, and Azariah, "Please test your servants for ten days, and let them give us vegetables to eat and water to drink. Then let our appearance be examined before you, and the appearance of the young men who eat the portion of the king's delicacies; and as you see fit, so deal with your servants." So he consented with them in this matter, and tested them ten days.

And at the end of ten days their features appeared better and fatter in flesh than all the young men who ate the portion of the king's delicacies. Thus the steward took away their portion of delicacies and the wine that they were to drink, and gave them vegetables.

As for these four young men, God gave them knowledge and skill in all literature and wisdom; and Daniel had understanding in all visions and dreams.

Now at the end of the days, when the king had said that they should be brought in, the chief of the eunuchs brought them in before Nebuchadnezzar. Then the king interviewed them, and among them all none was found like Daniel, Hananiah, Mishael, and Azariah; therefore they served before the king. And in all matters of wisdom and understanding about which the king examined them, he found them ten times better than all the magicians and astrologers who were in his entire realm. Thus Daniel continued until the first year of King Cyrus.

This is the first clinical trial that compared delicacies and wine to vegetables and water. The conclusion is that vegetables and water are better to build muscle than delicacies and wine (alcoholic beverages in general). To lose weight and build muscle and think better, it is imperative to start a diet of vegetables (organic vegetables are highly recommended) and plenty of water.

Eat for Your Hormone Type

Progesterone deficiency causes estrogen dominance that leads to decreased thyroid function and an increase in insulin. Increased insulin leads to craving for carbohydrates and to obesity. Obesity leads to leptin resistance and insulin resistance that may lead to diabetes and hypertension; leptin resistance causes a decrease in serotonin production that leads to depression, anxiety, and panic attacks. Progesterone deficiency also leads to estrogen dominance that leads to decrease in thyroid function as a result of increased thyroid binding globulin. Increased thyroid binding globulin causes increased thyroid hormones T4 and T3 binding to this protein and not relinquishing them to cells for metabolism. The end result is more weight gain. This explains why women gain weight when they go on birth control pills.

Note that progestins which are artificial progesterone have similar effects. Some researchers advocate looking into thyroid supplementation when a women starts on birth control pills. One notorious effect of birth control pills is blood clots that can lead to pulmonary embolism and stroke; thyroid deficiency can lead to blood clots as well. Progesterone deficiency will therefore cause low thyroid function and weight gain. Women would be expected to have more of these diseases. In an interview with CBS in 2006, Steven Hotze, MD, made the statement that by age fifty, many women will develop hypothyroidism. He was heavily criticized by the Endocrinology Society of Houston for lack of evidence. But results from the HCUP data analysis seem to corroborate his statement. As women get older they have more hypothyroidism discharges and they have higher rates than men.

If it is true that progesterone deficiency often leads to estrogen dominance and underactive thyroid, then women should increasingly have hypothyroidism as they age and also should have more obesity. This is because they tend to have more estrogen surges than progesterone surges. Remember that some women are born with a low progesterone gene, and many others acquire low progesterone starting from their late twenties secondary to anovulatory menstrual cycles. Increased estrogen should also produce more menstrual disturbances in women between the ages eighteen to forty four due to benign tumors and other related comorbidities. Fibroid tumors, ovarian cysts, fibrocystic breast disease, endometriosis, heavy menstrual bleeding, and irregular menstrual periods will prevail in this age group. Obesity associated comorbidities such as hypertension, diabetes, and hyperlipidemia should also prevail in women. Leptin resistance causes serotonin production to decrease. If women have more obesity and, hence, more leptin resistance, then they should have depressive episodes, anxiety, and panic attacks more than men. Where is the evidence of all these statements? In the era of statistics and clinical trials, statements made in vacuum are quickly dismissed.

The analysis encompassed data from hospital discharges and ED visits and discharges. The results show that women actually have more obesity than men and more of the associated comorbidities such as hypertension, hyperlipidemia, diabetes, and their related comorbidities. The results show that women have low thyroid function with increasing age.

It is intriguing not only that obesity is more prevalent in women but especially that morbid obesity is a disease of women. From the HCUP database, more than eighty percent of all morbid obesity related discharges occurred in women in 2006. From 1997 to 2009 the HCUP discharges for hypothyroidism and obesity patterns remained the same for women and men and for the four major regions in the US.

Low Progesterone and Thyroid Insufficiency

Patients with low progesterone most often have a concomitant thyroid insufficiency. In some cases, a thyroid boost will be necessary to overcome weight problems. However, an adequate progesterone replacement may also correct the thyroid problem in the long run. Beware of patients who are on Synthroid and are still obese. It may be because the Synthroid (T4) is not converting to (T3). After measuring the hormones including thyroid function test that measure TSH, free T4, and free T3, if FT3 is low and TSH is greater than two, then a combination of Synthroid and Cytomel can be used. I have used armour thyroid with good results, but patients should be followed regularly. I usually see the patient back in clinic in about eight weeks and reorder the thyroid function test. If all are in acceptable ranges, then the patient returns to clinic in three months. This frequent visit schedule allows me to keep an eye on patients' weight loss efforts and to correct any hormone abnormalities that may still hinder their progress.

If the patient has low progesterone and high estrogen and consumes foods rich in phytoestrogens and xenoestrogens, then she is helping to perpetuate the vicious cycle of chronic weight gain. In addition, foods high on the glycemic index will only turn into more fat and perpetuate leptin resistance, insulin resistance, high blood pressure, diabetes, and high cholesterol levels.

Remember that high glucose level, high insulin level, and high fatty acid state (obesity) are the fuels for synthesis of cholesterol. It is therefore imperative to know the patient's hormone status prior to their embarking on any weight loss programs. If the patient has insulin resistance and estrogen dominance and weight problems, she will be better off not eating proteins that contain glucogenic amino acids. These proteins will eventually break down to their basic amino acids, which will be converted to glucose and stored as fat. It is therefore false that a high-protein, low-carbohydrate diet will help with weight loss. Patients need to know what foods are low on the glycemic index and which proteins contain less glucogenic amino acids.

Weight Loss Steps

1. Measure the patient's hormones.
2. If the patient has low progesterone, start with bioidentical progesterone.
3. If the patient has low free T4 and free T3 and TSH greater than two, then add thyroid boosting medication or supplement.
4. If the estradiol level is high, then tell the patient to avoid phytoestrogens and xenoestrogens, and recommend foods with low glycemic index and glycemic load and proteins low in glucogenic amino acids. Inositol-3-carbinol or DIM (diindolmethane) and bioflavonoids supplements should be added to reduce the estrogen level and potentiate weight loss. Hence, progesterone, I-3-C and/or DIM, bioflavonoids, and avoidance of phytoestrogens and xenoestrogens will help balance the estrogen level.

If the DHEA and progesterone are both low and the patient has leptin and/or insulin resistance and obesity, then start patient on DHEA and progesterone. It is important to monitor patients on progesterone and DHEA because both the DHEA and progesterone can convert to estradiol, estrone, and testosterone. The progesterone can also convert to cortisol. If you use a high-dose progesterone and do not titrate or reassess, the patient can gain more weight due to the conversion into cortisol, estradiol, and estrone. Recall that too much estrogen leads to increased insulin that leads to craving sweets, which in turn leads to weight gain. To prevent the DHEA and progesterone from converting to estradiol and estrone, weak aromatase inhibitors such as zinc and chrysin should be added to the progesterone and DHEA regimen. If both DHEA and progesterone are low, then the precursor for both, pregnenolone, might also be low, and pregnenolone supplementation should be added to the hormone replacement regimen. Make sure to follow patients closely to avoid androgen excess with this regimen. You can also use 7-keto-DHEA for a better weight control and avoidance of the androgen-excess side effects of plain DHEA. You will not run into this problem if the patient has low testosterone to begin with. Most patients have testosterone deficiency. Remember that if the patient has low testosterone, using 7-keto-DHEA alone will make the low testosterone worse because 7-keto-DHEA does not convert to estrogens or testosterone. It will be useful, therefore, to combine regular DHEA with 7-keto-DHEA to promote weight loss and to prevent the decline in the testosterone level. I usually consider this regimen if the patient has low testosterone. You should note that low testosterone tends to cause an increase in insulin and, therefore, ventral obesity. As mentioned above, this may explain why men develop ventral obesity starting in their forties and beyond. Most men who drink beer also develop the ventral obesity sooner because some beers contain hops, which is a phytoestrogen. Hence, beer abuse can lead to hyperestrogen, hyperinsulinemia and ventral obesity. For effective weight loss, beer abuse should be addressed. Alcohol abuse in general should be addressed.

Gluten Sensitivity or Estrogen Dominance Effect?

It is well known that eating certain wheat products such as white bread can lead to weight gain. Many women complain of gluten sensitivity, and therefore health food stores have multiple gluten-free products to satisfy the needs of these individuals. This gluten sensitivity has reached epidemic proportions and it is more common in women. This gluten sensitivity may be due to estrogen dominance in women. Wheat is a weak phytoestrogen. Women who already have too much estrogen will have bloating, as well as many of the other estrogen-dominance symptoms reported at pages 111–115, when they consume wheat products. Since Celiac Disease is due to gluten sensitivity, these women with estrogen dominance who experience estrogen related symptoms, often undergo gluten sensitivity evaluation that turns out to be negative. The symptoms persist despite the negative test results, and many physicians cannot figure it out. These patients are referred to allergists in the hope that a skin testing will reveal an IgE-mediated wheat allergy. A skin test in these cases is always negative. The patients will insist that they have wheat allergy and will not eat wheat products, preferring to go on a gluten-free diet that helps alleviate their symptoms. Balancing the hormone may help resolve this gluten sensitivity problem.

Nutritional Supplements Recommendations for Weight Loss

To help patients in their weight loss effort, I often recommend the following nutritional supplements that seem to work.

Supplements Useful in Weight Loss

1. Leptin boosters are necessary. Bios Life Slim® (a leptin booster described in the *Physicians' Desk Reference*) may help
2. Super Citrimax
3. 7-Keto-DHEA
4. Chromemate
5. CLA
6. Growth Hormone Support
7. Thyroid Support
8. Bioflavonex
9. DIM (Diindolmethane derived from Indol-3-Carbinol, I-3-C)

These supplements will be described later in the appendix.

High Cholesterol Solution

High cholesterol is usually a signal that the hormones are out of balance and therefore need to be checked and corrected. Since LDL cholesterol is the principal ingredient used by the body to manufacture our good hormones, it may be a mistake to try to lower it. Many researchers are now arguing that it is not the high LDL in itself that causes atherosclerosis and therefore myocardial infarction (heart attack) and cerebral vascular accidents (strokes). It is well known that it is the oxidation of the LDL cholesterol that represents the danger, and the LDL does not have to be high to oxidize. The solution to the oxidation problem should therefore be prevention of the oxidation itself and not lowering the cholesterol level. Lowering the cholesterol level can be detrimental to health and may even lead to decreased longevity. Remember that DHEA is known as the longevity hormone. It is produced from pregnenolone, which in turn comes from cholesterol. Lowering the LDL or total cholesterol levels may lead to lowering our good hormone levels, and the hormone disequilibrium can lead to worse problems. It is known that more people with low cholesterol die of myocardial infarction than people with high cholesterol. The cholesterol, if channeled to the right hormones, may be life saving (I highly recommend Uffe Ravnskov's book, *"Ignore the Awkward! How the Cholesterol Myths Are Kept Alive"*). If oxidation is the problem, why don't we prevent this oxidation? It is rare to see healthcare providers recommending therapy that will prevent oxidation.

I recommend to all my patients, as young as sixteen, that if they have obesity problems and high cholesterol, they should start on high-dose antioxidants, vitamin D and minerals. I usually recommend:

1. B-complex vitamins
2. Buffered vitamin C

3. CoQ10
4. Vitamin E (make sure to use mixed tocopherols)
5. Omega-3 fish oil (EPA/DHA)
6. L-carnitine
7. Vitamin D
8. Multi-minerals such as calcium, magnesium, potassium, zinc, manganese, iron, boron, iodine, chromium, selenium, vanadium, molybdenum. I try to avoid copper in patients with obesity, estrogen dominance, and hypothyroidism.

For patients with diabetes (remember that diabetics tend to have high cholesterol and high blood pressure due to the hyperinsulinemia and high blood glucose levels), I also recommend:

9. Alpha Lipoic Acid
10. Cinnamon
11. Chromium and
12. Benfotiamine
13. Broad spectrum digestive enzymes and probiotics

Remember that there are many other nutritional supplements out there that help in optimal blood glucose, lipid and blood pressure control.

Supplementation with antioxidants such as vitamins C and L-carnitine has been growing rapidly in the past few years as research on harmful free radicals intensifies. Free radicals are atoms, ions, or molecules with one or more unpaired electrons that bind to and destroy cellular compounds. Dietary antioxidants disarm free radicals through a number of different mechanisms. Foremost, they bind to the free electrons, "pairing up" with them, creating an innocuous cellular compound that the body can eliminate as waste. The antioxidants in this formula also support and enhance the body's natural defense mechanisms against free radicals: the enzymes superoxide dismutase, catalase, and glutathione peroxidase. Recent research points to the fact that a synergistic combination of antioxidants is more effective than the total effect of each antioxidant taken alone. In addition to antioxidants, vitamin D and minerals are also recommended. The benefit of antioxidants, minerals and vitamin D go beyond oxidation and encompass better blood pressure, glucose and lipid controls.

Heavy Metal Decontamination Recommendations

From the CDC report and many other accounts, heavy metal contamination is a real threat to the health of the US population. Many healthcare providers, especially members of the anti-aging and regenerative medicine group, are recommending heavy metal decontamination via chelation and liver detoxification. Since the CDC has started biomonitoring, I suspect that patient care will soon incorporate measurement of toxins in the blood and decontamination will be offered. To antagonize estrogens, bio-identical progesterone will be administered and nutritional supplements that can reduce estrogen load will be recommended. Heavy metal chelation and liver and other detoxification procedures will be offered. Thyroid and androgen supplementation will be offered and all these treatment procedures will lead to increased life span with quality and healthy aging. Let us all remember that in biblical times, humans lived up to 350 years and women were able to give birth at ninety. What if we rediscover the secret of longevity tomorrow? Increased longevity and quality of life will not happen if healthcare professionals and the whole scientific community do not get outside the box to contemplate, observe and discover new technologies that will positively impact our health. This will require coordination of efforts of all private and governmental institutions, and working together to save the precious human life. Discovering environmental woes and offering viable solutions seems small in front of the mountain of problems that are getting worse. However, this step is a necessary beginning toward the path of better living now and tomorrow. We have failed to achieve the healthy people goal of 2010 but by changing course now, this goal might be achievable by 2050.

HORMONE IMBALANCE SYNDROME

This book set out to demonstrate empirically with data from the Healthcare Cost and Utilization Project (HCUP), the Centers for Disease Control (CDC) and US Geological Survey (USGS), that obesity is the number one killer in America today. It has multiple comorbidities that cause human misery in the US and the rest of the world. The journey took us to the roots of obesity and its comorbidities and the roots were found in hormone disruption. The bulk of hormone disruption roots were found in pesticides and herbicides sprayed in farmlands, but also found in daily chemicals, cosmetics and cosmeceuticals used by all households. Pesticides, cosmetics and cosmeceuticals cause three major problems: hyperestrogenism, hypothyroidism and hypoandrogenism. These three hormone disruptions are responsible for the obesity epidemic and the obesity comorbidities that lead to increasing death in the US and the rest of the world. The USGS pesticides maps and the CDC obesity maps put side by side allowed a visual representation of the correlation between pesticides used in farmlands and the obesity epidemic. Data analyses from the HCUP database allowed the multiple estrogenic comorbidities to translate into quantitative numbers that reflect the enormity of the estrogen epidemic. Estrogen not only is at the core of the obesity epidemic, but may also explain the rising mast cell diseases such as allergic rhinitis, asthma, urticaria/angioedema, atopic dermatitis, and even food allergy. Atopy was thought to start in childhood, but the increasing xenoestrogens and phytoestrogens effects have led to increasing adult-onset allergies in general. Hypothyroidism and hypoandrogenism relation to agrichemicals was exposed. Based on this body of evidence, I suggested that the roots of obesity be addressed for a lasting impact on the obesity epidemic. Solutions that encompassed professional intervention such as evaluation and treatment of hormone imbalance, adequate lifestyle changes, and nutritional supplementations were offered. Currently, the only hormone measured routinely is the thyroid stimulating hormone (TSH). Other important hormones are completely ignored by the healthcare system. If hyperestrogenism, hypothyroidism and hypoandrogenism cause the bulk of diseases in America, then choosing a comprehensive hormone panel that reflects the status of these hormones to measure, may be optimal and should be the standard of care. Estrogen alone is responsible for multiple cancers in women and men and by correcting the high estrogen levels, many cancers will be averted. Hence, negative opportunity cost will be incurred in terms of cancer related surgeries, chemotherapy, and radiation therapy averted. More cost will be saved for cardiac catheterization, stent placements and cardiac bypass surgeries that will be averted. Correcting estrogen and averting most conditions related to estrogen dominance will save billions in healthcare cost yearly and increase productivity in America. Many of the missed work days and missed school days will be averted.

Going to the roots of the epidemic necessitates adopting green chemicals and technology for agriculture. Research in this area should therefore be a priority for the government and all scientists should be engaged in finding viable solutions. Soil biodiversity that is natural and offers promise should be carefully studied for adaptation to various environments. If America wants to feed her population, keep everyone healthy, and help feed the rest of the world, then pollution issues should be addressed with all our might. Here again, I can say "Si Vis Sanitas Para Bellum." We should prepare for war on all undesirable chemicals and replace with desirable bio-compatible chemicals. This means that all chemicals should be scrutinized to meet safe standard criteria established not only by the US but also by the whole international community.

The CDC report on measurement of environmental chemicals in blood and urine of a sampled Americans is a noble start. A scientific committee should be appointed by the government to evaluate bio-identical hormone replacement therapy and natural progesterone effect on endogenous estrogens, xenoestrogens and phytoestrogens. If natural progesterone can balance high estrogen levels and neutralize their ill effects, then all individuals who test positive for the environmental chemicals in the blood and urine, known to cause hyperestrogenism should start on natural progesterone and nutritional supplements known to antagonize estrogens. Individuals who test positive for chemicals that cause low thyroid, such as the perchlorates, should start on thyroid supplementation if they show trends toward obesity regardless of whether they are euthyroid or not. Individuals who test for hypo-androgenism should start on androgen therapy. In some cases, the hyperestrogenism causes hyperandrogenism and hence correcting the estrogen problem also will help with the hyper-androgenism. All obese patients who have sequestered estrogen in adipocytes should automatically be candidate for bio-identical progesterone therapy and for thyroid replacement therapy. The TSH, free T4 and free T3 ranges may be too rigid and may not pick up the endocrine disrupting chemicals effects on the thyroid. All individuals with TSH greater than two have some thyroid impairment. Obesity alone should signal that metabolism has slowed and that thyroid and, especially T3, is not working. Underactive thyroid that goes along with progesterone deficiency and estrogen dominance may be minimized by thyroid supplementation. The HCUP data analysis showed that women in their fifties and beyond tended to have low thyroid and therefore should be monitored for thyroid supplementation. DHEA and testosterone and androstenedione should be evaluated and testosterone and DHEA should be replaced with bio-identical testosterone and DHEA for optimal weight loss and hence, optimal avoidance of the obesity comorbidities.

Since chemical overload seems to be the problem, all chemicals including household cosmetics should be treated as bio-hazards and the utmost precautions observed. Farmers and populations living in areas with high farming intensity should be educated about the dangers of the pesticides and they should exercise the highest precautions. Areas with highest pesticides spray intensity should be labeled with pesticide codes: red (very high), orange (high), yellow (medium), and green (low) for protection of individuals living in these communities. This will help individuals in these areas to exercise proper precautions such as using water filtering systems, insulation of houses for cleaner indoor air, and for choosing household chemicals that are bio-compatible. In the case of household chemicals and cosmetics choice, everyone should read labels to avoid chemicals with parabens, triclosan and other bio-hazards mentioned in the books cited at page 185.

What should we eat?

Those who can afford organic foods should go organic. Children should avoid peanut, soy, non-organic eggs, non-organic milk and non-organic wheat until age five or older to prevent early sensitization to these foods and allergic reactions. These foods are the most common allergenic foods for children. Multiple pesticides are used in the production of these foods and therefore may contribute to the rising food allergy epidemic. Do not assume that pasture-fed animal meat is safe. Pastures need to grow and 2 4-D and other pesticides are often used on these grasses for better growth; and 2 4-D and most of the other pesticides used are either potential or known to be endocrine-disrupting. Animals with high fat content will therefore sequester the chemicals in fat that will be transferred to humans through diet. The litany of reasons for exercising caution around chemicals, foods, water is long and will fit in another book.

In the end, let us all know that our beloved Earth is in peril and we are all in the same boat and contributing to her demise. Greed should be set aside as a human trait and humanity should prevail. In time of tragedy, human bond becomes stronger. We should all ask ourselves where our sense of humanity is today. Are we part of the destructive forces around us or are we inno-cent bystanders? Our global health is failing daily and pushing us slowly and silently toward our final demise. We should there-fore bond together to fight our common enemy which is greed. Globalization should mean taking care of the most vulnerable populations on our planet and as Rawls puts it, we should maxi-mize the utility of the least fortunate in society if we want to honor the global social contract. Health is the wealth of nations and therefore no human should be denied the right to be healthy. Chemicals in our midst are contributing to the fulfillment of the limits to growth prophecy. Are we going to watch and wait for doom's day to strike and then act in unison to grieve for our losses or are we going to take action today to prevent doom's day? Chemicals just do not land on farms and in households by themselves. We have the choice to manufacture them, buy them, and use them. All these processes may involve our idiosyncratic conceptions of life and the intrinsic value we attach to our self worth and our insecurities and anxiety about the idea of not having. Having by investing in companies that pollute and turn our foods and water sources into poison for us does not seem smart. Endocrine-disrupting chemicals are our choice and we can also chose to get rid of them. Meanwhile, the race to have continues and I suspect will continue until the end of our time which may not be too far if we do not change course today.

DESCRIPTION OF ANTIOXIDANTS, VITAMINS AND MINERALS (WITH PERMISSION FROM PURE ENCAPSULATIONS)

1. B-Complex

What is It?

B-Complex Plus is an exceptional combination of B vitamins, including vitamins B1, B2, B3, B5, B6, B12, biotin, and folic acid (as Metafolin® L-5-MTHF), all of which are provided in their optimal bioavailable and functional forms.*

Features Include:

- Vitamin B6 (pyridoxine HCl and pyridoxal 5′ phosphate), supporting amino acid metabolism, nervous system health, and neurotransmitter (i.e., GABA and serotonin) synthesis, which studies have reported may help promote menstrual comfort. Furthermore, pyridoxine supports healthy red blood cells by participating in hemoglobin synthesis, and some studies indicate that it supports wrist nerve comfort.*

- Vitamin B1 (thiamine HCl), processes carbohydrates, fat, and protein via its coenzyme form of thiamine pyrophosphate (TPP). Vitamin B1 is required to form adenosine triphosphate (ATP), the key source of energy for the body. Thiamine also promotes neural health.*

- Vitamin B2 (riboflavin and riboflavin 5′ phosphate), metabolizing nutrients and participating in electron transport to form ATP. Riboflavin is an integral part of fatty acid catabolism or β-oxidation and helps convert folic acid and vitamins B6 to their active states.*

- Vitamin B3 (niacinamide and inositol hexaniacinate), supporting cardiovascular health by mediating healthy lipid and carbohydrate metabolism.*

- Vitamin B5 (calcium pantothenate), supporting cardiovascular health. Pantothenic acid is vital in the healthy production, transportation, and breakdown of lipids. Furthermore, this B vitamin promotes the production of the neurotransmitter acetylcholine.*

- Vitamin B12 (methylcobalamin), supporting healthy nerve cell activity and DNA replication. Vitamin B12 is a vital component of the methionine synthase pathway which, along with folic acid and vitamin B6, supports healthy homocysteine metabolism and S-adenosylmethionine (SAMe) production.*

- Folic acid, promoting the production of healthy DNA and chromosomes. Adequate folate is critical for nucleic acid synthesis and neurotransmitter synthesis. At the molecular level, the main function of folate is to donate methyl groups in key biochemical reactions occurring in blood cells, neurons, the vasculature and many other tissues. It is provided in this formula as Metafolin®, the naturally-occurring universally-metabolized form of folate. Metafolin® is chemically identical to the active folate metabolite, 5-methyltetrahydrofolate (L-5-MTHF). L-5-MTHF is the predominant naturally occurring form of folate in food. Through bypassing several enzymatic activation steps, it is directly usable by the body and provides all of the benefits of folic acid regardless of functional or genetic variations. In conjunction with vitamins B12 and B6, folic acid helps to support healthy homocysteine metabolism. Additionally, this B vitamin is important for the growth and reproduction of red and white blood cells.*

- Biotin, acting as a coenzyme for the metabolism of fat, carbohydrates, and protein.*

Uses for B-Complex

These B vitamins play important roles in nearly all of the physiological systems in the body. Some of the key supportive roles include the maintenance of muscle tone in the GI tract, the functioning of the nervous system, and the integrity of skin, hair, and the liver. Furthermore, these compounds are essential for hemoglobin formation, nerve impulse transmissions, mood, hormone synthesis, and energy metabolism.*

Recommendations

1–2 capsules per day, in divided doses with meals.

Are There Any Potential Side Effects or Precautions?

At this time, there are no known side effects or precautions.

If pregnant or lactating, consult your physician before taking this product.

Are There Any Potential Drug Interactions?

Folic acid may adversely interact with chemotheraputic agents.

B-Complex Plus

Each vegetable capsule contains v 1:

thiamine HCl (B1) .... 100 mg
riboflavin (B2) .... 5 mg
riboflavin 5' phosphate (activated B2).................. 10 mg
niacinamide... 100 mg
inositol hexaniacinate (no-flush niacin)................ 10 mg
pyridoxine HCl (B6).. 10 mg
pyridoxal 5' phosphate (activated B6).................. 10 mg
pantothenic acid (calcium pantothenate) (B5) .... 100 mg
methylcobalamin (B12).................................... 400 mcg
folate (as Metafolin®, L-5-MTHF) .... 400 mcg
biotin .... 400 mcg
vitamin C (as ascorbyl palmitate) .... 16 mg

1–2 capsules per day, in divided doses, with meals.

2. BUFFERED VITAMIN C (Ascorbic Acid)

What is It?

Buffered ascorbic acid combines calcium ascorbate, magnesium ascorbate, and potassium ascorbate to create a neutral pH vitamin C. This special form of ascorbic acid lessens possible gastric irritation in sensitive individuals.*

Uses for Buffered Ascorbic Acid Various Physiological Support Properties:

Vitamin C offers a wide range of support for the human body. It is a potent antioxidant and free radical scavenger supporting cellular and vascular health. Vitamin C has been reported to promote nitric oxide activity as well as to help maintain healthy platelet function. It supports the body's defense system by enhancing white blood cell function and activity, as well as by increasing interferon levels, antibody responses, and secretion of thymic hormones. Furthermore, this antioxidant has histamine-lowering properties and increases lymphocyte formation. It is also essential for the formation and maintenance of intercellular ground substance and collagen, important for joint health. Vitamin C aids in the absorption of iron and the formation of red blood cells and converts folic acid to its active forms.*

What is the Source?

The ascorbic acid in this formula is derived from corn dextrose fermentation. The minerals in this formula are naturally derived from limestone. Ascorbyl palmitate in buffered ascorbic acid capsules is also derived from corn dextrose fermentation and palm oil.

Recommendations

Two to eight capsules (2–8 g), in divided doses, with or between meals, or more per day, as needed.

3. COQ10

What is It?

The essential nutrient Coenzyme Q10 (CoQ10) is a necessary component of cellular energy production. It is a component of the mitochondrial electron transport system in cells, which supplies energy required for all physiological functions.

Uses for CoQ10

Support for Cellular Energy Production

CoQ10 is a core component of cellular energy production and respiration, shuttling electrons down the electron transport chain to produce the key energy-rich molecule adenosine triphosphate (ATP). It provides support to all cells of the body and is especially supportive of tissues that require a lot of energy, such as the heart muscle, periodontal tissue, and the cells of the body's natural defense system.*

Cardiovascular Support

By enhancing energy levels and promoting cellular and tissue health, CoQ10 provides optimal nutritional support for the cardiovascular system. Numerous clinical studies suggest that CoQ10 supports healthy blood flow and heart muscle function. Furthermore, it acts as an antioxidant, providing cellular protection from free radicals, helps to maintain the integrity of vitamin E, and promotes healthy lipid metabolism.

What is the Source?

Pure Encapsulations CoQ10 is obtained naturally by fermentation from microorganisms. Pure Encapsulations CoQ10 also contains hypoallergenic plant fiber (pine cellulose).

Recommendations

60 to 1,000 mg per day, in divided doses, with meals.

Are There Any Potential Side Effects or Precautions?

At this time, there are no known side effects or precautions. If pregnant or lactating, consult your physician before taking this product.

Are There Any Potential Drug Interactions?

CoQ10 may react with blood thinning medications. Consult your physician for more information.

For educational purposes only. Consult your physician for any health problems.

CoQ10 500 mg
Each vegetable capsule contains:
coenzyme Q10... 500 mg
(hypo-allergenic plant fiber added to complete capsule volume requirement)
1–2 capsules per day, in divided doses, with meals.

CoQ10 250 mg
Each vegetable capsule contains:
coenzyme Q10... 250 mg
(hypo-allergenic plant fiber added to complete capsule volume requirement)
1–2 capsules per day, in divided doses, with meals.

CoQ10 120 mg
Each vegetable capsule contains:
coenzyme Q10... 120 mg
(hypo-allergenic plant fiber added to complete capsule volume requirement)
1–2 capsules per day, in divided doses, with meals.

CoQ10 60 mg
Each vegetable capsule contains:
coenzyme Q10... 60 mg
(hypo-allergenic plant fiber added to complete capsule volume requirement)
1–2 capsules per day, in divided doses, with meals.

CoQ10 30 mg
Each vegetable capsule contains:
coenzyme Q10... 30 mg
(hypo-allergenic plant fiber added to complete capsule volume requirement)
2–4 capsules per day, in divided doses, with meals.

4. VITAMIN E

What is It?

Vitamin E is a fat-soluble vitamin that contains a family of compounds called tocopherols, including d-alpha, beta, delta, and gamma.*

Uses for Vitamin E:

Antioxidant Support and Protection: Vitamin E is a powerful chain-breaking antioxidant and free radical scavenger and is considered the first line of defense against lipid peroxidation. It protects the integrity of the body's cellular membranes, and has the ability to unite with oxygen and prevent it from being converted into toxic peroxides.*

Cardiovascular Support: Vitamin E plays a beneficial role in the cellular respiration of muscles, especially cardiac and skeletal muscles. It also supports platelet function and blood vessel health.*

Cellular Function: protein metabolism, mitochondrial function, and hormone production.*

What Is the Source?

Vitamin E is derived from soy. There is no detectable GMO material in this product.

Recommendations

Pure Encapsulations recommends 1–2 capsules per day, with meals.

Are There Any Potential Side Effects or Precautions?

At this time, there are no known side effects or precautions. If pregnant or lactating, consult your physician before taking this product.

Are There Any Potential Drug Interactions?

Vitamin E may react with aspirin and blood thinning medications. Consult your physician for more information.

For educational purposes only. Consult your physician for any health problems.

Vitamin E

Each softgel capsule contains:

natural vitamin E (mixed tocopherols) providing (typical):

d-alpha tocopherol............................ (400 i.u.) 268 mg

other tocopherols... 67 mg

(other ingredients: soybean oil)

1–2 capsules per day, with meals.

5. FISH OIL

What is It?

Supercritical CO_2 extracted fish oil concentrate providing 840 mg DHA per serving. The omega-3 essential fatty acid DHA is well recognized for its ability to support neural and cognitive function. Fish oil containing DHA has also been associated with healthy lipid metabolism, platelet function, vascular health, joint function, and skin health.*

Features Include:

- High DHA concentrate for advanced support*
- Solvent-free, supercritical CO_2 based extraction
- Low temperature, oxygen-free processing prevents oxidation reactions
- Stringent purity guidelines established by the CRN and WHO are followed
- Each batch of fish oils tested for environmental contaminants, oxidation and rancidity, and microbial contamination

- Acid value (< 3 mg KOH/g)
- Peroxides (< 5 meq/kg)
- Anisidine (< 20)
- TOTOX (< 26)
- Heavy metals (< 0.1 ppm)
- Dioxins/furans (< 2 ppt WHO-TEQ)
- Dioxin-like PCBs (< 3 ppt WHO-TEQ)
- PCBs (< 0.09 ppm)

Uses For DHA Ultimate

Cognitive Support

Epidemiological studies indicate that a high intake of DHA is associated with healthy cognitive function. DHA-rich diets have been shown to support healthy neuron and cell membrane function in the brain as well as healthy gene expression, cell cycle function, arachidonic acid metabolism, and inflammation balance. These actions are associated with the ability of DHA to help with mild memory problems associated with aging and to help lessen occasional absentmindedness. Omega-3 fatty acids have also demonstrated the potential to support emotional well being.*

Heart Health

EPA and DHA from fish oil promote cardiovascular health by supporting healthy triglyceride and lipid metabolism, promoting healthy blood flow and vascular function, and maintaining healthy platelet function.*

Joint Function

Fish oil moderates the production of prostaglandins and leukotrienes, helping to maintain connective tissue health and comfort.*

Gastrointestinal Tract Comfort

Studies suggest that omega-3 fatty acids may play a role in maintaining healthy gastrointestinal function and comfort by supporting healthy eicosanoid production.*

Skin Health

Omega-3 fatty acids protect keratinocytes and skin fibroblasts from free radicals and immune mediators generated by sun exposure. Additionally, they help promote elasticity and hydration for smoother looking skin.*

What is the Source?

DHA Ultimate is sourced from sardines and anchovies from the Pacific Ocean off the coast of Chile. The fish oil is produced in a low-temperature, oxygen-free, solvent-free, supercritical CO_2-based extraction process using advanced "green technology." This process produces seventy five percent less carbon emissions than other methods of fatty acid extraction and purification.

Recommendations

Pure Encapsulations recommends two softgels per day, with meals.

Are There Any Potential Side Effects or Precautions?

If pregnant or lactating, consult your physician before taking this product. At this time, there are no known side effects or precautions. Consult your physician for more information.

Are There Any Potential Drug Interactions?

At this time, there are no known adverse reactions when taken in conjunction with medications, though some health professionals caution against taking with blood thinning medications due to a potential synergistic action. Consult your physician for more information.

DHA Ultimate two softgels contain 11 sg:

calories... 10
calories from fat 10
total fat .... 1,000 mg
vitamin E (mixed tocopherols) .... 2 i.u.
fish oil concentrate (anchovies, sardines)......... 1,400 mg
providing:
DHA (docosahexaenoic acid) .... 840 mg
EPA (eicosapentaenoic acid) .... 140 mg
other ingredients: gelatin capsule
2 softgels per day, with meals.

6. CALCIUM WITH VITAMIN D

Highly absorbable calcium, reduces risk of osteoporosis; combined with vitamin D to support bone, cardiovascular, and colon health.

Several clinical trials reveal the positive effects of combined supplemental calcium and vitamin D for bone health. Vitamin D is important for its ability to promote intestinal calcium and phosphorous absorption, reduce urinary calcium loss and enhance healthy bone composition. In a large trial published in the *New England Journal of Medicine* involving over 3,000 women, supplementation with calcium and vitamin D daily for one and a half years supported bone composition of the femur. In another study, calcium and vitamin D supplementation promoted calcium utilization and maintained healthy bones in postmenopausal women. Calcium citrate malate combined with vitamin D moderated the rate of bone loss for a separate group of postmenopausal women, maintaining support for the spine. Calcium and vitamin D also play roles in cardiovascular and colon health.

†*Risk factors for osteoporosis include sex, race, age and inadequate calcium intake. Populations at highest risk for osteoporosis include Caucasian, Asian, postmenopausal women, and the elderly. Adequate calcium intake throughout life is linked to a reduced risk of osteoporosis, as calcium helps to optimize peak bone mass during adolescence and early adulthood in conjunction with exercise and healthy diet. Calcium intake greater than 2,000 mg per day has no further known benefit to bone health.*

What is It?

Vitamin D3 enhances calcium absorption and retention, a key nutritional role in supporting healthy bones, and may play a potential role in cardiovascular, colon, and cellular health. Vitamin D levels have been shown to decline with age, due primarily to a reduction in either absorption or metabolism by the liver. Decreased exposure to sunlight, a vegetarian diet, or a low intake of vitamin D fortified foods also play a role in inadequate vitamin D levels.

Uses for Vitamin D3
Bone Health

Vitamin D promotes intestinal calcium and phosphorous absorption and reduces urinary calcium loss, essential mechanisms for maintaining proper calcium levels in the body and for healthy bone composition. Clinical studies involving vitamin D supplementation suggest the importance of vitamin D in addition to calcium for bone health. Vitamin D supplementation alone may also support bone health.

Cardiovascular Support: Vitamin D may also provide cardiovascular support for some individuals, which may be attributed to its effect on calcium metabolism or possibly by helping to maintain healthy plasma renin function in the islet cells of the pancreas.

Cellular Health

Studies suggest that vitamin D supports colon health by promoting healthy cellular function. Vitamin D is also believed to provide general cellular support potential, including breast and prostate cells, in part by helping to maintain healthy angiogenesis balance, supporting immune cell activity, and maintaining healthy cell metabolism. Preliminary evidence suggests that vitamin D may also play a role in maintaining healthy glucose metabolism, since vitamin D receptors are present on the islet cells of the pancreas.

What Is the Source?

Vitamin D3 is derived from the cholesterol in lanolin, the fat found in wool. Hypoallergenic plant fiber is derived from pine cellulose. Medium chain triglycerides (Vitamin D3 liquid only) are derived from coconut and palm oil.

Recommendations

Pure Encapsulations provides vitamin D3 capsules in four amounts (400 i.u., 1,000 i.u., 5,000 i.u. and 10,000 i.u.) and vitamin D3 liquid. Recommendations are as follows:
Vitamin D3 400 i.u. = 1–2 capsules per day, in divided doses, with meals.
Vitamin D3 1,000 i.u. = 1–5 capsules per day, in divided doses, with meals.
Vitamin D3 5,000 i.u. = 1 capsule per day, with a meal.
Vitamin D3 10,000 i.u. = 1 capsule per day, with a meal.
Vitamin D3 liquid = 1 or more drops daily, with a meal.

Are There Any Potential Side Effects or Precautions?

It is recommended that individuals using more than 2,000 i.u. of vitamin D per day have their blood levels monitored. Large doses of vitamin D can cause hypercalcemia, signs of which include headache, weakness, nausea, vomiting, and constipation. Individuals with hyperparathyroidism or kidney disease are at particular risk. Vitamin D3 10,000 i.u., Vitamin D3 5,000 i.u. and vitamin D3 1,000 i.u. are not to be taken by pregnant or lactating women. If pregnant or lactating, consult your physician before taking vitamin D3 400 i.u.

Are There Any Potential Drug Interactions?

Vitamin D may result in hypercalcemia in certain individuals taking digoxin or thiazide diuretics. Consult your physician for more information.

Vitamin D3 10,000 i.u.

One vegetable capsule contains:
vitamin D3.. 10,000 i.u
(hypoallergenic plant fiber added to complete capsule volume requirement)

Not to be taken by pregnant or lactating women. It is recommended that individuals taking more than 2,000 i.u. vitamin D per day have their blood levels monitored.

1 capsule daily for up to five days per week, with a meal, or as directed by a health professional.

Vitamin D3 5,000 i.u. each vegetable capsule contains:

vitamin D3.. 5,000 i.u.
(hypoallergenic plant fiber added to complete capsule volume requirement)

Not to be taken by pregnant or lactating women. It is recommended that individuals taking more than 2,000 i.u. vitamin D per day have their blood levels monitored.

1 capsule per day, with a meal Vitamin D3 1,000 i.u.

Each vegetable capsule contains:
vitamin D3.. 1,000 i.u.
(hypoallergenic plant fiber added to complete capsule volume requirement)

It is recommended that individuals taking more than 2,000 i.u. vitamin D per day have their blood levels monitored. If pregnant or lactating, consult your physician before use.

1–5 capsules per day, in divided doses, with meals
Vitamin D3 400 i.u.

Each vegetable capsule contains:
vitamin D3.. 400 i.u.
(hypoallergenic plant fiber added to complete capsule volume requirement)

1–2 capsules per day, in divided doses, with meals.
Vitamin D3 liquid

1 drop contains:
vitamin D3.. 1,000 i.u.
(other ingredients: medium chain triglycerides)

It is recommended that individuals taking more than 2,000 i.u. vitamin D per day have their blood levels monitored. If pregnant or lactating, consult your physician before use.

1 or more drops per day, with meals, as directed by a health professional.

7. MAGNESIUM

What is It?

Magnesium in aspartate, citrate, citrate/malate, and glycinate forms are highly bioavailable magnesium chelates, supporting the metabolism and utilization of many essential nutrients. Additionally, magnesium plays an important role in the proper functioning of numerous enzymatic and physiological functions, including neuromuscular contractions, cardiac function, and regulation of the acid-alkaline balance in the body.*

Uses for Magnesium
Nutrient Utilization

Magnesium is essential in the metabolism of macronutrients, energy production and the utilization of calcium, phosphorus, sodium, and potassium. This vital mineral also helps utilize B-complex vitamins, vitamin C, and vitamin E.*

Bone Health

Magnesium is an essential bone matrix mineral that promotes healthy bone metabolism. A trial involving 2,038 older individuals indicated that higher intakes of magnesium were positively associated with bone mineralization for certain individuals.*

Cardiovascular Support

Magnesium provides broad spectrum cardiovascular support, including arterial function, endothelial function, c-reactive protein metabolism, and lipid metabolism. A meta-analysis of twenty randomized trials suggest that it also promotes healthy systolic and diastolic function. In addition, magnesium promotes healthy glucose metabolism.

In one fifteen-year study involving 4,637 young adults, higher intakes of magnesium were associated with healthy cardiovascular function and glucose utilization. Magnesium also plays important roles in muscle function, mood and calming, and cranial vessel comfort.

What is the Source?

Magnesium is naturally derived from limestone. Citrate is produced by corn dextrose fermentation. Aspartate, glyincate, and malate are synthetic. Ascorbyl palmitate is derived from corn dextrose fermentation and palm oil.

Recommendations

Pure Encapsulations recommends 1–4 capsules per day, in divided doses, with meals.

Are There Any Potential Side Effects or Precautions?

Adverse effects from magnesium supplementation are rare when taken as directed but can include gastrointestinal upset and diarrhea. Individuals with kidney disease should not take magnesium supplements without consulting a doctor. Magnesium glycinate is less likely to cause loose stools. If pregnant or lactating, consult your physician before taking this product.

Are There Any Potential Drug Interactions?

Magnesium should be taken separately from bisphosphonate medications. Caution should be taken with concurrent use of potassium-sparing diuretics. It may also be contraindicated with certain antibiotics. Consult your physician for more information

Magnesium (aspartate)

Each vegetable capsule contains:
magnesium (aspartate) .... 75 mg
vitamin C (as ascorbyl palmitate) .... 9 mg
1–4 capsules per day, in divided doses, with meals.

Magnesium (citrate)

Each vegetable capsule contains:
magnesium (citrate) .... 150 mg
vitamin C (as ascorbyl palmitate) .... 11 mg

1–4 capsules per day, in divided doses, with meals.

Magnesium (citrate/malate)
Each vegetable capsule contains:

magnesium (citrate/malate) .... 120 mg

vitamin C (as ascorbyl palmitate) .... 10 mg

1–4 capsules per day, in divided doses, with meals.

Magnesium (glycinate)
Each vegetable capsule contains:

magnesium (glycinate) .... 120 mg

vitamin C (as ascorbyl palmitate) .... 10 mg

1–4 capsules per day, in divided doses, with meals.

Magnesium (powder)
One scoop (4.4 g) contains:

magnesium (citrate)... 150 mg

magnesium (glycinate) .... 150 mg

stevia.. 20 mg

other ingredients: xylitol, natural pineapple, banana and coconut flavors

1 scoop 1–2 times per day, in divided doses, with meals, mixed with 8 oz. water.

8. ZINC

What is It?
Zinc is essential for a wide range of physiological functions, including support of the body's defense system and tissue development and repair. Picolinate and citrate are both highly absorbable zinc chelates.*

Uses for Zinc Nutrient Metabolism
Zinc is a constituent of over two dozen enzymes involved in digestion and metabolism, including healthy storage and

metabolism of carbohydrates. It is also related to the normal absorption and actions of the B vitamins.*

Immune Support
Zinc plays an important role in supporting the body's defense system, promoting healthy neutrophil, natural killer cell, and T-lymphocyte function.*

Tissue Development and Repair
Zinc plays a fundamental role in collagen formation and healthy tissue development, including enzymes vital to tissue respiration. It is also essential for normal fetal and reproductive development, and contributes to healthy prostatic function as well.*

What is the Source?
Zinc is derived from earthen ore. Citrate is derived from corn dextrose fermentation. Picolinate is synthetic. Gluconate is derived from corn dextrose fermentation. Ascorbyl palmitate is derived from corn dextrose fermentation and palm oil. Hypo-allergenic plant fiber is derived from pine cellulose.

Recommendations
Pure Encapsulations recommends:
- Zinc 30 = 1–2 capsules per day, in divided doses, with meals.
- Zinc 15 = 1–4 capsules per day, in divided doses, with meals.
- Zinc (citrate) = 1–2 capsules per day, in divided doses, with meals.
- Zinc liquid (adults) = 4 ml (2 full droppers), with a meal.
- Zinc liquid (children ages 4 and up) = 2 ml (1 full dropper), with a meal.

Are There Any Potential Side Effects or Precautions?

If pregnant or lactating, consult your physician before taking this product. In rare cases, zinc can cause nausea, vomiting or a metallic taste. High intakes of zinc can cause fever, diarrhea or fatigue and may impair immune response. Consult your physician for more information.

Are There Any Potential Drug Interactions?

Zinc may be contraindicated with certain antibiotics. Consult your physician for more information.

Zinc liquid 15 mg 4 ml (0.13 fl oz) (2 full droppers) contains:

zinc (gluconate.. 15 mg
other ingredients: purified water, apple juice concentrate, cranberry juice concentrate, purified stevia extract, potassium sorbate, citric acid
serving size: 4 ml (0.13 fl oz) (2 full droppers) servings per container: 30
Adults, take 4 ml (2 full droppers), with a meal.
Children ages 4 and up, take 2 ml (1 full dropper), with a meal.

Zinc (citrate)

Each vegetable capsule contains;
zinc (citrate)... 30 mg
vitamin C (as ascorbyl palmitate) .... 4 mg
(hypoallergenic plant fiber added to complete capsule volume requirement)
1–2 capsules per day, in divided doses, with meals.

Zinc 30

Each vegetable capsule contains:

zinc (picolinate) .... 30 mg

vitamin C (as ascorbyl palmitate) .... 4 mg

(hypoallergenic plant fiber added to complete capsule volume requirement)

1–2 capsules per day, in divided doses, with meals.

Zinc 15

Each vegetable capsule contains:

zinc (picolinate) .... 15 mg

(hypoallergenic plant fiber added to complete capsule volume requirement)

1–4 capsules per day, in divided doses, with meals.

9. DHEA

What is It?

DHEA, dehydroepiandrosterone, is the most abundant adrenal steroid hormone in the body. After it is made by the adrenal glands, it travels into cells throughout the body where it is converted into androgens, estrogens, and other hormones. These hormones regulate fat and mineral metabolism, endocrine and reproductive function, and energy levels. The amount of each hormone that DHEA converts to depends on an individual's biochemistry, age, and sex. DHEA levels peak around age twenty five and then decline steadily.*

Uses for DHEA
Immune Function

DHEA supplementation has been shown to support healthy immune cell activity and immune system function in several trials.*

Emotional Well-Being

Several studies suggest that DHEA can enhance an overall sense of well-being. In one randomized placebo-controlled cross-over trial, DHEA supplementation for six months supported healthy physical and psychological outlook in men and women between the ages of forty to seventy years.*

Lean Body Mass

Some studies involving men and postmenopausal women suggest that DHEA administration may support a healthy ratio of lean muscle to fat mass.*

Sexual Function Support

In a six-month prospective, double blind, randomized, placebo-controlled study, DHEA supplementation supported healthy male sexual function.*

What Is the Source?

The compound diosgenin is extracted from wild yam and undergoes a proprietary synthetic process to develop DHEA. The human body cannot metabolize wild yam into DHEA. This process can only take place in a laboratory. Pure Encapsulations DHEA is micronized to increase absorption. It is made with 99.38% pure, pharmaceutical grade DHEA. Vitamin C (ascorbyl palmitate) is derived from corn dextrose fermentation and palm oil. Hypoallergenic plant fiber is derived from pine cellulose.

Are There Any Precautions or Potential Side Effects?

Precautions:

NOT FOR USE BY INDIVIDUALS UNDER THE AGE OF 18.
DO NOT USE IF PREGNANT OR NURSING.
KEEP OUT OF REACH OF CHILDREN.

Consult a physician or licensed qualified healthcare professional before using this product if you have, or have a family history of, prostate cancer, prostate enlargement, heart disease, low "good" cholesterol (HDL), or if you are using any other dietary supplement, prescription drug, or over-the-counter drug.

- Individuals with hypertension should avoid this product.
- Do not exceed the recommended serving. Exceeding the recommended serving may cause serious adverse health effects.

Potential Side Effects:

- Possible side effects include acne, hair loss, hair growth on the face (in women), aggressiveness, irritability, and increased levels of estrogen.
- Discontinue use and call a physician or licensed qualified health care professional immediately if you experience rapid heartbeat, dizziness, blurred vision, or other similar symptoms.
- To report any adverse event call 1-800-332-1088.

Are There Any Potential Drug Interactions?

Because calcium channel blockers may increase DHEA levels in some individuals, concurrent DHEA supplementation is not recommended unless closely monitored by a healthcare professional

DHEA 25 mg (micronized) ach vegetable capsule contains:

DHEA (dehydroepiandrosterone, C19H28O2)
    (micronized)...25 mg
ascorbyl palmitate (fat-soluble vitamin C) ....3 mg
(hypo-allergenic plant fiber added to complete capsule volume requirement)
Not to be taken by pregnant or lactating women. See full warning. 1 capsule per day, with a meal.

DHEA 10 mg (micronized) each vegetable capsule contains:

DHEA (dehydroepiandrosterone, C19H28O2)
(micronized)... 10 mg
(hypoallergenic plant fiber added to complete capsule
volume requirement)
*Not to be taken by pregnant or lactating women. See full
warning.* 1 capsule per day, with a meal.

DHEA 5 mg (micronized) each vegetable capsule contains:

DHEA (dehydroepiandrosterone, C19H28O2)
(micronized)... 5 mg
(hypoallergenic plant fiber added to complete capsule
volume requirement)
*Not to be taken by pregnant or lactating women. See
full warning.* 1–2 capsules per day, in divided doses, with
meals, or as directed by your physician

10. 7-KETO DHEA

What is It?

7-KETO™ DHEA, a safe and natural metabolite of DHEA,
was the subject of research for over a decade at the University of
Wisconsin, Madison. Of over 150 DHEA compounds tested, 7-KETO
proved to be the most promising form. Researchers discovered that
7-KETO does not convert to testosterone or estrogen and supports
various physiological processes. 7-KETO DHEA is also known as
DHEA-Acetate-7-one or 3-acetoxy-androst-5-ene-7,17-dione.

Uses for 7-KETO™ DHEA Metabolic Support and Weight Management

7-KETO is several times more potent than DHEA in stimulating the thermogenic enzymes of the liver, promotes basal
metabolism, and helps to increase the lean/adipose ratio. These

actions safely support a leaner BMI (Body Mass Index) and healthy weight control. In a double-blind study involving thirty overweight adults, 7-KETO supported healthy body composition and BMI when combined with exercise.

Other Patented Applications

Research on the role of 7-KETO in immune, cognitive and other areas of support similar to DHEA has proven promising, but is preliminary.

What is the Source?

7-KETO is made from pharmaceutical grade DHEA. DHEA is produced when diosgenin is extracted from wild yam and modified in a laboratory process to achieve the final structure. Hypo-allergenic plant fiber is derived from pine cellulose.

Recommendations

Pure Encapsulations recommends 25–200 mg per day, in divided doses, with meals. For weight loss support, 100 mg twice daily is recommended.

Are There Any Potential Side Effects or Precautions?

Not to be taken by pregnant or lactating women. Vivid dreams have been reported if taken too close to bedtime. Individuals with breast, prostate, or other hormonally linked cancers (or a family history of these conditions) should avoid this product as 7-KETO has not been studied in these contexts.

Are There Any Potential Drug Interactions?

7-KETO has been shown to promote healthy platelet function. As a result, it may be contraindicated for individuals using Coumadin due to a potential synergistic blood-thinning effect.

7-Keto™ DHEA 100 mg
Each vegetable capsule contains:
DHEA-Acetate-7-one....................................... 100 mg
(hypoallergenic plant fiber added to complete capsule volume requirement)
Not to be taken by pregnant or lactating women. 1–2 capsules per day, in divided doses, with meals.

7-Keto™ DHEA 50 mg
Each vegetable capsule contains:
DHEA-Acetate-7-one... 50 mg
(hypoallergenic plant fiber added to complete capsule volume requirement)
Not to be taken by pregnant or lactating women. 1–4 capsules per day, with a meal.

7-Keto™ DHEA 25 mg
Each vegetable capsule contains:
DHEA-Acetate-7-one... 25 mg
(hypoallergenic plant fiber added to complete capsule volume requirement)
Not to be taken by pregnant or lactating women. 1–8 capsules per day, in divided doses, with meals.

In addition to these vitamins and minerals, I also recommend for men supplements for prostate health:
1. Beta-sistosterol
2. Lycopene
3. Lysine
4. N-Acetyl-Cysteine
5. Arginine

11. BETA-SISTOSTEROL

What is It?

Beta-sitosterol is a naturally occurring plant sterol. Plant sterols are a family of compounds similar in structure to cholesterol that have positive effects on prostate health.*

Uses for Beta-Sitosterol Supports Prostate Health:

In a six-month randomized, double-blind, placebo-controlled, multicenter study with 200 male subjects, it was proposed that a mixed phytosterol complex providing beta-sitosterol supported healthy urinary flow. In an eighteen-month follow-up trial, beta-sitosterol maintained healthy urinary function. These results have been supported in other clinical trials as well.*

What is the Source?

Beta-sitosterol is sourced from a soy-based phytosterol complex. Vitamin C (ascorbyl palmitate) is derived from corn dextrose fermentation. Hypoallergenic plant fiber is derived from pine cellulose. There is no detectable GMO material in this product.

Recommendations

Pure Encapsulations recommends 1–2 capsules per day, in divided doses, with meals.

Are There Any Potential Side Effects or Precautions?

This product may not be desirable for individuals with a sensitivity to soy. If pregnant or lactating, consult your physician before taking this product.

Are There Any Potential Drug Interactions?

At this time, there are no known adverse reactions when taken in conjunction with medications.

Beta-sitosterol

Each vegetable capsule contains:

beta-sitosterol (from 150 mg of a phytosterol
    complex)... 68 mg
vitamin C (as ascorbyl palmitate)....................... 20 mg
(hypoallergenic plant fiber added to complete capsule
volume requirement)
1–2 capsules per day, in divided doses, with meals.

12. LYCOPENE

What is It?

Lycopene is a member of the carotenoid family and provides
the rich red pigments found in tomatoes, watermelon, pink
grapefruit, pink guava and papaya. Lycopene is a lipophilic
molecule that contains eleven conjugated double bonds. These
conjugated double bonds are what enables lycopene to be a
powerful antioxidant. Pure Encapsulations Lycopene provides
a natural tomato extract rich in lycopene, various carotenoids,
vitamin E and other important phytochemicals.*

Uses for Lycopene Prostate Support

In one study involving thirty male subjects, supplementation
with lycopene promoted healthy prostate function. This was one
of the first randomized, prospective clinical trials to show that a
lycopene supplement, rather than dietary tomato consumption,
supported prostate health.*

Cardiovascular Support Potential

Research compiled in a multicenter study involving ten
European countries revealed that the antioxidant properties of
dietary lycopene supported cardiovascular health.*

Support for Cellular Health

Fifty-seven epidemiological studies indicate that lycopene from tomato consumption or tomato-based products may help digestive, lung, stomach, cervical, and breast cell health.*

Ocular Support: Lycopene has also demonstrated potential for promoting retinal and macular health.*

What is the Source?

Pure Encapsulations Lycopene is derived from natural tomato concentrate. Fresh tomatoes contain lycopene almost exclusively in the trans conformation, although a variety of cis isomers are possible. When exposed to light and heat, such as during food processing, trans isomers will convert to cis as it is the more stable form of lycopene.

Pure Encapsulations Lycopene is naturally extracted by a proprietary method, which preserves the trans conformation of the molecule.

Recommendations

Pure Encapsulations recommends up to 40 mg per day, in divided doses, with meals.

Are There Any Potential Side Effects or Precautions?

At this time, there are no known side effects or precautions. If pregnant or lactating, consult your physician before taking this product.

Are There Any Potential Drug Interactions?

At this time, there are no known adverse reactions when taken in conjunction with medications.

Lycopene 20 mg

Each softgel capsule contains:

lycopene ....20 mg

(in a base of rice bran oil and beeswax)

1–2 capsules per day, in divided doses, with meals.

Lycopene 10 mg

Each softgel capsule contains:

lycopene .... 10 mg

(in a base of rice bran oil and beeswax)

1–3 capsules per day, in divided doses, with meals.

13. DIM

What is It?

Diindolylmethane is a metabolite of indole-3-carbinol (I3C). Both are found naturally in cruciferous vegetables like broccoli, kale, and brussel sprouts. Upon contact with gastric acid in the stomach, I3C is converted to a number of active compounds in varying amounts, predominantly diindolylmethane. Therefore, it may be more supportive than I3C in cases of low gastric acidity. Diindolylmethane provides support for healthy breast, cervical and prostate cells.*

Uses For DIM-PRO® 100 Promotes Breast, Cervical and Prostate Cell Health

Animal and cell studies have found that diindolylmethane supports healthy breast cell metabolism in part by promoting healthy cytochrome P450 detoxification, maintaining healthy gene expression, and supporting healthy cell cycle function and enzyme activity. A doubleblind, randomized clinical trial involved nineteen postmenopausal women who supplemented with BioResponse-DIM® (diindolylmethane) for thirty days.

Results suggest that it promoted healthy breast cell function. Furthermore, an additional double blind randomized clinical trial of fifty two women found that BioResponse-DIM® supported cervical cell health. Animal and cell studies have also indicated that diindolylmethane enhances prostate cell health by maintaining healthy gene expression.*

Promotes Breast Comfort

Another randomized placebo-controlled crossover trial including thirty three pre-menopausal women found that supplementing with BioResponse DIM® for three months promoted statistically significant breast comfort.*

What is the Source?

Diindolylmethane in its pure form is highly insoluble. Patented, microencapsulated BioResponse DIM® has been specially developed for enhanced absorption. BioResponse DIM® is a complex of starch (derived from corn), diindolylmethane, d-alpha tocopheryl succinate, phosphatidylcholine (derived from soy) and silica, standardized to contain twenty five percent diindolylmethane. BioResponse DIM® and DIM-PRO® are trademarks of BioResponse, L.L.C., Boulder, CO. U.S. Patent 6,086,915. Vitamin C (ascorbyl palmitate) is derived from corn dextrose fermentation and palm oil. Hypoallergenic plant fiber is derived from pine cellulose.

Recommendations

Pure Encapsulations recommends 1–3 capsules per day, in divided doses, with or between meals.

Are There Any Potential Side Effects or Precautions?

If pregnant or lactating, consult your physician before taking this product.

Are There Any Potential Drug Interactions?

At this time, there are no known adverse reactions when taken in conjunction with medications.

DIM-PRO® 100

Each vegetable capsule contains:
diindolylmethane complex**............................. 100 mg
(complex of starch, diindolylmethane, d-alpha tocopheryl succinate, phosphatidylcholine and silica)
(standardized to contain 25%
  diindolylmethane)..25 mg
vitamin C (as ascorbyl palmitate)........................20 mg
(hypoallergenic plant fiber added to complete capsule volume requirement)
Contains soy
Not to be taken by pregnant or lactating women.
Natural color variations may occur.
1–3 capsules per day, in divided doses, with or between meals.

14. L-CARNITINE

What is It?

L-Carnitine is an amino acid found abundantly in skeletal and heart muscle. It functions primarily to support fat utilization by acting as a carrier of fatty acids into the mitochondria, where they are oxidized and converted to energy. L-Carnitine also facilitates the removal of short and medium chain fatty acids from the mitochondria that accumulate during normal metabolic processes. In studies, l-carnitine has demonstrated the ability to promote oxygenation of heart muscle and maintain healthy enzyme activity, support cardiovascular energy, enhance exercise recovery, and maintain healthy lipid metabolism. Fumarate, or fumaric acid, is an important compound, which is also naturally present in the body. As a component of the Krebs cycle (Citric Acid Cycle), fumaric acid plays a key role in generating energy. Combined, l-carnitine and fumarate provide dual support for energizing the heart and skeletal muscles.*

Uses for L-Carnitine Fumarate Cardiovascular Support:

A randomized double-blind placebo-controlled trial involving 101 volunteers indicated that l-carnitine maintained healthy lipid peroxide and lactate dehydrogenase cardiac enzyme activity. L-Carnitine may also support ventricular function and superoxide dismutase enzyme activity. Long-term l-carnitine supplementation has demonstrated positive support for cardiovascular health after a three-year follow-up in adult subjects. In a recent six-month, randomized, double-blind placebo-controlled trial, l-carnitine supplementation supported healthy lipid metabolism in volunteers. In a metabolic analysis performed at George Washington University Medical Center, carnitine and fumarate provided synergistic cardioprotective support.*

Support for Exercise Recovery

In a prospective double-blind placebo-controlled trial, carnitine supplementation supported training for elite athletes. Additional studies suggest that l-carnitine promotes exercise recovery by moderating tissue damage, decreasing production of free radicals and reducing muscle soreness following exercise.*

What is the Source?

L-Carnitine fumarate is synthetically produced. It is patented worldwide by BIOSINT SpA (58.5% l-carnitine, 41.5% fumaric acid, US patent number 4,602,039). Vitamin C (ascorbyl palmitate) is derived from corn dextrose fermentation and palm oil. Hypo-allergenic plant fiber is derived from pine cellulose.

Recommendations

Pure Encapsulations recommends 2–4 capsules per day, in divided doses, between meals.

Are There Any Potential Side Effects or Precautions?

At this time, there are no known side effects or precautions. If pregnant or lactating, consult your physician before taking this product.

Are There Any Potential Drug Interactions?

At this time, there are no known adverse reactions when taken in conjunction with medications.

L-Carnitine Fumarate

Each vegetable capsule contains:
L-carnitine (free-form) .... 340 mg
(from 586 mg l-carnitine fumarate) (hypoallergenic plant fiber added to complete capsule volume requirement)
2–4 capsules per day, in divided doses, between meals.

15. ACETYL-L-CARNITINE

What is It?

Acetyl-l-carnitine is the acetylated form of l-carnitine. The two compounds share similar energy and metabolism promoting properties. Found naturally in the body, acetyl-l-carnitine supports the availability of acetyl-CoA, an important energy generating metabolite. In addition, it supports proper mitochondrial function and cell membrane stability. The acetyl group from acetyl-l-carnitine is also responsible for the production of acetylcholine, an important neurotransmitter for optimal mental functioning.*

Uses for Acetyl-L-Carnitine Support for Cognitive Function, Memory, and Emotional Well-Being:

The efficacy of long-term acetyl-l-carnitine supplementation was determined in a double-blind, placebo-controlled, randomized trial involving 130 elderly individuals for a one-year period. In this trial, acetyl-l-carnitine demonstrated the ability to slow negative cognitive changes, and supported memory and attention. In another randomized double-blind study, three-month acetyl-l-carnitine supplementation provided statistically significant support for mental function, including memory and attention, compared to placebo. A multicenter trial of 481 volunteers showed significant memory, behavioral and emotional support with acetyl-l-carnitine supplementation. In an evaluation of twenty eight elderly individuals using acetyl-l-carnitine or placebo, the supplemented group experienced enhanced emotional well-being.

What is the Source?

Pure Encapsulations Acetyl-l-carnitine consists of acetyl-l-carnitine HCl, a synthetically derived amino acid.

Recommendations

Pure Encapsulations recommends 500–1,000 mg acetyl-lcarnitine per day, in divided doses, between meals.

Are There Any Potential Side Effects or Precautions?

If pregnant or lactating, consult your physician before taking this product. Gastrointestinal upset and skin rash have been reported in sensitive individuals.

Are There Any Potential Drug Interactions?

At this time, there are no known adverse reactions when taken in conjunction with medications.

Acetyl-l-Carnitine 500 mg
Each vegetable capsule contains:
acetyl-l-carnitine HCl .... 500 mg
vitamin C (as ascorbyl palmitate) .... 8 mg
(hypoallergenic plant fiber added to complete capsule
volume requirement)
1–2 capsules per day, in divided doses, between meals.

Acetyl-l-Carnitine 250 mg
Each vegetable capsule contains:
acetyl-l-carnitine HCl .... 250 mg
vitamin C (as ascorbyl palmitate) .... 4 mg
(hypoallergenic plant fiber added to complete capsule
volume requirement)
2–4 capsules per day, in divided doses, between meals.

16. ALPHA-LIPOIC ACID

What is It?
Sodium R-alpha-lipoic acid is a highly bioavailable and stabilized form of R-lipoic acid. Regular R-lipoic acid is heat sensitive and may polymerize extensively, decreasing its absorption
significantly. In real-time stability tests, sodium R-lipoic remained
stable for twelve months. The natural R isomer of alpha-lipoic
acid may provide enhanced antioxidant activity, energy production, and general metabolic function.*

Uses for R-lipoic acid (stabilized) Nerve Health
In a recent in vitro study at the Buck Institute for Aging in
California, R-lipoic acid moderated oxidative stress in neurons. A
related study demonstrates the ability of R-lipoic acid to support
memory tasks in animals by supporting mitochondrial function
and protecting cells from free radicals.*

Glucose Metabolism

An animal study suggested that R-lipoic acid supported healthy glucose metabolism. Additional studies suggest that R-lipoic acid promotes glucose metabolism in skeletal muscle.*

Antioxidant Support

A University of California Berkeley study indicates that R-lipoic acid may be protective against age-related oxidative stress in the liver. Furthermore, a study at Oregon State University established a potential role for R-lipoic acid in protecting the heart from age-related oxidative stress.*

What is the Source?

Pure Encapsulations R-Lipoic Acid (stabilized) delivers 100 mg of actual R-lipoic acid per capsule from 143 mg of synthetically derived sodium R-alpha-lipoic acid. Sodium is from sodium carbonate. Hypoallergenic plant fiber is derived from pine cellulose.

Recommendations

Pure Encapsulations recommends 1–2 capsules per day, in divided doses, with meals.

Are There Any Potential Side Effects or Precautions?

If pregnant or lactating, consult your physician before taking this product. R-lipoic acid may cause gastrointestinal discomfort in some individuals and should always be taken with meals. In rare cases, R-lipoic acid may also cause skin rash in sensitive individuals.

Are There Any Potential Drug Interactions?

People taking anti-diabetic medications or medications for thyroid disease should be monitored by a healthcare professional.

For educational purposes only. Consult your physician for any health problems.

17. R-LIPOIC ACID

Each vegetable capsule contains v 2:
sodium .... 14 mg
R-lipoic acid (from 143 mg sodium R-alpha-lipoic
acid) .... 100 mg
vitamin C (as ascorbyl palmitate) .... 5 mg
(hypoallergenic plant fiber added to complete capsule
volume requirement)
other ingredients: sodium carbonate
1–2 capsules per day, in divided doses, with meals

What is It?

Alpha lipoic acid is an exceptionally versatile nutrient. Being both water and fat soluble, it is able to function in almost any part of the body. It is a potent antioxidant which enhances the activity of vitamins C and E. It is a multifunctional compound providing protection from free radicals and supporting various metabolic processes. It has been associated with supporting nerve health, cardiovascular function, and glucose metabolism.*

Uses for Alpha Lipoic Acid Nerve Health

At this time, as many as fifteen clinical trials have examined the role of alpha lipoic acid in maintaining healthy nerve function. The results of these trials have typically demonstrated that alpha lipoic acid administration provides neuroprotection. In part, this may be due to alpha lipoic acid's ability to modulate nitric oxide metabolite activity and to promote healthy microcirculation.*

Glucose Metabolism

Alpha lipoic acid supports healthy glucose uptake and helps to maintain healthy glucose utilization. It also plays a role in moderating the formation of advanced glycation end products.*

Cardiovascular Support

In addition to supporting healthy glucose metabolism, the antioxidant properties of alpha lipoic acid also promote healthy vascular and blood vessel function.*

What is the Source?

Alpha lipoic acid is synthetically produced and has a minimum purity of 99%. Vitamin C (ascorbyl palmitate) is derived from corn dextrose fermentation. Hypoallergenic plant fiber is derived from pine cellulose.

Recommendations

Pure Encapsulations recommends 100–1200 mg per day, in divided doses, with meals.

Are There Any Potential Side Effects or Precautions?

If pregnant or lactating, consult your physician before taking this product. Alpha lipoic acid may cause gastrointestinal discomfort in some individuals and should always be taken with meals. In rare cases, alpha lipoic acid may also cause skin rash in sensitive individuals.

Are There Any Potential Drug Interactions?

At this time, there are no known adverse reactions when taken in conjunction with medications.

Alpha Lipoic Acid 400 mg

Each vegetable capsule contains:
alpha lipoic acid (thioctic acid)..........................400 mg
vitamin C (as ascorbyl palmitate)........................ 16 mg
(hypoallergenic plant fiber added to complete capsule
volume requirement)
1–2 capsules per day, in divided doses, with meals.

Alpha Lipoic Acid 200 mg
Each vegetable capsule contains:
alpha lipoic acid (thioctic acid)..........................200 mg
vitamin C (as ascorbyl palmitate).........................16 mg
(hypoallergenic plant fiber added to complete capsule volume requirement)
1–4 capsules per day, in divided doses, with meals.

Alpha Lipoic Acid 100 mg
Each vegetable capsule contains:
alpha lipoic acid (thioctic acid)..........................100 mg
vitamin C (as ascorbyl palmitate)..........................8 mg
(hypoallergenic plant fiber added to complete capsule volume requirement)
1–8 capsules per day, in divided doses, with meals.

18. L-CARNOSINE

What is It?

L-Carnosine (beta-alanyl-L-histidine) occurs naturally in the body's muscle and nervous tissues and is formed by the amino acids alanine and histidine. Levels of this dipeptide can decline with age. The primary context of support for l-carnosine involves cellular longevity support.*

Uses For L-Carnosine Antioxidant Support

L-Carnosine is a water-soluble antioxidant with well-documented free-radical scavenging activity and is believed to promote cell health and cell longevity. In vitro experiments show carnosine to be a potent scavenger of peroxyl and hydroxyl radicals. Carnosine may also help to maintain superoxide dismutase (SOD) activity. SOD is an important antioxidant enzyme.*

Cellular Support

In vitro, it helps to protect proteins from the formation of advanced glycosylation end-products. These end-products are formed when aldehydes (such as aldose and ketose sugars) and lipid peroxidation by-products bind to vital proteins and compromise their function. L-Carnosine also plays a role in protecting DNA from the effects of acetaldehyde and formaldehyde.*

Nervous System Support

L-Carnosine may help to maintain healthy peptide metabolism in the brain, supporting neuronal cell health.*

Cardiovascular Support

Its membrane-stabilizing properties maintain healthy lactate dehydrogenase activity of cardiovascular cells, providing a protective effect.*

Muscular Support

The concentration of l-carnosine in muscle may prove to be an important factor in high-intensity exercise performance based on a recent human study.*

Liver Support

A preliminary animal study shows carnosine has the potential to support healthy liver function.*

What is the Source?

L-Carnosine is synthetically produced.

Recommendations

Pure Encapsulations recommends between 500–1500 mg daily (1–3 capsules), in divided doses, between meals.

Are There Any Potential Side Effects or Precautions?

Not to be taken by pregnant or lactating women. At this time, there are no known side effects or precautions.

Are There Any Potential Drug Interactions?

In animal studies, carnosine has been shown to inhibit intestinal uptake of several antibiotics. This has not been shown in humans, but it might be wise for those taking antibiotics to make sure they don't take carnosine at the same time.

L-Carnosine

Each vegetable capsule contains:
l-carnosine (beta-alanyl-L-histidine).................. 500 mg
Not to be taken by pregnant or lactating women.
1–3 capsules per day, in divided doses, between meals

19. NITTOKINASE

What is It?

A traditional Japanese vegetable-derived cheese used for over 1,000 years, natto has been prized for both its popular taste and vascular support properties. Nattokinase, a fibrinolytic enyzme isolated from natto, helps to maintain healthy activity of the body's natural clotting and fibrinolytic processes. This enzyme has demonstrated enhanced oral fibrinolytic potential when compared with other fibrinolytic enzymes from over 200 foods.

Uses For NSK-SD™

Supports Healthy Fibrinolytic Activity And Clotting Function: Fibrinolysis is a natural physiological process.

As the body ages, however, endogenous fibrinolytic activity declines. One study suggested that nattokinase inactivates plasminogen activator inhibitor, maintaining healthy fibrinolytic activity. Nattokinase may also directly degrade fibrin in much the same way as plasmin. Furthermore, researchers from JCR Pharmaceuticals, Oklahoma State University and Miyazaki Medical College examined the effect of nattokinase from natto food consumption in twelve healthy Japanese participants. The results suggested that natto supported healthy clotting function compared to placebo.*

Promotes Healthy Circulation And Blood Flow

In another study, nattokinase provided positive support for healthy circulation in animals. In an additional animal study conducted by Biotechnology Research Laboratories and JCR Pharmaceuticals of Kobe, Japan, nattokinase promoted healthy blood flow.*

Maintains Blood Vessel Function: In 1995, scientists at the Miyazaki Medical College and Kurashiki University in Japan demonstrated the potential for nattokinase to support blood vessel health in human subjects.*

What is the Source?

Natto is produced by a fermentation process when *Bacillus natto (also known as Bacillus subtilis natto) is* added to boiled soybeans. Nattokinase, a fibrinolytic enzyme, is isolated from natto. NSK-SD™ is a registered trademark of Japan Bio Science Laboratories.

Recommendations

Pure Encapsulations recommends 1–2 capsules 2 times per day, 12 hours apart, with or between meals.

Are There Any Potential Side Effects or Precautions?

This product is contraindicated for individuals with a history of bleeding tendency or with conditions associated with bleeding. If pregnant or lactating, consult your physician before taking this product.

Are There Any Potential Drug Interactions?

Due to potential synergistic effects, concurrent use with anticoagulant and blood pressure medications should be closely supervised by a health professional.

NSK-SD™ (Nattokinase)

NSK-SD™ 100 mg

Each vegetable capsule contains:

nattokinase (2000 FU) (soy)............................ 100 mg

vitamin C (as ascorbyl palmitate) .... 5 mg

(hypoallergenic plant fiber added to complete capsule volume requirement)

1 capsule 2 times per day, 12 hours apart, with or between meals.

NSK-SD™ 50 mg

Each vegetable capsule contains:

nattokinase (1000 FU) (soy).............................. 50 mg

(hypoallergenic plant fiber added to complete capsule volume requirement)

1–2 capsules 2 times per day, 12 hours apart, with or between meals.

20. NUTRIENT 950

What is It?

Nutrient 950® is a complete hypoallergenic, nutrient rich, highly bioavailable multi-vitamin, multi-mineral and trace element supplement. It contains superior mineral cofactors and activated vitamins, and provides an excellent antioxidant profile. Nutrient 950 is also available in the following formulas: without iron;

without copper and iron; without copper, iron and iodine; with Vitamin K; with N-acetyl-l-cysteine (NAC); and as the reduced potency formula, Nutrient 280®. Nutrient 950 was formulated exclusively for nutritionally oriented doctors who demand the highest quality multi-vitamin and mineral formula available for their patients.*

Uses For Nutrient 950®

Optimal Health: Nutrient 950 provides a high profile of free radical scavenging antioxidants important for cardiovascular, immune, and cellular health. The vitamins and minerals in this formula also support various physiological functions, including nervous system health, bone health, nutrient and hormone metabolism, and glucose utilization. Nutrient 950 provides fully chelated minerals for optimal absorption and activated vitamins, including Metafolin®, the naturally occurring universally metabolized form of folate. Metafolin® is chemically identical to the active folate metabolite, 5 methyltetrahydrofolate (L-5-MTHF), the predominant, naturally occurring form of folate in food. Through bypassing several enzymatic activation steps, it is directly usable by the body and provides all of the benefits of folic acid regardless of functional or genetic variations. This is a gentle, hypoallergenic formula, which is well tolerated by sensitive individuals.*

What is the Source?

The nutrients found in Nutrient 950® are derived from the following:

- Beta carotene: *Blakeslea trispora*
- Lycopene: natural tomato concentrate
- Lutein: marigold flower extract
- Zeaxanthin: synthetic

- Vitamin C: corn dextrose fermentation
- Vitamin E: soybean
- Vitamin K (only Nutrient 950® with Vitamin K):
- Synthetic (vitamin K1 and vitamin K2 (menaquinone-4))
- and natto (vitamin K2 (MK-7))
- Vitamin D3: cholesterol from wool fat (lanolin)
- Vitamin B1 (thiamine HCl): synthetic
- Vitamin B2 (riboflavin): corn dextrose fermentation
- Niacinamide and Inositol hexaniacinate: synthetic
- Vitamin B5 (calcium pantothenate): synthetic
- Vitamin B6 (pyridoxal HCl): synthetic
- Vitamin B12 (methylcobalamin): corn dextrose fermentation
- Folic acid (Metafolin®, L-5-MTHF): synthetic
- Biotin: synthetic
- Minerals: naturally derived from limestone
  Sources of the mineral chelates include:
  - Aspartate: synthetic
  - Citrate: corn dextrose fermentation
  - Glycinate: synthetic
  - Picolinate: synthetic
  - Nutrient 950 mixed carotenoid profile typically contains 9,000 mcg beta carotene, 250 mcg lycopene, 500 mcg lutein and 100 mcg zeaxanthin. Nutrient 280 mixed carotenoid profile typically contains 2,700 mcg beta carotene, 75 mcg lycopene, 150 mcg lutein and 30 mcg zeaxanthin.
  - There is no detectable GMO material in this product.

Recommendations

Pure Encapsulations recommends per 4–6 capsules per day, in divided doses, with meals.

Are There Any Potential Side Effects or Precautions?

At this time, there are no known side effects or precautions. If pregnant or lactating, consult your physician before taking this product.

Are There Any Potential Drug Interactions?

Nutrient 950 contains vitamin E, which may react with blood thinning medications. Consult your physician for more information. Vitamin K may be contraindicated for individuals taking Coumadin/warfarin blood thinning medication.

Nutrient 950®

Six vegetable capsules contain:

ascorbic acid.. 1,000 mg

vitamin C (as ascorbyl palmitate)...................... 120 mg

mixed carotenoids .... 15,000 i.u.
  (providing beta carotene, lycopene, lutein and zeaxanthin)

vitamin D3.. 800 i.u.

d-alpha tocopherol succinate (vitamin E)........... 400 i.u.

thiamine HCl (B1) .... 100 mg

riboflavin (B2) .... 50 mg

riboflavin 5' phosphate (activated B2)................. 25 mg

pyridoxine HCl (B6)... 25 mg

pyridoxal 5' phosphate (activated B6).................. 25 mg

niacinamide.. 100 mg

inositol hexaniacinate (no-flush niacin)............... 90 mg

folate (as Metafolin®, L-5-MTHF) .... 800 mcg

biotin .... 800 mcg

pantothenic acid (calcium pantothenate) (B5) .... 400 mg

methylcobalamin (B12)................................ 1,000 mcg

calcium (citrate)... 300 mg

magnesium (citrate).. 200 mg

potassium (aspartate).. 99 mg
zinc (picolinate) ....25 mg
manganese (aspartate)....................................... 10 mg
iron (glycinate) .... 10 mg
boron (glycinate)..2 mg
copper (glycinate) ....2 mg
iodine (potassium iodide).............................. 200 mcg
chromium (polynicotinate)............................. 200 mcg
selenium (selenomethionine)........................... 200 mcg
vanadium (aspartate) .... 200 mcg
molybdenum (aspartate)................................. 100 mcg

WARNING: Accidental overdose of iron-containing products is a leading cause of fatal poisoning in children under 6. Keep this product out of the reach of children. In case of accidental overdose, call a doctor or poison control center immediately.

4–6 capsules per day, in divided doses, with meals.

Also available:
* **Nutrient 950 without iron**
* **Nutrient 950 without copper and iron**
* **Nutrient 950 without copper, iron and iodine**

Nutrient 950 with NAC
* Offers the vitamin/mineral profile of Nutrient 950 (without boron, copper, iron or iodine) combined with 1,000 mg NAC per 8 capsule serving
* NAC supports immune defense and detoxification*

Nutrient 950 with Vitamin K
* Offers the vitamin/mineral profile of Nutrient 950 without iron with the addition of 250 mcg vitamin K1, 500 mcg

vitamin K2 (menaquinone-4) and 15 mcg vitamin K2 (MK-7) per 6 capsule serving

- Also contains the most vitamin D of all our multivitamins at 1,000 i.u per serving.
- Vitamin K1, K2 and D provide synergistic support for bone health and healthy arterial calcium metabolism

21. SUPER CITRIXMAX PLUS

What is It?

Super CitriMax® Plus is an all-natural, non-stimulating clinically studied formula consisting of *Garcinia cambogia* fruit extract (standardized for hydroxycitric acid, or HCA), chromium polynicotinate, and *Gymnema sylvestre* extract.*

Features Include:

- *Garcinia cambogia* extract, supporting natural weight management without stimulating the central nervous system. This extract influences appetite and energy levels naturally by redirecting calories from fat production toward increasing glycogen production and storage. In addition, (-)HCA inhibits the pathway of fatty acid biosynthesis and promotes healthy blood lipid levels.*
- Chromium polynicotinate, enhancing the effectiveness of (-)HCA, chromium inhibits the synthesis of new fat from carbohydrates, thus freeing the mitochondria to burn already stored fat. This mineral also is important for enzyme activation and may potentially promote Glucose Tolerance Factor (GTF) activity, helping to maintain healthy glucose metabolism and supporting body composition.*
- Gymnema sylvestre, supporting pancreas function and healthy glucose metabolism. Studies report that this extract is supportive of enzyme activity for glucose utilization

and helps moderate glucose uptake into the intestines. Furthermore, Gymnema also has the potential to support healthy lipid and triglyceride metabolism.*

Uses For Super CitriMax® Plus

Support For Lean Body Composition: A recent randomized, double-blind, placebo-controlled clinical trial conducted by researchers at Georgetown University Medical Center and Creighton University School of Pharmacy, examined the effects of Super CitriMax® on various aspects of body composition. The results indicated support for lean body composition, healthy serotonin levels, and improved body mass index. This concentrated formula also increased output of urinary fat metabolites, indicating increased fat degradation. In addition, it decreased serum leptin levels, improving signals that moderate food intake in the brain. Researchers at the University of California, Berkeley, have recently confirmed that HCA is absorbed and retained by overweight subjects. At Creighton University, Super Citrimax increased the release and availability of serotonin in brain tissue. ChromeMate® chromium (polynicotinate) supports healthy weight in combination with exercise for overweight females, as indicated by a study at the University of Texas, Austin. In a separate, randomized, placebo-controlled trial, ChromeMate® promoted healthy body composition in overweight women.*

What is the Source?

Garcinia cambogia extract is derived from the fruit and standardized to contain sixty percent (-)hydroxycitric acid. Chromium polynicotinate is synthetically derived. *Gymnema sylvestre* extract is derived from the leaf and standardized to contain seventy five percent gymnemic acids. Vitamin C is derived from corn dextrose fermentation and palm oil. Super Citrimax® and ChromeMate®

chromium (polynicotinate) are trademarks of InterHealth, NI ChromeMate® brand chromium (polynicotinate)

Recommendations

3 capsules 3 times per day, 30–60 minutes before meals.

Are There Any Potential Side Effects or Precautions?

At this time, there are no known side effects or precautions. If pregnant or lactating, consult your physician before taking this product.

Are There Any Potential Drug Interactions?

Super CitriMax® Plus may enhance the effects of drugs for diabetes (e.g., insulin, blood sugar-lowering agents) and possibly lead to hypoglycemia. Therefore, diabetics taking these medications should use this supplement only under the supervision of a doctor.

Super CitriMax® Plus

Three vegetable capsules contain:

Garcinia cambogia (fruit) extract.................... 1,500 mg
   (standardized to contain 60% (-)hydroxycitric acid)
   providing (typical):

calcium (as hydroxycitrate) (min.) .... 150 mg

potassium (as hydroxycitrate) (min.).................. 210 mg

chromium (polynicotinate)............................. 200 mcg

Gymnema sylvestre (leaf) extract...................... 133 mg
   (standardized to contain 75% gymnemic acids)

vitamin C (as ascorbyl palmitate) ....30 mg

3 capsules 3 times per day, 30–60 minutes before meals.

22. CARBCRAVE COMPLEX

What is It?

CarbCrave Complex is designed to help lessen appetite and curb excessive carbohydrate intake by supporting healthy brain chemistry and mood.*

Uses for CarbCrave Complex

Lessens Cravings: CarbCrave Complex supports healthy neurotransmitter metabolism, affecting the appetite and mood centers of the brain. 5-HTP is a precursor for serotonin, the same neurotransmitter released by the consumption of carbohydrates and associated with enhanced mood. At the same time, dl-phenylalanine supports dopamine and epinephrine production, responsible for the sensation of well-being. Vitamin B6 is integral as a cofactor for neurotransmitter synthesis. Rhodiola and ashwagandha are believed to encourage the activities of these neurotransmitters while strengthening the body's resistance to stress and fatigue, common triggers for undesirable eating behaviors. Research indicates that Sensoril®Trim ashwagandha promotes relaxation and maintains healthy cortisol levels. It is these actions that may be responsible for its supportive effects on glucose and fat metabolism. Both chromium picolinate and Relora® have demonstrated the potential to promote more healthful patterns of carbohydrate and energy intake in adult subjects. In one study involving forty nine volunteers prone to eating under stress, Relora® helped reduce stress-related snacking of sweets by seventy six percent. In another trial, chromium picolinate supplementation helped reduce carbohydrate intake and mood fluctuations.*

Cravings and appetite are influenced by many factors, only some of which may be affected by the ingredients in this formula.

What is the Source?

Chromium is derived from the lime of rock. 5-Hydroxytryptophan is derived from *Griffonia simplicifolia* seed. Pyridoxal 5'phosphate (activated B6) and dl-phenylalanine are synthetic. Relora® is derived from a proprietary blend of patented extracts from *Magnolia officinalis* bark and *Phellodendron amurense* bark. Sensoril®Trim ashwagandha extract is derived from *Withania somnifera* root and leaf. *Rhodiola rosea* extract is derived from the root and standardized to contain three percent total rosavins and min. one percent salidrosides. Ascorbyl palmitate is derived from corn dextrose fermentation and palm oil. Hypo-allergenic plant fiber is derived from pine cellulose. Relora® is a trademark of Next Pharmaceuticals.

Recommendations

Pure Encapsulations recommends 2 capsules 3 times per day, in divided doses, with or before meals.

Are There Any Potential Side Effects or Precautions?

Not to be taken by pregnant or lactating women. Ingredients in this formula can cause gastrointestinal side effects such as heartburn, stomach pain, belching and flatulence, nausea, vomiting and diarrhea. Chromium has have been associated with headaches, sleep disturbances, mood changes or painful joints. Consult your physician for more information.

Are There Any Potential Drug Interactions?

This formula may be contraindicated with SSRI medications or MAO inhibitors. Avoid taking phenylalanine with Levadopa and neuroleptic medications. Chromium may alter the absorption of thyroid medications. This formula should be taken at least thirty minutes after thyroid medications. Consult your physician for more information.

CarbCrave Complex

Two vegetable capsules contain:

pyridoxal 5'phosphate (activated B6)..................... 5 mg

chromium (picolinate)..................................... 200 mcg

5-hydroxytryptophan (griffonia simplicifolia)...... 50 mg

dl-phenylalanine .... 250 mg

Relora®.. 175 mg
  proprietary blend of patented extracts from:
  magnolia officinalis (bark)
  phellodendron amurense (bark)

Sensoril®Trim ashwagandha (withania
  somnifera)... 75 mg
  extract (root and leaf)

rhodiola rosea extract (root) .... 75 mg
  (standardized to contain 3% total rosavins and
  min. 1% salidrosides)

vitamin C (as ascorbyl palmitate)...................... 20 mg

other ingredients: modified food and corn starch, silicon dioxide

2 capsules three times per day, in divided doses, with or before meals.

Not to be taken by pregnant or lactating women. Consult your physician before use if taking SSRI medications or MAO inhibitors. Consult a physician if you are taking any other prescription medications.

23. CLA (CONJUGATED LINOLEIC ACID)

What is It?

CLA is a naturally occurring trans isomer of linoleic acid. It is unique in structure because of the location of the double bonds in the linoleic acid molecule. Pure Encapsulations concentrated CLA provides an average of 77% total CLA, and contains the main isomers c9,t11 and t10,c12.*

Uses for CLA

Promotes Lean Body Composition: CLA may benefit body composition and support weight control. Recent research shows that the specific isomers c9,t11 and t10,c12 play key roles in many of CLA's physiological properties. In a preliminary human study involving sixty overweight subjects, conjugated linoleic acid reduced body fat mass. Several animal studies explore possible mechanisms of CLA, including the ability to moderate fat deposition, increase lipolysis in adipocytes, reduce energy intake, increase energy expenditure and support metabolic rate.*

What is the Source?

This product is derived from safflower oil using a patented process and is Tonalin® brand CLA.

Recommendations

Pure Encapsulations recommends 3–5 grams per day, in divided doses, before meals.

Are There Any Potential Side Effects or Precautions?

If pregnant or lactating, consult your physician before taking this product. CLA may cause gastrointestinal upset in sensitive individuals.

Are There Any Potential Drug Interactions?

At this time, there are no known adverse reactions when taken in conjunction with medications.

CLA 1,000 mg

Each softgel capsule contains 22 sg:
conjugated linoleic acid .... 1,000 mg
providing:
pure conjugated linoleic acid (CLA) .... 770 mg

(This plant sourced CLA is derived from safflower oil using a patented process.)
other ingredients: carob (to darken capsules), gelatin capsule

3–5 capsules per day, in divided doses, before meals.

24. THYROID SUPPORT COMPLEX

What is It?

Thyroid Support Complex is a comprehensive formula containing vitamins, minerals and herbal extracts to nourish and support healthy thyroid cell metabolism and thyroid gland function.*

Uses for Thyroid Support Complex

Thyroid Function: Healthy vitamin A, vitamin D, zinc and selenium status have been associated with maintaining healthy thyroid cell metabolism as well as triioidothyronine (T3) and thyroxine (T4) hormone function. Kelp contains nutrients and minerals that support the thyroid, particularly iodine. Iodine and l-tyrosine are key components in the synthesis of thyroid hormones. Coleus extract contains forskolin, which has been shown to promote adenylate cyclase activity, supporting thyroid hormone metabolism. Research indicates that ashwagandha and guggul are also key factors for helping to sustain healthy thyroid function. Doubling as powerful antioxidants, vitamins A and C, selenium and guggul combine with curcumin to neutralize free radicals that affect iodothyronine 5'-monodeiodinase enzyme activity, the limiting factor in the conversion of T4 to the more active T3 hormone.*

What is the Source?

Vitamin A (acetate) is synthetic. Ascorbic acid is derived from corn dextrose fermentation. Vitamin D3 is derived from lanolin. Zinc and selenium are derived from the lime of rock. Kelp is derived from *Ascophyllum nodosum* and standardized to contain 0.5% iodine (150 mcg). l-Tyrosine (free-form) is derived from soy. Ashwagandha extract is derived from *Withania somnifera* root and standardizd to contain five percent withanolides. *Coleus forskohlii* extract is derived from the root and standardized to provide ten percent forskolin. Guggul extract is derived from *Commiphoramukul* gum resin and standardized to contain two point five percent guggulsterones. Turmeric is derived from *Curcuma longa* root and standardized to contain ninety five percent curcuminoids. Ascorbyl palmitate is derived from corn dextrose fermentation and palm oil.

Recommendations

Pure Encapsulations recommends 2 capsules daily, with meals.

Are There Any Potential Side Effects or Precautions?

In rare cases, certain ingredients may cause nausea, vomiting, diarrhea, headache or fatigue. Guggul may cause a skin rash in certain sensitive individuals. Not to be taken by pregnant or lactating women.

Are There Any Potential Drug Interactions?

Certain ingredients may be contraindicated for individuals taking benzodiazepines or CNS depressants. Ashwagandha is not recommended for individuals taking immunosuppressant medications. Certain ingredients may interact with blood thinning medications. Ashwagandha, guggul and l-tyrosine may have an additive effect with thyroid medications. Consult your physician for more information.

Thyroid Support Complex

Two vegetable capsules contain:

vitamin A (acetate)..2,500 i.u.

ascorbic acid.. 150 mg

vitamin D3 ....200 i.u.

Ascophyllum nodosum (kelp) (whole plant).........30 mg

(standardized to contain 0.5% iodine)...............150 mcg

zinc (citrate)..20 mg

selenium (selenomethionine)............................ 200 mcg

l-tyrosine (free-form).. 500 mg

ashwagandha *(Withania somnifera)*

   extract (root)...400 mg
    (standardized to contain 5% withanolides)

Coleus forskohlii extract (root)[†] .... 100 mg
    (standardized to contain 10% forskolin)

guggul *(Commiphora mukul)* extract

   (gum resin)... 150 mg
    (standardized to contain 2.5% guggulsterones)

turmeric *(Curcuma longa)* extract (root) .... 100 mg
    (standardized to contain 95% curcuminoids)

ascorbyl palmitate (fat-soluble vitamin C) ....30 mg

Not to be taken by pregnant or lactating women.

2 capsules per day, with meals.

25. GROWTH HORMONE SUPPORT

What is It?

Growth Hormone Support contains the amino acids arginine and ornithine. These amino acids may synergistically support healthy growth hormone production. Growth hormone is naturally released by the pituitary gland in response to sleep and exercise in order to help replenish tissues. It supports muscle protein synthesis, moderates the breakdown of muscle tissue and promotes fat utilization for energy.*

Uses for Growth Hormone Support Supports Growth Hormone Production And Protein

Synthesis: Arginine supports healthy growth hormone synthesis and is also a precursor for protein synthesis. Ornithine alpha-ketoglutarate (OKG) is composed of two molecules of ornithine and one molecule of alpha-ketoglutarate. OKG has demonstrated the ability to support healthy nitrogen balance, important for healthy muscle function. OKG also promotes healthy polyamine, Arginine and glutamine levels, important metabolites for muscle protein support. One study demonstrated the potential for arginine and ornithine in combination to support lean muscle mass when combined with physical training. A second study also suggests a possible role of Arginine and ornithine in supporting lean muscle mass and strength training when combined with a high intensity exercise program.*

What is the Source?

L-Arginine HCl is derived from the fermentation of soy and other vegetable sources and is ultra-filtered and highly purified. Ornithine alpha-ketoglutarate is synthetically produced.

Recommendations

Pure Encapsulations recommends 2–4 capsules per day, on an empty stomach, with juice or water, before bedtime or 1 hour before a workout, or as directed by your physician.

Are There Any Potential Side Effects or Precautions?

If pregnant or lactating, consult your physician before taking this product. Because of its effect on nitric oxide production, l-arginine is theoretically best avoided by individuals with migraines, depression, autoimmune disorders, and kidney or liver disease. Arginine is contraindicated for individuals with the herpes virus.

Are There Any Potential Drug Interactions?

At this time, there are no known adverse reactions when taken in conjunction with medications.

Growth Hormone Support

Each vegetable capsule contains:

l-arginine HCl.. 500 mg

ornithine alpha-ketoglutarate ....250 mg

2–4 capsules per day, on an empty stomach, with juice or water, before bedtime or 1 hour before a workout, or as directed by your physician.

26. CHROMEMATE

What is It?

Chromium is important for fat and carbohydrate metabolism, as well as enzyme activation. ChromeMate provides all the benefits of chromium and enhances this with the additional benefits of nicotinic acid.*

Uses for ChromeMate® GTF:

Glucose and Fat Metabolism: Optimal levels of chromium are essential for proper glucose and lipid metabolism. It is a critical component of Glucose Tolerance Factor (GTF). The potential for ChromeMate to promote GTF activity accounts for its roles in maintaining healthy glucose metabolism and supporting body composition.*

Body Composition: One study showed that when combined with modest diet and exercise, ChromeMate® supported lean body composition in overweight women.

A similar study at Georgetown University also suggested that ChromeMate may support lean muscle mass in overweight women.*

What is the Source?

ChromeMate is synthetically produced through a specialized process from the highest quality chromium chloride (trivalent chromium) and niacin. Hypoallergenic plant fiber is derived from pine cellulose. ChromeMate® brand niacin-bound chromium.

Recommendations

- ChromeMate® GTF 600: 1 capsule per day, with a meal.
- ChromeMate® GTF 200: 1–3 capsules per day, in divided doses, with a meal.

Are There Any Potential Side Effects or Precautions?

If pregnant or lactating, consult your physician before taking this product. Chromium is generally well tolerated, however has been associated with headaches, sleep disturbances, irritability and mood changes. There have also been rare reports of cognitive, perceptual, and motor dysfunction. Consult your physician for more information.

Are There Any Potential Drug Interactions?

Chromium may inhibit thyroid medication absorption. Concurrent administration is not recommended. Individuals on insulin or anti-diabetes medication should have blood glucose levels monitored. Consult your physician for more information.

ChromeMate® GTF 600

Each vegetable capsule contains:

chromium (from chromium polynicotinate)..... 600 mcg
(hypoallergenic plant fiber added to complete capsule volume requirement)

1 capsule per day, with a meal.

ChromeMate® GTF 200

Each vegetable capsule contains:

chromium (from chromium polynicotinate)..... 200 mcg
  (hypoallergenic plant fiber added to complete
  capsule volume requirement)

1–3 capsules per day, in divided doses, with meals.

27. BIOFLAVONEX

What is It?

Bioflavonex is a bioflavonoid formula combining concentrated, standardized extracts of grape seed, green tea, milk thistle, and resveratrol. Bioflavonoids are water-soluble plant pigments with powerful antioxidant properties.*

Features Include:

- Grape seed polyphenols and oligomeric proanthocyanidins provide protective support for capillaries and blood vessels. These compounds are among the most powerful antioxidants known in nature, as laboratory studies have shown them to be twenty times more powerful than vitamin C and fifty times more powerful than vitamin E in antioxidant capability. Oligomeric proanthocyanidins have also been shown to inhibit collagenase, elastase and hyaluronidase enzyme activity, supporting blood vessel integrity.*

- Resveratrol, promoting cardiovascular health through its antioxidant action and its ability to maintain healthy platelet function and arachidonic acid metabolism. Furthermore, this polyphenol most commonly associated with the health benefits of red wine provides additional antioxidant support for blood vessel integrity.*
- Green tea, containing catechins, a class of polyphenols that promote cardiovascular, immune and cellular function. The antioxidant activity of green tea catechins, specifically epigallocatechin gallate, also protects cells from lipid peroxidation and preserves and promotes vitamin E levels in the body.*
- Silymarin, stabilizing hepatic cell membranes and scavenging free radicals and toxins in the liver. Two of silymarin's mechanisms involve promoting superoxide dismutase antioxidant enzyme activity and increasing glutathione concentrations in the liver.*

Uses For Bioflavonex:

Bioflavonex combines natural, concentrated bioflavonoid extracts for cardiovascular, liver, and cellular antioxidant protection.*

What is the Source?

This formula contains: grape (*Vitis vinifera*) seed extract (standardized to contain ninety two percent polyphenols); green tea extract (standardized to contain a minimum of sixty five percent total tea catechins, providing twenty three percent epigallocatechin gallate (EGCg)); milk thistle (*Silybum marianum*) extract (standardized to contain eighty percent silymarin); resveratrol (*Polygonum cuspidatum*) extract (standardized to contain twenty percent trans resveratrol and ten percent emodin); and vitamin C ascorbyl palmitate) (corn dextrose fermentation).

Recommendations
1–4 capsules per day, in divided doses, between meals.

Are There Any Potential Side Effects Or Precautions?
If pregnant or lactating, consult your physician before taking this product. Frequent use of green tea may impede the absorption of non-heme iron (the form of iron in plant foods).

Are There Any Potential Drug Interactions?
This formula may potentially inhibit the absorption of certain medications, including: codeine, as well as asthma, allergy, antidiarrheals, blood thinning and other heart medications. Consult your physician for more information.

Bioflavonex
Each vegetable capsule contains:

grape (Vitis vinifera) seed extract........................ 50 mg
    (standardized to contain 92% polyphenols)

green tea extract.. 100 mg
    (standardized to contain a minimum of 65% total tea catechins)

providing:

epigallocatechin gallate (EGCg) (min.) .... 23 mg

caffeine .... 7 mg

milk thistle *(Silybum marianum)* extract........... 100 mg
    (standardized to contain 80% silymarin)

resveratrol *(Polygonum cuspidatum)* extract..... 100 mg
    (standardized to contain 20% trans resveratrol and 10% emodin)

vitamin C (as ascorbyl palmitate) .... 6 mg

1–4 capsules per day, in divided doses, between meals.

28. BIOSLIFE SLIM®

Unicity International is pleased to announce that Bios Life Slim is included in the *2010 Physicians' Desk Reference®* (PDR).

Bios Life Slim® is a natural supplement designed to help burn fat and to increase energy level. It also helps the body to naturally regulate the amount of fat stored and helps to control cholesterol and blood sugar levels. Slim trains your body to burn away excess fat without the jitters, hunger of other weight-loss products—creating a slimmer, more active and more attractive you! Bios Life Slim has helped hundreds of people on their journey to weight loss. Check out our Slim Winners to learn more about their success with Slim.

- Bios Life Slim—A Leptin Booster
- Leptin resistance markedly contributes to the obesity cycle as shown above
- Bios Life Slim contains a patented proprietary state-of-the art nutritional component that helps to restore the connection between leptin and the brain
- With Bios Life Slim, the abundant leptin signal in blood is heard again by the brain so that a stronger "full" signal is received over time.
- High cholesterol and lipids, reduction total cholesterol, reduction LDL cholesterol, increased HDL cholesterol lowering triglycerides
- Significant cardiovascular risks
- Strong family risk (high risk)
- Known coronary disease (high risk)
- Slowing progression or reversing coronary arteriosclerosis
- Appetite control (weight management)
- Regulation of glucose metabolism (diabetes, pre-diabetes), reduction of blood pressure

- Reducing risks of breast, prostate, and colorectal cancer (maybe, ovarian, uterine, vaginal, and cervical cancers)
- Prevention of constipation
- Prevention of diverticular disease of the colon
- Bios Life Slim works in two ways:
  - Has a direct filling effect in the digestive tract by the unique fiber mix
  - Has a subtle effect by causing the brain to realize again that we have enough food.
- Bios Life Slim decreases appetite and as a result, less fat and cabohydrates are consumed
- Increased leptin sensitivity is the key to Bios Life Slim miracle!
- The benefits of Bios Life have been clinically proven in eight scientific trials and clinical studies at some of the top universities, hospitals, and research institutions around the world, including the Cleveland Clinic, recognized as the leading heart research institution in the United States.
- On average, Bios Life reduces bad cholesterol (LDL) by thirty one percent in only eight weeks and over fifty percent in participants with very high LDL levels. It improves good cholesterol levels (HDL) by an average twenty nine percent in the same eight weeks and up to eighty percent in those with very low HDL levels. Continued use showed further improvement in both LDL and HDL levels. It also reduces triglyceride levels an average of forty percent. There is no known clinically proven drug or natural product in the world that offers these three combined benefits to help reduce one's risk of cardiovascular disease. Unlike prescription drugs, Bios Life is a true cholesterol optimization product.
- In addition, a recent study presented at the American Heart Association Annual Conference concluded Bios Life reduced

the post-prandial glucose levels twenty eight percent and HbA1c levels fifteen percent; indicating Bios Life provides a natural option to improve diabetes management.

* Please note: All marked (*) statements in Appendix A have not been evaluated by the Food & Drug Administration. This product is not intended to diagnose, treat, cure or prevent any disease.

For educational purposes only. Consult your physician for any health problems.

BIBLIOGRAPHICAL NOTES

Introduction

Carson R. *Silent Spring,* 1962. Houghton Mifflin.

Colborn T, Dumanoski D and Meyers JP. *Our Stolen Future: Are we Threatening our Fertility, Intelligence and Survival? A scientific Detective Story,* March 1, 1996. The Penguin Group.

Keynes, John Maynard. 1936. *The General Theory of Employment, Interest and Money.* London: Macmillan.

Chapter I: THE OBESITY MODEL

http://water.usgs.gov/nawqa/pnsp/usage/maps/

Epstein SS, Fitzgerald R. *Toxic Beauty: How Cosmetics and Personal Care Products Endanger Your Health... And What You Can Do About It,* 2009. Ben Bella Books.

Winter R. *A Consumer's Dictionary of Cosmetic Ingredients. Complete Information About the Harmful and Desirable Ingredients Found in Cosmetics and Cosmeceuticals.* 7th Edition, 2009. New York: Three Rivers Press.

Chapter II: MAKING SENSE OF OBESITY STATISTICS

The HCUP statistics are obtained from data published at:
http://hcupnet.ahrq.gov/

HCUPnet is a free, online query system based on data from the Healthcare Cost and Utilization Project (HCUP). It provides access to health statistics and information on hospital inpatient and emergency department utilization.

To find out more about CDC Mortality facts for 2007 go to:
http://www.cdc.gov/NCHS/data/nvsr/nvsr58/nvsr58_19.pdf

Chapter III: FARMING AND OBESITY IN THE UNITED STATES

Centers for Disease Control and Prevention (CDC). Behavioral Risk Factor Surveillance System Survey Data. Atlanta, Georgia: US Department of Health and Human Services, Centers for Disease Control and Prevention, 1985–2009.

The USGS pesticide maps are found in the following link:
http://water.usgs.gov/nawqa/pnsp/usage/maps/
http://ks.water.usgs.gov/pubs/fact-sheets/fs.022-98.pdf
http://hcupnet.ahrq.gov/
HCUPnet is a free, online query system based on data from the Healthcare Cost and Utilization Project (HCUP). It provides access to health statistics and information on hospital inpatient and emergency department utilization.

A complete listing of the seventy five new chemicals is given in What's New. A full listing of all the chemicals included in the *Fourth Report* is available at:
http://www.cdc.gov/exposurereport/pdf/
NER_CHEMICALlist

Abstracts and links to full-text articles are available at:
http://www.cdc.gov/exposurereport/

Information is available at:

http://www.cdc.gov/exposurereport/chemical_selection.html
For the most up-to-date biomonitoring information, users can view the National Exposure Report Web site *http://www.cdc.gov/exposurereport/,* a one-stop source that contains the most recent version of the report as well as the biomonitoring publications.

Jones RL, Homa DM, Meyer PA, Brody DJ, Caldwell KL, Pirkle JL, Brown MJ. Trends in blood lead levels and blood lead testing among US children aged 1 to 5 Years, 1988–2004. *Pediatrics 2009,* Mar;123(3):e376–e385.

Caldwell KL, Mortensen ME, Jones RL, Caudill SP, Osterloh JD. Total blood mercury concentrations in the US population: 1999–2006. *Int J Hyg Environ Health,* 2009.

Chapter IV: THE ESTROGEN EPIDEMIC AND ASSOCIATED DISEASES

http://hcupnet.ahrq.gov/
HCUPnet is a free, online query system based on data from the Healthcare Cost and Utilization Project (HCUP). It provides access to health statistics and information on hospital inpatient and emergency department utilization.

Epstein, SS, Fitzgerald, R. *Toxic Beauty: How Cosmetics and Personal Care Products Endanger Your Health... And What You Can Do About It,* 2009. Ben Bella Books.

Winter, R. *A Consumer's Dictionary of Cosmetic Ingredients. Complete Information About the Harmful and Desirable Ingredients Found in Cosmetics and Cosmeceuticals.* 7th Edition, 2009. New York: Three Rivers Press.

Endocrine Disruptors (Environmental Estrogens) Enhance Autoantibody Production by B1 Cells

Hideaki Yurino,* Sho Ishikawa,* Taku Sato,* Kenji Akadegawa,* Toshihiro Ito,* Satoshi Ueha,* Hidekuni Inadera,† and Kouji Matsushima*,[1]

*Department of Molecular Preventive Medicine, School of Medicine, The University of Tokyo, Tokyo, 113-0033, Japan; and †Department of Public Health, Toyama Medical and Pharmaceutical University, 930-0194, Japan Received March 19, 2004; accepted May 18, 2004.

Abstract:

Accumulating data suggest that endocrine disruptors affect not only the reproductive system, but also the immune system. We demonstrate here that endocrine disruptors including diethylstilbestrol (DES) and bisphenol-A (BPA) enhance autoantibody production by B1 cells both in vitro and in vivo. BWF1 mice, a murine model for systemic lupus erythematosus (SLE), implanted with Silastic tubes containing DES after orchidectomy developed murine lupus characterized by immunoglobulin G (IgG) anti-DNA antibody production and IgG deposition in the glomeruli in the kidney as well as those implanted with 17b-estradiol (E2). Plaque-forming cells (PFC) producing autoantibodies specific for bromelain-treated blood cells were significantly increased in mice implanted with DES and BPA. IgM antibody production by B1 cells in vitro was also enhanced in the presence of endocrine disruptors including DES and BPA. Estrogen receptor (ER) expression was upregulated in B1 cells in aged BWF1 mice that developed lupus nephritis. These results suggest that endocrine disruptors are involved in autoantibody production by B1cells and maybe an etiologic factor in the development of autoimmune diseases.

Ahmed SA. The immune system as a potential target for environmental estrogens (endocrine disrupters): A new emerging field. *Toxicology* 2000;150, 191–296.

Ahmed SA, Dauphinee MJ, Montoya AI and Talal N. Estrogen induces normal murine CD51 B cells to produce autoantibodies *J Immunol* 1989;142, 2647–2653.

Arcaro KF, Yi L, Seegal RF, Vakharia DD, Yang Y, Spink DC, Brosch K, and Gierthy JF. 2,20,6,60-tetrachlorobiphenyl is estrogenic in vitro and in vivo. *J Cell Biochem* 1999;72, 94–102.

Bjorksten, B. Environment and infant immunity. *Proc Nutr Soc* 1999;58, 729–732.

Burr M, Butland B, King S, and Vaughan-Williams E. Changes in asthmatic prevalence: Two surveys 15 years apart. *Arch Dis Child* 1989;64, 1452–1456.

Carlsten H, Holmdahl R, Tarkowski A, Nilsson LA. Oestradiol- and testosterone-mediated effects on the immune system in normal and autoimmune mice are genetically linked and inherited as dominant traits. *Immunology* 1989;68, 209–214.

Cunningham AJ. Large numbers of cells in normal mice produce antibody components of isologous erythrocytes. *Nature* 1974;252, 749–752.

Das SK, Taylor JA, Korach KS, Pari, BC, Dey SK, Lubahn DB. Estrogenic responses in estrogen receptor-alpha deficient mice reveal a distinct estrogen signaling pathway. *Proc Natl Acad Sci USA.* 1997;94, 12786–12791.

Dauphinee M, Tovar Z, and Talal N. B cells expressing CD5 are increased in Sjögren's syndrome. *Arthritis Rheum* 1988;31, 642–647.

Eaton RB, Schneider G, and Schur PH. Enzyme immunoassay for antibodies to native DNA. Specificity and quality of antibodies. *Arthrits Rheum* 1983;26, 52–60.

Erlandsson MC, Jonsson CA, Islander U, Ohlsson C, Carlsten H. Oestrogen receptor specificity in oestradiol-mediated effects on B lymphopoiesis and immunoglobulin production in male mice. *Immunology* 2003;108, 346–351.

Forsberg JG. Neonatal estrogen treatment and its consequences for thymus development, serum level autoantibodies to cardiolipin, and the delayed-type hypersensitivity response. *J Toxicol Environ Health A* 2000;60, 185–213.

Fujimaki H, Nohara O, Ichinose T, Watanabe N, and Saito S. IL-4 production in mediastinal lymph node cells in mice intratracheally instilled with diesel exhaust particles and antigen. *Toxicology* 1994;92, 261–268.

Gilmore W, Weiner LP, and Correale J. Effect of estradiol on cytokine secretion by proteolipid protein-specific T cell clones isolated from multiple sclerosis patients and normal control subjects. *J Immunol* 1997;158, 446–451.

Grossman C. Regulation of the immune system by sex steroids. *Endocrinol Rev 5* 1984; 435–454.

Hardy RR, and Hayakawa K. B cell developmental pathways. *Annu Rev Immunol* 2001;19, 595–621.

Hayakawa K, Hardy RR, Parks DR, and Herzenberg LA. The "Ly-1 B" cell subpopulations in normal, immunodefective, and autoimmune mice. *J Exp Med* 1983;157, 202–218.

Homo-Delarche F, Fitzpatrick F, Christeff N, Nunez EZ, Bach JF, Dardenne M. Sex steroids, glucocorticoids, stress and autoimmunity. *J Steroid Biochem Mol Biol* 1991;40, 619–637.

Inadera H, Hashimoto S, Dong HY, Suzuki T, Nagai S, Yamashita T, Toyoda N, and Matsushima K. WISP-2 as a novel estrogenresponsive gene in human breast cancer cells. *Biochem Biophys Res Commun* 2000;275, 108–114.

Ishida H, Hastings R, Kearney J, and Howard M. Continuous antiinterleukin 10 antibody administration depletes mice of Ly-1 B cells but not conventional B cells. *J Exp Med* 1992;175, 1213–1220.

Ishida H, Muchamuel T, Sakaguchi S, Andrade S, Menon S, and Howard M. Continuous administration of anti-interleukin 10 antibodies delays onset of autoimmunity in NZB/W F1 mice. *J Exp Med* 1994;179, 305–310.

Kotzin BL. Systemic lupus erythematosus. *Cell* 1996;85, 303–306.

Medina KL, Stasser A, Kincade PW. Estrogen influences the differentiation, proliferation, and survival of early B-lineage precursors. *Blood* 2000;95, 2059–2067.

Merucolino TJ, Arnold LW, Haskins LA, and Haughton G. Normal mouse peritoneum contains a large population of Ly-11 (CD51) B cells that recognize phosphatidyl choline. *J Exp Med* 1988;168, 687–698.

Murakami M, Tsubata T, Okamoto M, Shimizu A, Kumagai S, Imura H, and Honjo T. Antigen-induced apoptotic death of Ly-1 B cells responsible for autoimmune disease in transgenic mice. *Nature* 1992;357, 77–80.

Murakami M, Tsubata T, Shinkura R, Nishitani S, Okamoto M, Yoshioka H, Usui T, Miyawaki S, and Honjo T. Oral administration of lipopolysaccharides activates B-1 cells in the peritoneal cavity and lamina propria of the gut and induces autoimmune symptoms in an autoantibodytransgenic mice. *J Exp Med* 1994;180, 111–121.

Murakami M, Yoshioka H, Shirai T, Tsubata T, and Honjo T. Prevention of autoimmune symptoms in autoimmune-prone mice by elimination of B-1 cells. *Int Immunol* 1995;7, 877–882.

Nel AE, Diaz-Sanchez D, Ng D, Hiura T, and Saxon A. Enhancement of allergic inflammation by the interaction between diesel exhaust particles and the immune system. *J Allergy Clin Immunol* 1998;102, 539–554.

Nishikawa J, Saito K, Goto J, Dakeyama F, Matsuo M, Nishihara T. New screening methods for chemicals with hormonal activities using interaction of nuclear hormone receptor with coactivator. *Toxicol Appl Pharmacol* 1999;154, 76–83.

Noller KL, Offord JR, Blair PB, Kaufman RH, O'Brien PC, Colton T, and Melton LJ. Increased occurrence of autoimmune disease among women exposed in utero to diethylstilbestrol. *Fertil Steril* 1988;49, 1080–1082.

Ohno Y. Annual Report of Research Committee on Epidemiology of Intractable Diseases. The Ministry of Health and Welfare of Japan, 1999;246–254.

Plater-Zyberk C, Maini RN, Lam K, Kennedy TD, and Janossy G. A rheumatoid arthritis B cell subset expresses a phenotype similar to that in chronic lymphocytic leukemia. *Arthritis Rheum* 1985;28, 971–976.

Roubinian JR, Talal N, Greenspan JS, Goodman JR, and Siteri PK. Effect of castration and sex hormone treatment on survival, antinucleic acid antibodies and glomerulonephritis in NZB/NZW F1 mice. *J Exp Med* 1978;147, 1568–1583.

Shirai T, Hirose S, Okada T, and Nishimura H. Immunology and immunopathology of the autoimmune disease of NZB and related mouse strains. In *Immunological Disorders in*

Mice. Rihova EB and Vetvicka V, editors. 1991 CRC Press Inc., Boca Raton, FL, 95–136.

Soto AM, Sonnenschein C, Chung KL, Fernandez MF, Olea N, Serrano FO. The E-SCREEN assay as a tool to identify estrogens: an update on estrogenic environmental pollutants. *Environ Health Perspect* 1995;103, 113–122.

Takano H, Yoshikawa T, Ichinose T, Miyabara Y, Imaoka K, and Sugai M. Diesel exhaust particles enhance antigen-induced airway inflammation and local cytokine expression in mice. *Am J Respir Crit Care Med* 1997;156, 36–42.

Theofilopoulos AN. Murine models of systemic lupus erythematosus. *Adv Immunol* 1985;37, 269–390.

von Mutius E. The environmental predictors of allergic disease. *J Allergy Clin Immunol* 2000;105, 9–19.

Wingard DL, Turiel J. Long-term effects of exposure to diethylstilbestrol. *West J Med* 1988;149, 551–554.

Wira CR, Sandoe CP. Specific IgA and IgG antibodies in the secretions of the female reproductive tract: Effects of immunization and estradiol on expression of this response in vivo. *J Immunol* 1987;138, 4159–4164.

Chapter V: PROGESTERONE DEFICIENCY, ESTROGEN DOMINANCE, LEPTIN RESISTANCE, INSULIN RESISTANCE AND OBESITY

http://hcupnet.ahrq.gov/

HCUPnet is a free, online query system based on data from the Healthcare Cost and Utilization Project (HCUP). It provides access to health statistics and information on hospital inpatient and emergency department utilization.

Chapter VI: ESTROGEN DOMINANCE AND ATOPIC DISEASE

The Estrogen Effect on Mast Cells is captured in the following articles and their references

Estradiol activates mast cells via a non-genomic estrogen receptor-α and calcium influx
Zaitsu M, Narita S, Lambert KC, Grady JJ, Estes DM, et al. (2007) Estradiolactivates mast cells via a non-genomic estrogen receptor-alpha and calcium influx. Mol Immunol 44(8): 1977–85.

References:

Barr RG, Wentowski CC, Grodstein F, Somers SC, Stampfer MJ, Schwartz J, Speizer FE, Camargo CA Jr. Prospective study of postmenopausal hormone use and newly diagnosed asthma and chronic obstructive pulmonary disease. *Arch Intern Med* 2004;164:379–386. [PubMed: 14980988]

Bulayeva NN, Gametchu B, Watson CS. Quantitative measurement of estrogen-induced ERK 1 and 2 activation via multiple membrane-initiated signaling pathways. *Steroids* 2004;69:181–192. [PubMed: 15072920]

Bulayeva NN, Wozniak AL, Lash LL, Watson CS. Mechanisms of membrane estrogen receptor-alphamediated rapid stimulation of Ca2+ levels and prolactin release in a pituitary cell line. *Am J Physiol Endocrinol Metab* 2005;288:E388–E397. [PubMed: 15494610]

Butterfield JH, Weiler D, Dewald G, Gleich GJ. Establishment of an immature mast cell line from a patient with mast cell leukemia. *Leuk Res* 1988;12:345–355. [PubMed:3131594] Cary, NC. SAS Publishing. 2000.

Cocchiara R, Albeggiani G, Di Trapani G, Azzolina A, Lampiasi N, Rizzo F, Diotallevi L, Gianaroli L, Geraci D. Oestradiol enhances in vitro the histamine release induced by embryonic histamine-releasing factor (EHRF) from uterine mast cells. *Hum Reprod* 1992;7:1036–1041. [PubMed: 1383260]

Cocchiara R, Albeggiani G, Di Trapani G, Azzolina A, Lampiasi N, Rizzo F, Geraci D. Modulation of rat peritoneal mast cell and human basophil histamine release by estrogens. *Int Arch Allergy Appl Immunol* 1990;93:192–197. [PubMed: 1712002]

Collins P, Webb C. Estrogen hits the surface. *Nat Med* 1999;5:1130–1131. [PubMed: 10502813]

Dastych J, Walczak-Drzewiecka A, Wyczolkowska J, Metcalfe DD. Murine mast cells exposed to mercuric chloride release granule-associated N-acetyl-beta-D-hexosaminidase and secrete IL-4 and TNF-alpha. *J Allergy Clin Immunol* 1999;103:1108–1114. [PubMed: 10359893]

De Marco R, Locatelli F, Cerveri I, Bugiani M, Marinoni A, Giammanco G. Incidence and remission of asthma: a retrospective study on the natural history of asthma in Italy. *J Allergy Clin Immunol* 2002;110:228–235. [PubMed: 12170262]

Dijkstra A, Howard TD, Vonk JM, Ampleford EJ, Lange LA, Bleecker ER, Meyers DA, Postma DS. Estrogen receptor 1 polymorphisms are associated with airway hyperresponsiveness and lung function decline, particularly in female subjects with asthma. *J Allergy Clin Immunol* 2006;117:604–611. [PubMed: 16522460]

Doolan CM, Condliffe SB, Harvey BJ. Rapid non-genomic activation of cytosolic cyclic AMP-dependent protein kinase activity and [Ca(2+)](i) by 17-beta-oestradiol in female rat distal colon. *Br J Pharmacol* 2000;129:1375–1386. [PubMed: 10742293]

Doolan CM, Harvey BJ. A Galphas protein-coupled membrane receptor, distinct from the classical oestrogen receptor, transduces rapid effects of oestradiol on [Ca2+]i in female rat distal colon. *Mol Cell Endocrinol* 2003;199:87–103. [PubMed: 12581882]

Durstin M, Durstin S, Molski TF, Becker EL, Sha'afi RI. Cytoplasmic phospholipase A2 translocates to membrane fraction in human neutrophils activated by stimuli that phosphorylate mitogen-activated protein kinase. *Proc Natl Acad Sci* USA 1994;91:3142–3146. [PubMed: 7512725]

Fiorini S, Ferretti ME, Biondi C, Pavan B, Lunghi L, Paganetto G, Abelli L. 17Beta-eEstradiol stimulates arachidonate release from human amnion-like WISH cells through a rapid mechanism involving a membrane receptor. *Endocrinology* 2003;144:3359–3367. [PubMed: 12865314]

Harnish DC, Albert LM, Leathurby Y, Eckert AM, Ciarletta A, Kasaian M, Keith JC Jr. Beneficial effects of estrogen treatment in the HLA-B27 transgenic rat model of inflammatory bowel disease. *Am J Physiol Gastrointest Liver Physiol* 2004;286:G118–G125. [PubMed: 12958017]

Improta-Brears T, Whorton AR, Codazzi F, York JD, Meyer T, McDonnell DP. Estrogen-induced activation of mitogen-activated protein kinase requires mobilization of intracellular calcium. *Proc Natl Acad Sci USA* 1999;96:4686–4691. [PubMed: 10200323]

Ishizaka T, Hirata F, Ishizaka K, Axelrod J. Stimulation of phospholipid methylation, Ca2+ influx, and histamine release by bridging of IgE receptors on rat mast cells. *Proc Natl Acad Sci USA* 1980;77:1903–1906. [PubMed: 6154940]

Jiang YA, Zhang YY, Luo HS, Xing SF. Mast cell density and the context of clinicopathological parameters and expression of p185, estrogen receptor, and proliferating cell nuclear antigen in gastric carcinoma. *World J Gastroenterol* 2002;8:1005–1008. [PubMed: 12439914]

Lambert KC, Curran EM, Judy BM, Lubahn DB, Estes DM. Estrogen receptor-{alpha} deficiency promotes increased TNF-{alpha} secretion and bacterial killing by murine macrophages in response to microbial stimuli in vitro. *J Leukoc Biol* 2004;75:1166–1172. [PubMed: 15020652]

Lambert KC, Curran EM, Judy BM, Milligan GN, Lubahn DB, Estes DM. Estrogen receptor {alpha} (ER{alpha}) deficiency in macrophages results in increased stimulation of CD4+ T cells while 17 {beta}-estradiol acts through ER{alpha} to increase IL-4 and GATA-3 expression in CD4+ T cells independent of antigen presentation. *J Immunol* 2005;175:5716–5723. [PubMed: 16237062]

Mannino DM, Homa DM, Akinbami LJ, Moorman JE, Gwynn C, Redd SC. Surveillance for asthma— United States, 1980–1999. MMWR Surveill Summ 2002;51:1–13.

Morita Y, Siraganian RP. Inhibition of IgE-mediated histamine release from rat basophilic leukemia cells and rat mast cells by inhibitors of trans-methylation. *J Immunol* 1981;127:1339–1344. [PubMed: 6168684]

Nadal A, Ropero AB, Laribi O, Maillet M, Fuentes E, Soria B. Nongenomic actions of estrogens and xenoestrogens by binding at a plasma membrane receptor unrelated to estrogen receptor alpha and estrogen receptor beta. *Proc Natl Acad Sci USA* 2000;97:11603–11608. [PubMed: 11027358]

Nakasato H, Ohrui T, Sekizawa K, Matsui T, Yamaya M, Tamura G, Sasaki H. Prevention of severe premenstrual asthma attacks by leukotriene receptor antagonist. *J Allergy Clin Immunol* 1999;104:585–588. [PubMed: 10482831]

Nicovani S, Rudolph MI. Estrogen receptors in mast cells from arterial walls. *Biocell* 2002;26:15–24. [PubMed: 12058378]

Odom S, Gomez G, Kovarova M, Furumoto Y, Ryan JJ, Wright HV, Gonzalez-Espinosa C, Hibbs ML, Harder KW, Rivera J. Negative regulation of immunoglobulin E-dependent allergic responses by Lyn kinase. *J Exp Med* 2004;199:1491–1502. [PubMed: 15173205]

Pouliot M, McDonald PP, Krump E, Mancini JA, McColl SR, Weech PK, Borgeat P. Colocalization of cytosolic phospholipase A2, 5-lipoxygenase, and 5-lipoxygenase-activating protein at the nuclear membrane of A23187-stimulated human neutrophils. *Eur J Biochem* 1996;238:250–258. [PubMed: 8665944]

Schatz M, Camargo CA Jr. The relationship of sex to asthma prevalence, health care utilization, and medications in a large managed care organization. *Ann Allergy Asthma Immunol* 2003;91:553–558. [PubMed: 14700439]

Simoncini T, Mannella P, Fornari L, Caruso A, Varone G, Genazzani AR. Genomic and non-genomic effects of estrogens on endothelial cells. *Steroids* 2004;69:537–542. [PubMed: 15288766]

Skobeloff EM, Spivey WH, Silverman R, Eskin BA, Harchelroad F, Alessi TV. The effect of the menstrual cycle on asthma presentations in the emergency department. *Arch Intern Med* 1996;156:1837–1840. [PubMed: 8790078]

Skobeloff EM, Spivey WH, St Clair SS, Schoffstall JM. The influence of age and sex on asthma admissions. *JAMA* 1992;268:3437–3440. [PubMed: 1460733]

Smith GD, Lee RJ, Oliver JM, Keizer J. Effect of Ca2+ influx on intracellular free Ca2+ responses in antigen-stimulated

RBL-2H3 cells. *Am J Physiol* 1996;270:C939–C952. [PubMed: 8638649]

Song RX, Barnes CJ, Zhang Z, Bao Y, Kumar R, Santen RJ. The role of Shc and insulin-like growth factor 1 receptor in mediating the translocation of estrogen receptor alpha to the plasma membrane. *Proc Natl Acad Sci USA* 2004;101:2076–2081. [PubMed: 14764897]

Spanos C, el Mansoury M, Letourneau R, Minogiannis P, Greenwood J, Siri P, Sant GR, Theoharides TC. Carbachol-induced bladder mast cell activation: augmentation by estradiol and implications for interstitial cystitis. *Urology* 1996;48:809–816. [PubMed: 8911535]

Stefano GB, Prevot V, Beauvillain JC, Fimiani C, Welters I, Cadet P, Breton C, Pestel J, Salzet M, Bilfinger TV. Estradiol coupling to human monocyte nitric oxide release is dependent on intracellular calcium transients: evidence for an estrogen surface receptor. *J Immunol* 1999;163:3758–3763. [PubMed: 10490972]

Suzuki Y, Yoshimaru T, Matsui T, Inoue T, Niide O, Nunomura S, Ra C. Fc epsilon RI signaling of mast cells activates intracellular production of hydrogen peroxide: role in the regulation of calcium signals. *J Immunol* 2003;171:6119–6127. [PubMed: 14634127]

Vliagoftis H, Dimitriadou V, Boucher W, Rozniecki JJ, Correia I, Raam S, Theoharides TC. Estradiol augments while tamoxifen inhibits rat mast cell secretion. *Int Arch Allergy Immunol* 1992;98:398–409. [PubMed: 1384869]

Vrieze A, Postma DS, Kerstjens HA. Perimenstrual asthma: a syndrome without known cause or cure. *J Allergy Clin Immunol* 2003;112:271–282. [PubMed: 12897732]

Wang HQ, Kim MP, Tiano HF, Langenbach R, Smart RC. Protein kinase C-alpha coordinately regulates cytosolic phospholipase A(2) activity and the expression of cyclooxygenase-2 through different mechanisms in mouse keratinocytes. *Mol Pharmacol* 2001;59:860–866. [PubMed: 11259631]

Watson CS, Norfleet AM, Pappas TC, Gametchu B. Rapid actions of estrogens in GH3/B6 pituitary tumor cells via a plasma membrane version of estrogen receptor-alpha. *Steroids* 1999;64:5–13. [PubMed: 10323667]

Wozniak AL, Bulayeva NN, Watson CS. Xenoestrogens at pico-molar to nanomolar concentrations trigger membrane estrogen receptor-alpha-mediated Ca2+ fluxes and prolactin release in GH3/B6 pituitary tumor cells. *Environ Health Perspect* 2005;113:431–439. [PubMed: 15811834]

Zhao XJ, McKerr G, Dong Z, Higgins CA, Carson J, Yang ZQ, Hannigan BM. Expression of oestrogen and progesterone receptors by mast cells alone, but not lymphocytes, mac-rophages or other immune cells in human upper airways. *Thorax* 2001;56:205–211. [PubMed: 11182013]

Zivadinovic D, Gametchu B, Watson CS. Membrane estro-gen receptor-alpha levels in MCF-7 breast cancer cells pre-dict cAMP and proliferation responses. *Breast Cancer Res* 2005;7:R101–R112. [PubMed: 15642158]

Environmental Estrogens Induce Mast Cell Degranulation and Enhance IgE-Mediated Release of Allergic Mediators

Shin-ichiro Narita,[1] Randall M. Goldblum,[1] Cheryl S. Watson,[2] Edward G. Brooks,[1] D. Mark Estes,[1] Edward M. Curran,[1] and Terumi Midoro-Horiuti[1]

[1]Department of Pediatrics, Child Health Research Center; and [2]Department of Biochemistry and Molecular Biology, University of Texas Medical Branch, Galveston, Texas, USA

References:

Aravindakshan J, Gregory M, Marcogliese DJ, Fournier M, Cyr DG. Consumption of xenoestrogen-contaminated fish during lactation alters adult male reproductive function. *Toxicol Sci* 2004;81:179–189.

Ayotte P, Muckle G, Jacobson JL, Jacobson SW, Dewailly É. Assessment of pre- and postnatal exposure to polychlorinated biphenyls: lessons from the Inuit Cohort Study. *Environ Health Perspect* 2003;111:1253–1258.

Bologa CG, Revankar CM, Young SM, Edwards BS, Arterburn JB, Kiselyov AS, et al. Virtual and biomolecular screening-converge on a selective agonist for GPR30. *Nat Chem Biol* 2003;2:207–212.

Bulayeva NN, Watson CS. Xenoestrogen-induced ERK-1 and ERK-2 activation via multiple membrane-initiated signaling pathways. *Environ Health Perspect* 2004;112:1481–1487.

Bulayeva NN, Wozniak AL, Lash LL, Watson CS. Mechanisms of membrane estrogen-α-mediated rapid stimulation of Ca2+ levels and prolactin release in a pituitary cell line. *Am J Physiol Endocrinol Metab* 2005;288:E388–E397.

Burr ML, Wat D, Evans C, Dunstan FD, Doull IJ. Asthma prevalence in 1973, 1988 and 2003. *Thorax* 2006;61:296–299.

Butterfield JH, Weiler D, Dewald G, Gleich GJ. Establishment of an immature mast cell line from a patient with mast cell leukemia. *Leuk Res* 1988;12:345–355.

Dastych J, Walczak-Drzewiecka A, Wyczolkowska J, Metcalfe DD. Murine mast cells exposed to mercuric chloride release granule-associated N-acetyl-β-Dhexosaminidase and secrete IL-4 and TNF-α. *J Allergy Clin Immunol* 1999;103:1108–1114.

De Marco R, Locatelli F, Cerveri I, Bugiani M, Marinoni A, Giammanco G. Incidence and remission of asthma: a retrospective study on the natural history of asthma in Italy. *J Allergy Clin Immunol* 2002;110:228–235.

Dewailly É, Ayotte P, Bruneau S, Laliberté C, Muir DCG, Norstrom RJ. Inuit exposure to organochlorines through the aquatic food chain in arctic Quebec. *Environ Health Perspect* 1993;101:618–620.

Dijkstra A, Howard TD, Vonk JM, Ampleford EJ, Lange LA, Bleecker ER, et al. Estrogen receptor 1 polymorphisms are associated with airway hyperresponsiveness and lung function decline, particularly in female subjects with asthma. *J Allergy Clin Immunol* 2006;117:604–611.

Falconer IR, Chapman HF, Moore MR, Ranmuthugala G. Endocrine-disrupting compounds: a review of their challenge to sustainable and safe water supply and water reuse. *Environ Toxicol* 2006;21:181–191.

Ibarluzea JJ, Fernandez MF, Santa-Marina L, Olea-Serrano MF, Rivas AM, Aurrekoetxea JJ, et al. Breast cancer risk and the combined effect of environmental estrogens. *Cancer Causes Control* 2004;15:591–600.

Kos M, Denger S, Reid G, Korach KS, Gannon F. Down but not out? A novel protein isoform of the estrogen receptor α is expressed in the estrogen receptor α knockout mouse. *J Mol Endocrinol* 2002;29:281–286.

Lambert KC, Curran EM, Judy BM, Milligan GN, Lubahn DB, Estes DM. Estrogen receptor α (ERα) deficiency in macrophages results in increased stimulation of CD4+ T cells while 17β-estradiol acts through ERα to increase IL-4 and GATA-3 expression in CD4+ T cells independent of antigen presentation. *J Immunol* 2005;175:5716–5723.

Metcalfe CD, Metcalfe TL, Kiparissis Y, Koenig BG, Khan C, Hughes RJ, et al. Estrogenic potency of chemicals detected in sewage treatment plant effluents as determined by in vivo assays with Japanese medaka (Oryzias latipes). *Environ Toxicol Chem* 2001;20:297–308.

Newbold RR, Padilla-Banks E, Jefferson WN. Adverse effects of the model environmental estrogen diethylstilbestrol are transmitted to subsequent generations. *Endocrinology* 2006;147(suppl 6):S11–S17.

Odom S, Gomez G, Kovarova M, Furumoto Y, Ryan JJ, Wright HV, et al. Negative regulation of immunoglobulin Edependent allergic responses by Lyn kinase. *J Exp Med* 2004;199:1491–1502.

Solomon GM, Weiss PM. Chemical contaminants in breast milk: time trends and regional variability. *Environ Health Perspect* 2002;110:A339–A347.

Thomas P, Pang Y, Filardo EJ, Dong J. Identity of an estrogen membrane receptor coupled to a G protein in human breast cancer cells. *Endocrinology* 2005;146:624–632.

Vartiainen T, Saarikoski S, Jaakkola JJ, Tuomisto J. PCDD, PCDF, and PCB concentrations in human milk from two areas in Finland. *Chemosphere* 1997;34:2571–2583.

Wang SL, Lin CY, Guo YL, Lin LY, Chou WL, Chang LW. Infant exposure to polychlorinated dibenzo-p-dioxins, dibenzofurans and biphenyls (PCDD/Fs, PCBs)—correlation between prenatal and postnatal exposure. *Chemosphere* 2004;54:1459–1473.

Watson CS, Campbell CH, Gametchu B. Membrane oestrogen receptors on rat pituitary tumour cells: immunoidentification and responses to oestradiol and xenoestrogens. *Exp Physiol* 1999;84:1013–1022.

Watson CS, Gametchu B. Membrane estrogen and glucocorticoid receptors—implications for hormonal control of immune function and autoimmunity. *Int Immunopharmacol* 2001;1:1049–1063.

Watson CS, Gametchu B. Proteins of multiple classes may participate in nongenomic steroid actions. *Exp Biol Med* 2003, (Maywood) 228:1272–1281.

Welshons WV, Thayer KA, Judy BM, Taylor JA, Curran EM, Vom Saal FS. Large effects from small exposures. I. Mechanisms for endocrine-disrupting chemicals with estrogenic activity. *Environ Health Perspect* 2003;111:994–1006.

Wozniak AL, Bulayeva NN, Watson CS. Xenoestrogens at picomolar to nanomolar concentrations trigger membrane estrogen receptor-α-mediated Ca2+ fluxes and prolactin release in GH3/B6 pituitary tumor cells. *Environ Health Perspect* 2005;113:431 439.

Yunginger JW, Reed CE, O'Connell EJ, Melton LJ III, O'Fallon WM, Silverstein MD. A community-based study of the epidemiology of asthma. Incidence rates, 1964–1983. *Am Rev Respir Dis* 1992;146:888–894.

Zaitsu M, Narita S, Lambert KC, Grady JJ, Estes DM, Curran EM, et al. Estradiol activates mast cells via a non-genomic estrogen receptor-α and calcium influx. *Mol Immunol* 2006, doi:10.1016/j.molimm.2006.09.030 [Online 3 November 2006].

Maternal Bisphenol A Exposure Promotes the Development of Experimental Asthma in Mouse Pups

Terumi Midoro-Horiuti,[1,2] *Ruby Tiwari,*[1] *Cheryl S. Watson,*[2] *and Randall M. Goldblum*[1,2]

[1]Department of Pediatrics, Child Health Research Center, and [2]Department of Biochemistry and Molecular Biology, University of Texas Medical Branch, Galveston, TX, USA

Abstract:

Background: We recently reported that various environmental estrogens induce mast cell degranulation and enhance IgE-mediated release of allergic mediators *in vitro*.

Objectives: We hypothesized that environmental estrogens would enhance allergic sensitization as well as bronchial inflammation and responsiveness. To test this hypothesis, we exposed fetal and neonatal mice to the common environmental estrogen bisphenol A (BPA) via maternal loading and assessed the pups' response to allergic sensitization and bronchial challenge.

Methods: Female BALB/c mice received 10 µg/mL BPA in their drinking water from one week before impregnation to the end of the study. Neonatal mice were given a single 5 µg intraperitoneal dose of ovalbumin (OVA) with aluminum hydroxide on postnatal day 4 and 3% OVA by nebulization for 10 minutes on days 13, 14, and 15. Forty-eight hours after the last nebulization, we assessed serum IgE antibodies to OVA by enzyme-linked immunosorbent assay (ELISA) and airway inflammation and hyperresponsiveness by enumerating eosinophils in bronchoalveolar lavage fluid, whole-body barometric plethysmography, and a forced oscillation technique.

Results: Neonates from BPA-exposed mothers responded to this "suboptimal" sensitization with higher serum IgE anti-OVA concentrations compared with those from unexposed mothers ($p < 0.05$), and eosinophilic inflammation in their airways was significantly greater. Airway responsiveness of the OVA-sensitized neonates from BPA-treated mothers was enhanced compared with those from unexposed mothers ($p < 0.05$).

Conclusions: Perinatal exposure to BPA enhances allergic sensitization and bronchial inflammation and responsiveness in a susceptible animal model of asthma.

Key words: airway hyperresponsiveness, asthma, bisphenol A, environmental estrogen, eosinophilia, experimental asthma, IgE, maternal exposure, perinatal sensitization. *Environ Health Perspect* 118:273–277 (2010). doi:10.1289/ehp.0901259 available via *http://dx.doi.org/* [Online 5 October 2009]

References:

Adler A, Cieslewicz G, Irvin CG. Unrestrained plethysmography is an unreliable measure of airway responsiveness in BALB/c and C57BL/6 mice. *J Appl Physiol* 2004;97:286–292.

Allam JP, Zivanovic O, Berg C, Gembruch U, Bieber T, Novak N. In search for predictive factors for atopy in human cord blood. *Allergy* 2005;60:743–750.

Anderson SC, Poulsen KB. White blood cells. In: *Anderson's Atlas of Hematology* 2003 Philadelphia:Lippincott Williams & Wilkins, 57–128.

Bulayeva NN, Watson CS. Xenoestrogen-induced ERK-1 and ERK-2 activation via multiple membrane-initiated signaling pathways. *Environ Health Perspect* 2004;112:1481–1487.

Castro SM, Guerrero-Plata A, Suarez-Real G, Adegboyega PA, Colasurdo GN, Khan AM, et al. Antioxidant treatment ameliorates respiratory syncytial virus-induced disease and lung inflammation. *Am J Respir Crit Care Med* 2006;174:1361–1369.

Curran EM, Judy BM, Newton LG, Lubahn DB, Rottinghaus GE, MacDonald RS, et al. Dietary soy phytoestrogens and ERα signalling modulate interferon gamma production in response to bacterial infection. *Clin Exp Immunol* 2004;135:219–225.

Dewailly É, Ayotte P, Bruneau S, Laliberte C, Muir DC, Norstrom RJ. Inuit exposure to organochlorines through the aquatic food chain in Arctic Quebec. *Environ Health Perspect* 1993;101:618–620.

Dirtu AC, Roosens L, Geens T, Gheorghe A, Neels H, Covaci A. Simultaneous determination of bisphenol A, triclosan, and tetrabromobisphenol A in human serum using solid-phase extraction and gas chromatography-electron capture negative-ionization mass spectrometry. *Anal Bioanal Chem* 2008;391:1175–1181.

Fedulov AV, Leme A, Yang Z, Dahl M, Lim R, Mariani TJ, et al. Pulmonary exposure to particles during pregnancy causes increased neonatal asthma susceptibility. *Am J Respir Cell Mol Biol* 2008;38:57–67.

Fernandez MF, Arrebola JP, Taoufiki J, Navalon A, Ballesteros O, Pulgar R, et al. Bisphenol-A and chlorinated derivatives in adipose tissue of women. *Reprod Toxicol* 2007;24:259–264.

Gern JE, Lemanske RF Jr, Busse WW. Early life origins of asthma. *J Clin Invest* 1999;104:837–843.

Hamada K, Suzaki Y, Leme A, Ito T, Miyamoto K, Kobzik L, et al. Exposure of pregnant mice to an air pollutant aerosol increases asthma susceptibility in offspring. *J Toxicol Environ Health A* 2007;70:688–695.

Holt PG, Jones CA. The development of the immune system during pregnancy and early life. *Allergy* 2000;55:688–697.

Iwata M, Eshima Y, Kagechika H, Miyaura H. The endocrine disruptors nonylphenol and octylphenol exert direct effects on T cells to suppress Th1 development and enhance Th2 development. *Immunol Lett* 2004;94:135–139.

Johnson CC, Ownby DR, Peterson EL. Parental history of atopic disease and concentration of cord blood IgE. *Clin Exp Allergy* 1996;26:624–629.

Kabuto H, Amakawa M, Shishibori T. Exposure to bisphenol A during embryonic/fetal life and infancy increases oxidative injury and causes underdevelopment of the brain and testis in mice. *Life Sci* 2004;74:2931–2940.

Kim YH, Kim CS, Park S, Han SY, Pyo MY, Yang M. Gender differences in the levels of bisphenol A metabolites in urine. *Biochem Biophys Res Commun* 2003;312:441–448.

Kuroda N, Kinoshita Y, Sun Y, Wada M, Kishikawa N, Nakashima K, et al. Measurement of bisphenol A levels in human blood serum and ascitic fluid by HPLC using a fluorescent labeling reagent. *J Pharm Biomed Anal* 2003;30:1743–1749.

Lambert KC, Curran EM, Judy BM, Milligan GN, Lubahn DB, Estes DM. Estrogen receptor α (ERα) deficiency in macrophages results in increased stimulation of CD4+ T cells while 17β-estradiol acts through ERα to increase IL-4 and GATA-3 expression in CD4+ T cells independent of antigen presentation. *J Immunol* 2005;175:5716–5723.

Lee MH, Chung SW, Kang BY, Park J, Lee CH, Hwang SY, et al. Enhanced interleukin-4 production in CD4+ T cells and elevated immunoglobulin E levels in antigen-primed mice by bisphenol A and nonylphenol, endocrine disruptors: involvement of nuclear factor-AT and Ca2+. *Immunology* 2003;109:76–86.

Leme AS, Hubeau C, Xiang Y, Goldman A, Hamada K, Suzaki Y, et al. Role of breast milk in a mouse model of maternal transmission of asthma susceptibility. *J Immunol* 2006;176:762–769.

McCoy L, Redelings M, Sorvillo F, Simon P. A multiple cause-of-death analysis of asthma mortality in the United States, 1990–2001. *J Asthma* 2005;42:757–763.

Nakano N, Nishiyama C, Yagita H, Koyanagi A, Akiba H, Chiba S, et al. Notch signaling confers antigen-presenting cell functions on mast cells. *J Allergy Clin Immunol* 2009;123:74–81.

Narita S, Goldblum RM, Watson CS, Brooks EG, Estes DM, Curran EM, et al. Environmental estrogens induce mast cell degranulation and enhance IgE-mediated release of allergic mediators. *Environ Health Perspect* 2007;115:48–52.

Ohshima Y, Yamada A, Tokuriki S, Yasutomi M, Omata N, Mayumi M. Transmaternal exposure to bisphenol A modulates the development of oral tolerance. *Pediatr Res* 2007;62:60–64.

Padmanabhan V, Siefert K, Ransom S, Johnson T, Pinkerton J, Anderson L, et al. Maternal bisphenol-A levels at delivery: a looming problem? *J Perinatol* 2008;28:258–263.

Prescott SL, Macaubas C, Holt BJ, Smallacombe TB, Loh R, Sly PD, et al. Transplacental priming of the human immune system to environmental allergens: universal skewing of initial T cell responses toward the Th2 cytokine profile. *J Immunol* 1998;160:4730–4737.

Prescott SL, Macaubas C, Smallacombe T, Holt BJ, Sly PD, Holt PG. Development of allergen-specific T-cell memory in atopic and normal children. *Lancet* 1999;353:196–200.

Sayed BA, Brown MA. Mast cells as modulators of T-cell responses. *Immunol Rev* 2007;217:53–64.

Schonfelder G, Wittfoht W, Hopp H, Talsness CE, Paul M, Chahoud I. Parent bisphenol A accumulation in the human maternal-fetal-placental unit. *Environ Health Perspect* 2002;110:A703–A707.

Shore SA, Rivera-Sanchez YM, Schwartzman IN, Johnston RA. Responses to ozone are increased in obese mice. *J Appl Physiol* 2003;95:938–945.

Siegrist CA. Neonatal and early life vaccinology. *Vaccine* 2001;19:3331–3346.

Solomon GM, Weiss PM. Chemical contaminants in breast milk: time trends and regional variability. *Environ Health Perspect* 2002;110:A339–A347.

Sudowe S, Rademaekers A, Kolsch E. Antigen dose-dependent predominance of either direct or sequential switch in IgE antibody responses. *Immunology* 1997;91:464–472.

Sun Y, Irie M, Kishikawa N, Wada M, Kuroda N, Nakashima K. Determination of bisphenol A in human breast milk by HPLC with column-switching and fluorescence detection. *Biomed Chromatogr* 2004;18:501–507.

Tsukioka T, Brock J, Graiser S, Nguyen J, Nakazawa H, Makino T. Determination of trace amounts of bisphenol A in urine by negative-ion chemical-ionization-gas chromatography/mass spectrometry. *Anal Sci* 2003;19:151–153.

Volkel W, Bittner N, Dekant W. Quantitation of bisphenol A and bisphenol A glucuronide in biological samples by high performance liquid chromatography-tandem mass spectrometry. *Drug Metab Dispos* 2005;33:1748–1757.

Vollmer WM, Osborne ML, Buist AS. 20-year trends in the prevalence of asthma and chronic airflow obstruction in an HMO. *Am J Respir Crit Care Med* 1998;157:1079–1084.

Wang SL, Lin CY, Guo YL, Lin LY, Chou WL, Chang LW. Infant exposure to polychlorinated dibenzo-p-dioxins, dibenzofurans and biphenyls (PCDD/Fs, PCBs)—correlation between prenatal and postnatal exposure. *Chemosphere* 2004;54:1459–1473.

Watson CS, Gametchu B. Membrane estrogen and glucocorticoid receptors—implications for hormonal control of immune function and autoimmunity. *Int Immunopharmacol* 2001;1:1049–1063.

Yang L, Hu Y, Hou Y. Effects of 17β-estradiol on the maturation, nuclear factor kappa B p65 and functions of murine spleen CD11c-positive dendritic cells. *Mol Immunol* 2006;43:357–366.

Ye X, Kuklenyik Z, Needham LL, Calafat AM. Quantification of urinary conjugates of bisphenol A, 2,5-dichlorophenol, and 2-hydroxy-4-methoxybenzophenone in humans by online solid phase extraction-high performance liquid chromatography-tandem mass spectrometry. *Anal Bioanal Chem* 2005;383:638–644.

Zaitsu M, Narita S, Lambert KC, Grady JJ, Estes DM, Curran EM, et al. Estradiol activates mast cells via a non-genomic estrogen receptor-α and calcium influx. *Μολ Ιμμυνολ* 2007;44:1987–1995.

Gender-medicine aspects in allergology

E. Jensen-Jarolim, E. Untersmayr

Department of Pathophysiology, Center of Physiology, Pathophysiology and Immunology, Medical University Vienna, Vienna, Austria

Abstract:

Despite the identical immunological mechanisms activating the release of mediators and consecutive symptoms in immediate-type allergy, there is still a clear clinical difference between female and male allergic patients. Even though the risk of being allergic is greater for boys in childhood, almost from adolescence onward it seems to be a clear disadvantage to be a woman as far as atopic disorders are concerned. Asthma, food allergies and anaphylaxis are more frequently diagnosed in females. In turn, asthma and hay fever are associated with irregular menstruation.

Pointing toward a role of sex hormones, an association of asthma and intake of contraceptives, and a risk for asthma exacerbations during pregnancy have been observed. Moreover, peri- and postmenopausal women were reported to increasingly suffer from asthma, wheeze and hay fever, being even enhanced by hormone replacement therapy. This may be on account of the recently identified oestradiol-receptor-dependent mast-cell activation. As a paradox of nature, women may even become hypersensitive against their own sex hormones, resulting in positive reactivity upon intradermal injection of oestrogen or progesterone. More importantly, this specific hypersensitivity is associated with recurrent miscarriages. Even though there is a striking genderspecific bias in IgE mediated allergic diseases, public awareness of this fact still remains minimal today.

References:

Almqvist C, Worm M, Leynaert B. Impact of gender on asthma in childhood and adolescence: a GA(2)LEN review. *Allergy* 2008;63:47–57.

Balzano G, Fuschillo S, Melillo G, Bonini S. Asthma and sex hormones. *Allergy* 2001;56:13–20.

Becklake MR, Kauffmann F. Gender differences in airway behavior over the human life span. *Thorax* 1999;54:1119–1138.

Bender AE, Matthews DR. Adverse reactions to foods. *Br J Nutr* 1981;46:403–407.

Benyamini Y, Leventhal EA, Leventhal H. Gender differences in processing information for making self-assessments of health. *Psychosom Med* 2000;62:354–364.

Binkley KE, Davis AE III. Estrogendependent inherited angioedema. *Transfus Apher Sci* 2003;29:215–219.

Birrell SN, Butler LM, Harris JM, Buchanan G, Tilley WD. Disruption of androgen receptor signaling by synthetic progestins may increase risk of developing breast cancer. *FASEB J* 2007; 21:2285–2293.

Burr ML, Merrett TG. Food intolerance: a community survey. *Br J Nutr* 1983;49:217–219.

Carroll KN, Gebretsadik T, Griffin MR, Dupont WD, Mitchel EF, Wu P et al. Maternal asthma and maternal smoking are associated with increased risk of bronchiolitis during infancy. *Pediatrics* 2007;119:1104–1112.

Chalubinski M, Kowalski ML. Endocrine disrupters—potential modulators of the immune system and allergic response. *Allergy* 2006;61:1326–1335.

Chhabra SK. Premenstrual asthma. *Indian J Chest Dis Allied Sci* 2005;47:109–116.

Ciray M, Mollard H, Duret M. Asthma et menstruation. *Presse Med* 1938;38:755–759.

Cocchiara R, Albeggiani G, Di Trapani G, Azzolina A, Lampiasi N, Rizzo F et al. Oestradiol enhances in vitro the histamine release induced by embryonic histamine releasing factor (EHRF) from uterine mast cells. *Hum Reprod* 1992;7:1036–1041.

Cocchiara R, Albeggiani G, Di Trapani G, Azzolina A, Lampiasi N, Rizzo F et al. Modulation of rat peritoneal mast cell and human basophil histamine release by estrogens. *Int Arch Allergy Appl Immunol* 1990;93:192–197.

Coogan PF, Palmer JR, et al. Body mass index and asthma incidence in the Black Women's Health Study. *J Allergy Clin Immunol* 2009;123(1): 89–95.

Cutolo M, Capellino S, Sulli A, Serioli B, Secchi ME, Villaggio B et al. Estrogens and autoimmune diseases. *Ann N Y Acad Sci* 2006;1089:538–547.

Da Silva JA. Sex hormones and glucocorticoids: interactions with the immune system. *Ann N Y Acad Sci* 1999;876:102–117.

Daeron M. Fc receptor biology. *Annu Rev Immunol* 1997;15:203–234.

Dean NL. Perimenstrual asthma exacerbations and positioning of leukotriene-modifying agents in asthma management guidelines. *Chest* 2001;120:2116–2117.

Dewyea VA, Nelson MR, Martin BL. Asthma in pregnancy. *Allergy Asthma Proc* 2005;26:323–325.

Dijkstra A, Howard TD, Vonk JM, Ampleford EJ, Lange LA, Bleecker ER et al. Estrogen receptor 1 polymorphisms are associated with airway hyperresponsiveness and lung function decline, particularly in female subjects with asthma. *J Allergy Clin Immunol* 2006;117:604–611.

DunnGalvin A, Hourihane JO, Frewer L, Knibb RC, Oude Elberink JN, Klinge I. Incorporating a gender dimension in food allergy research: a review. *Allergy* 2006;61:1336–1343.

Eisenberg SW, Cacciatore G, Klarenbeek S, Bergwerff AA, Koets AP. Influence of 17beta-oestradiol, nortestosterone and dexamethasone on the adaptive immune response in veal calves. *Res Vet Sci* 2008;84: 199–205.

Ford ES, Mannino DM, Homa DM, Gwynn C, Redd SC, Moriarty DG et al. Self reported asthma and health-related quality of life: findings from the behavioral risk factor surveillance system. *Chest* 2003;123:119–127.

Furuichi K, Rivera J, Isersky C. The receptor for immunoglobulin E on rat basophilic leukemia cells: effect of ligand binding on receptor expression. *Proc Natl Acad Sci USA* 1985;82:1522–1525.

Geiger E, Magerstaedt R, Wessendorf JH, Kraft S, Hanau D, Bieber T. IL-4 induces the intracellular expression of the alpha chain of the high-affinity receptor for IgE in in vitro-generated dendritic cells. *J Allergy Clin Immunol* 2000;105:150–156.

Gluck JC. The change of asthma course during pregnancy. *Clin Rev Allergy Immunol* 2004;26:171–180.

Gomez Real F, Svanes C, Bjornsson EH, Franklin KA, Gislason D, Gislason T et al. Hormone replacement therapy, body mass index and asthma in perimenopausal women: a cross sectional survey. *Thorax* 2006;61:34–40.

Grimaldi CM. Sex and systemic lupus erythematosus: the role of the sex hormones estrogen and prolactin on the regulation of autoreactive B cells. *Curr Opin Rheumatol* 2006;18:456–461.

Gruijthuijsen YK, Grieshuber I, Stocklinger A, Tischler U, Fehrenbach T, Weller MG et al. Nitration enhances the allergenic potential of proteins. *Int Arch Allergy Immunol* 2006;141:265–275.

Haggerty CL, Ness RB, Kelsey S, Waterer GW. The impact of estrogen and progesterone on asthma. *Ann Allergy Asthma Immunol* 2003;90:284–291; quiz 291–283, 347.

Hanania NA, Belfort MA. Acute asthma in pregnancy. *Crit Care Med* 2005;33:S319 S324.

Hantusch B, Schöll I, Harwanegg C, Krieger S, Becker WM, Spitzauer S et al. Affinity determinations of purified IgE and IgG antibodies against the major pollen allergens Phl p 5a and Betv 1a: discrepancy between IgE and IgG binding strength. *Immunol Lett* 2005;97:81–89.

Harnish DC, Albert LM, Leathurby Y, Eckert AM, Ciarletta A, Kasaian M et al. Beneficial effects of estrogen treatment in the HLA-B27 transgenic rat model of inflammatory bowel disease. *Am J Physiol Gastrointest Liver Physiol* 2004;286:G118 G125.

Hendler I, Schatz M, Momirova V, Wise R, Landon M, Mabie W et al. Association of obesity with pulmonary and nonpulmonary complications of pregnancy in asthmatic women. *Obstet Gynecol* 2006;108:77–82.

Itsekson AM, Seidman DS, Zolti M, Lazarov A, Carp HJ. Recurrent pregnancy loss and inappropriate local immune response to sex hormones. *Am J Reprod Immunol* 2007;57:160–165.

Jaakkola JJ, Ahmed P, Ieromnimon A, Goepfert P, Laiou E, Quansah R et al. Preterm delivery and asthma: a systematic review and meta-analysis. *J Allergy Clin Immunol* 2006;118:823–830.

Jakobsen CG, Bodtger U, Poulsen LK, Roggen EL. Vaccination for birch pollen allergy: comparison of the affinities of specific immunoglobulins E, G1 and G4 measured by surface plasmon resonance. *Clin Exp Allergy* 2005;35:193–198.

Jansen JJ, Kardinaal AF, Huijbers G, Vlieg-Boerstra BJ, Martens BP, Ockhuizen T. Prevalence of food allergy and intolerance in the adult Dutch population. *J Allergy Clin Immunol* 1994;93:446–456.

Jiang YA, Zhang YY, Luo HS, Xing SF. Mast cell density and the context of clinicopathological parameters and expression of p185, estrogen receptor, and proliferating cell nuclear antigen in gastric carcinoma. *World J Gastroenterol* 002;8:1005–1008.

Kinet JP. The high-affinity IgE receptor (Fc epsilon RI): from physiology to pathology. *Annu Rev Immunol* 1999;17:931–972.

Kiriyama K, Sugiura H, Uehara M. Premenstrual deterioration of skin symptoms in female patients with atopic dermatitis. *Dermatology* 2003;206:110–112.

Lang TJ. Estrogen as an immunomodulator. *Clin Immunol* 2004;113:224–230.

Lenoir RJ. Severe acute asthma and the menstrual cycle. *Anaesthesia* 1987;42:1287–1290.

Lovik M, Namork E, Faeste C, Egaas E. The Norwegian National Reporting System and Register of severe allergic reactions to food. In: Marone G, editor. *Clinical immunology and allergy in medicine.* Napoli: JGC Publishers, 2003:461–466.

Ma LJ, Guzman EA, DeGuzman A, Muller HK, Walker AM, Owen LB. Local cytokine levels associated with delayed-type hypersensitivity responses: modulation by gender, ovariectomy, and estrogen replacement. *J Endocrinol* 2007;193:291–297.

Maleki SJ, Chung SY, Champagne ET, Raufman JP. The effects of roasting on the allergenic properties of peanut proteins. *J Allergy Clin Immunol* 2000;106:763–768.

Maleki SJ, Kopper RA, Shin DS, Park CW, Compadre CM, Sampson H et al. Structure of the major peanut allergen Ara h 1 may protect IgE-binding epitopes from degradation. *J Immunol* 2000;164:5844–5849.

Maranghi F, Rescia M, Macri C, Di Consiglio E, De Angelis G, Testai E et al. Lindane may modulate the female reproductive development through the interaction with ER-beta: an in vivo-in vitro approach. *Chem Biol Interact* 2007;169:1–14.

Martinez-Moragon E, Plaza V, Serrano J, Picado C, Galdiz JB, Lopez-Vina A et al. Near-fatal asthma related to menstruation. *J Allergy Clin Immunol* 2004;113:242–244.

Masuch GI, Franz JT, Schoene K, Musken H, Bergmann KC. Ozone increases group 5 allergen content of Lolium perenne. *Allergy* 1997;52: 874–875.

Metcalfe D. Food allergy in adults. Chapter 10 from *Food Allergy: Adverse Reactions to Foods and Food Additives*, 3rd edn. USA: Blackwell Sciences, 2003:36–143.

Metzger H. The receptor with high affinity for IgE. *Immunol Rev* 1992;125:37–48.

Mitchell VL, Gershwin LJ. Progesterone and environmental tobacco smoke act synergistically to exacerbate the development of allergic asthma in a mouse model. *Clin Exp Allergy* 2007;37:276–286.

Möhrenschlager M, Schäfer T, Huss-Marp J, Eberlein-König B, Weidinger S, Ring J et al. The course of eczema in children aged 5–7 years and its relation to atopy: differences between boys and girls. *Br J Dermatol* 2006; 154:505–513.

Moneret-Vautrin DA, Morisset M. Adult food allergy. *Curr Allergy Asthma Rep* 2005;5:80–85.

Narita S, Goldblum RM, Watson CS, Brooks EG, Estes DM, Curran EM et al. Environmental estrogens induce mast cell degranulation and enhance IgE-mediated release of allergic mediators. *Environ Health Perspect* 2007;115:48–52.

Nicovani S, Rudolph MI. Estrogen receptors in mast cells from arterial walls. *Biocell* 2002;26:15–24.

Novak N, Tepel C, Koch S, Brix K, Bieber T, Kraft S. Evidence for a differential expression of the FcepsilonRIgamma chain in dendritic cells of atopic and nonatopic donors. *J Clin Invest* 2003;111:1047–1056.

Quarto R, Kinet JP, Metzger H. Coordinate synthesis and degradation of the alpha-, beta- and gamma-subunits of the receptor for immunoglobulin E. *Mol Immunol* 1985;22:1045–1051.

Rahimi R, Nikfar S, Abdollahi M. Meta-analysis finds use of inhaled corticosteroids during pregnancy safe: a systematic meta-analysis review. *Hum Exp Toxicol* 2006;25:447–452.

Regal JF, Fraser DG, Weeks CE, Greenberg NA. Dietary phytoestrogens have anti-inflammatory activity in a guinea pig model of asthma. *Proc Soc Exp Biol Med* 2000;223:372–378.

Riffo-Vasquez Y, Ligeiro de Oliveira AP, Page CP, Spina D, Tavares-de-Lima W. Role of sex hormones in allergic inflammation in mice. *Clin Exp Allergy* 2007;37:459 470.

Roby RR, Richardson RH, Vojdani A. Hormone allergy. *Am J Reprod Immunol* 2006;55:307–313.

Salam MT, Wenten M, Gilliland FD. Endogenous and exogenous sex steroid hormones and asthma and wheeze in young women. *J Allergy Clin Immunol* 2006;117:1001–1007.

Schäfer T, Bohler E, Ruhdorfer S, Weigl L, Wessner D, Heinrich J et al. Epidemiology of food allergy/food intolerance in adults: associations with other manifestations of atopy. *Allergy* 2001;56:1172–1179.

Schöll I, Kalkura N, Shedziankova Y, Bergmann A, Verdino P, Knittelfelder R et al. Dimerization of the major birch pollen allergen Bet v 1 is important for its in vivo IgE-crosslinking potential in mice. *J Immunol* 2005;175:6645–6650.

Searing DA, Zhang Y, et al. Decreased serum vitamin D levels in children with asthma are associated with increased corticosteroid use. *J Allergy Clin Immunol* 1 2010;25(5): 995–1000.

Siroux V, Curt F, Oryszczyn MP, Maccario J, Kauffmann F. Role of gender and hormone-related events on IgE, atopy, and eosinophils in the Epidemiological Study on the Genetics and

Environment of Asthma, bronchial hyperresponsiveness and atopy. *J Allergy Clin Immunol* 2004;114:491–498.

Skobeloff EM, Spivey WH, Silverman R, Eskin BA, Harchelroad F, Alessi TV. The effect of the menstrual cycle on asthma presentations in the emergency department. *Arch Intern Med* 1996;156:1837–1840.

Spanos C, el-Mansoury M, Letourneau R, Minogiannis P, Greenwood J, Siri P et al. Carbachol-induced bladder mast cell activation: augmentation by estradiol and implications for interstitial cystitis. *Urology* 1996; 48:809–816.

Sterk AR, Ishizaka T. Binding properties of IgE receptors on normal mouse mast cells. *J Immunol* 1982;128:838–843.

Stygar D, Masironi B, Eriksson H, Sahlin L. Studies on estrogen receptor (ER) alpha and beta responses on gene regulation in peripheral blood leukocytes in vivo using selective ER agonists. *J Endocrinol* 2007;194:101–119.

Suzuki K, Hasegawa T, Sakagami T, Koya T, Toyabe S, Akazawa K et al. Analysis of perimenstrual asthma based on question-naire surveys in Japan. *Allergol Int* 2007;56:249–255.

Svanes C, Real FG, Gislason T, Jansson C, Jogi R, Norrman E et al. Association of asthma and hay fever with irregular menstruation. *Thorax* 2005;60:445 450.

Tata LJ, Lewis SA, McKeever TM, Smith CJ, Doyle P, Smeeth L et al. A comprehensive analysis of adverse obstetric and pediatric complications in women with asthma. *Am J Respir Crit Care Med* 2007;175:991–997.

Temprano J. and Mannino DM. The effect of sex on asthma control from the National Asthma Survey. *J Allergy Clin Immunol* 2009;123(4): 854–860.

The British Dietetic Association. Paediatric group position statement on the use of soya protein for infants. *J Fam Health Care* 2003;13:93.

The pill, breast cancer risk and your age. Mayo Clin Health Lett 2007;25:4.

Thomas K, Herouet-Guicheney C, Ladics G, Bannon G, Cockburn A, Crevel R et al. Evaluating the effect of food processing on the potential human allergenicity of novel proteins: international workshop report. *Food Chem Toxicol* 2007;45:1116–1122.

Vasiadi M, Kempuraj D, Boucher W, Kalogeromitros D, Theoharides TC. Progesterone inhibits mast cell secretion. *Int J Immunopathol Pharmacol* 2006;19:787–794.

Vliagoftis H, Dimitriadou V, Boucher W, Rozniecki JJ, Correia I, Raam S et al. Estradiol augments while tamoxifen inhibits rat mast cell secretion. *Int Arch Allergy Immunol* 1992;98:398–409.

Vrieze A, Postma DS, Kerstjens HA. Perimenstrual asthma: a syndrome without known cause or cure. *J Allergy Clin Immunol* 2003;112:271–282.

Watson HG. Sex hormones and thrombosis. *Semin Hematol* 2007;44:98–105.

Webb LM, Lieberman P. Anaphylaxis: a review of 601 cases. *Ann Allergy Asthma Immunol* 2006;97:39–43.

Wizeman TM, Pardue ML. Exploring the biological contributions to human health: does sex matter? Institute of Medicine (IOM). Washington, D.C.: National Academic Press, 2003.

Young E, Stoneham MD, Petruckevitch A, Barton J, Rona R. A population study of food intolerance. *Lancet* 1994;343:1127–1130.

Zaitsu M, Narita S, Lambert KC, Grady JJ, Estes DM, Curran EM et al. Estradiol activates mast cells via a non-genomic estrogen receptor-alpha and calcium influx. *Mol Immunol* 2007;44:1977–1985.

Zhang Z, Lai HJ, et al. Early childhood weight status in relation to asthma development in high-risk children. *J Allergy Clin Immunol* 2010;126(6): 1157–1162.

Zhao XJ, McKerr G, Dong Z, Higgins CA, Carson J, Yang ZQ et al. Expression of oestrogen and progesterone receptors by mast cells alone, but not lymphocytes, macrophages or other immune cells in human upper airways. *Thorax* 2001;56:205–211.

Sensitization and immune cells response to allergen immunotherapy

Norman PS. Immunotherapy: 1999–2004. *J Allergy Clin Immunol* 2004;113(6): 1013–1023.

Mast cell and Basophil degranulation products

Simons FER, Frew AJ, et al. Risk assessment in anaphylaxis: Current and future approaches. *J Allergy Clin Immunol* 2007;120(1): S2–S24.

Chapter VII: OVERALL SUMMARY

Berkowitz A. Clinical Pathophysiology made Ridiculously Simple. *MedMaster Inc,* 2007 pp. 107–109.

Chapter VIII: OBESITY SOLUTIONS

Low Glycemic Index Eating popularized by Dr. Jennie Brand-Miller and her team from Sidney Australia

Brand-Miller J and Powell KA. *The New Glucose Revolution Shopper's Guide.* 2010 Da Capo Press

The Cholesterol Controversy is addressed by Dr. Uffe Ravnskov

Ravnskov U. *Ignore the Awkward! How the Cholesterol Myths Are Kept Alive.* 2010 CreateSpace.

The first clinical trial known to man was performed by the prophet Daniel

Nelson, Thomas Inc. *The Nelson Study Bible Bible, New King James Version.* 1997. Thomas Nelson Bibles. Book of Daniel Chapter 1: verse 1–18.

ACKNOWLEDGMENTS

I recently attended the 2011 USGS GIS Workshop and The National Map Users Conference in Denver, CO. I am not a geologist or geographer and I do not work for the USGS. I found out about this meeting because I wanted to recognize the work of NAWQA, a USGS group. I used the USGS pesticides maps in this book and wanted to give credit to the makers of the maps. While searching for the USGS-NAWQA group that published the maps, two names appeared with phone numbers. I called Jeff Dietterle, and he was just the right person I needed to connect with. Jeff was gracious and tried to connect me with the right group for proper citation and acknowledgments. When I told Jeff that I have written a book about obesity and used the USGS pesticides maps in my book, he asked if I wanted to submit an abstract for the USGS meeting in May 2011 and I did. Bill Carswell read the abstract and made insightful comments and I thank him for his comments. I then heard from Yvonne Baevsky, Geologist with USGS in Albany, NY, and organizer of the Health session of the conference. During this conference, I learned about the amount of time it takes to make a map and how much work goes into it. It is team effort all the way. I therefore would like to thank Jeff Dietterle and Yvonne Baevsky, for giving me the opportunity to attend this meeting which was informative and opened my eyes to medical geography. The abstract I presented was an excerpt from this book and I would like to thank the participants of our health session who after the presentation made insightful comments and encouraged me to go forward with the book. Now instead of thanking one individual on the NAWQA side, I know that I should thank everyone at NAWQA and at the USGS who contributed to the making of the maps that are so invaluable for the book and for understanding the roots of the US obesity epidemic. By the same token, I would like to thank all the contributors of the CDC obesity maps derived from the BRFSS survey. Without the work of the scientists and supporting staff, the book would not have been complete. I would like to also thank those at AhrQ, for the healthcare cost and utilization project data that provided a solid evidence about obesity and its comorbidities.

A book takes a long road from conception to publication. I have worked on this book since 2007, when I was first introduced to the idea that hormone imbalance may impact health and correction of the imbalance may solve many medical problems. I would like to thank my patients from the University of Texas Health Sciences Center at Tyler, those at the Center for Asthma, Allergy, Immunology & Hormone Health in Tyler, TX and Woodbridge, VA, those at Fort Belvoir, VA and finally my current patients at Altru Health System, who have taught me so much and continue to reveal to me the etiology of common diseases including atopic diseases. Many who have tried, have found that bioidentical hormone therapy and orthomolecular practice work well and have a future in healthcare. Those of you who have gone through my clinics and have seen the impact in your lives and have written to me about your satisfaction, I thank you for your comments, belief and trust in me. For those of you I could not connect with at any level, I still learned from your comments and say let's try it again. I would like to thank Adan Rios and Cynthia Kinsey, my nurses at Fort Belvoir, who were with me all the way in the care of our military and their family members at Fort Belvoir and who have continued to support my ideas and encouraged me along the way. Our teamwork and caring for the patients led to the Ace of Excellence award I received at Fort Belvoir and I appreciated that. I would like to thank my colleagues and the staff at Altru Health System, Fort Belvoir, and UTHSCT, who support my ideas and who are too many to list here, for their encouragements.

I would like to thank my copy editor, Doran Hunter for his systematic line-by-line editing and his contributions that have made this book a better finished product and Michele DeFilippo and her team at 1106 Design for the wonderful design of this book.

I would like to thank my children Jean-Yves, Colette, Melanie, and step-children Adam and Sam, who actively read the draft of the book or voted on the cover design and my younger ones, David, Yahmeah and Ezechiel, for their patience and unconditional love.

Finally, I would like to thank Fatima, my wife and companion, who has from start to end been the captive audience, for her support, encouragements and nurturing.

In the end, I must agree with Descartes that knowing that we know nothing is the beginning of real knowledge and if knowledge comes from a higher power, then all thanks and praise go to that higher power.

Benoit Tano, MD, PhD
Grand Forks, 2011

INDEX

Note: Italicized page numbers indicate tables and figures.

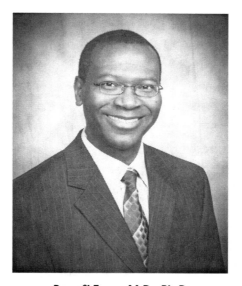

Benoît Tano, M.D., Ph.D

D r. Tano is currently a Clinical Associate Professor of Medicine with specialization in Allergy and Clinical Immunology at the University of North Dakota School of Medicine & Health Sciences and employed full-time as an allergist with the Altru Health System in Grand Forks, North Dakota.

Prior to joining Altru and UND, Dr. Tano completed a Ph.D. degree in Economics at the State University of New York at

Albany, with specialization in econometrics and labor economics (1988) and taught economics at the University of Toledo in Ohio (1988–1995). He then entered medical school and completed his MD degree at the Medical College of Ohio in 1999, followed by a three-year residency training in internal medicine at the Ohio State University Medical Center (1999–2002). In 2002, he engaged in two-year fellowship training in Pharmacoeconomics and outcomes research, sponsored by GlaxoSmithKline and Ohio State University Medical Center (2002–2004). The research fellowship was followed by a clinical fellowship in allergy and immunology at the Johns Hopkins Asthma and Allergy Center in Baltimore Maryland (July 2004–June 2006).

Dr. Tano is certified by the American Board of Internal Medicine, 2002, and by the American Board of Allergy and Immunology, 2006.

Dr. Tano's current research focuses on uncovering the roots of the American obesity epidemic for better diagnosis and treatment of the multiple associated comorbidities. He continues to conduct research in Pharmacoeconomics and Health Outcomes and Allergy/Clinical Immunology (uncovering the roots of the growing atopic diseases). Dr. Tano has presented his work nationally and internationally (UK, Brazil, Spain, Cote d'Ivoire). His publications have appeared in the *Journal of Allergy and Clinical Immunology, Respiratory Care, Value Health, Expert Review of Pharmacoeconomics and Outcomes Research, Hypertension, Journal of Urology, Scandinavian Journal of Work and Environmental Health, Economics Letters and Journal of Business and Economics.*

Dr. Tano is a member of the American Academy of Allergy, Asthma & Immunology, and The Academy of Anti-Aging and Regenerative Medicine

Dr. Tano can be contacted at:
PO Box 12117
Grand Forks, ND 58208
Tel: 855–DR-BTANO
Website: *www.drbtano.com* Email: *HIS@drbtano.com*

CPSIA information can be obtained at www.ICGtesting.com
Printed in the USA
LVOW040228231012

304033LV00001B/57/P